T0335932

Dynamics of Swarm Intelligence Health Analysis for the Next Generation

Arumugam Suresh Kumar
Jain University (Deemed), India

Utku Kose
Suleyman Demirel University, Turkey

Sachin Sharma
Graphic Era University (Deemed), India

S. Jerald Nirmal Kumar
Sharda University, India

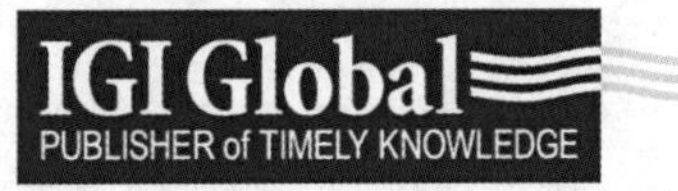

A volume in the Advances in Healthcare Information Systems and Administration (AHISA) Book Series

Published in the United States of America by
IGI Global
Medical Information Science Reference (an imprint of IGI Global)
701 E. Chocolate Avenue
Hershey PA, USA 17033
Tel: 717-533-8845
Fax: 717-533-8661
E-mail: cust@igi-global.com
Web site: http://www.igi-global.com

Library of Congress Cataloging-in-Publication Data

Names: Kumar Arumugam, Suresh, 1979- editor. | Kose, Utku, 1985- editor. | Sharma, Sachin, 1988- editor. | Nirmal Kumar, S. Jerald (Sujeet Jerald), 1981- editor.
Title: Dynamics of swarm intelligence health analysis for the next generation / edited by Suresh Kumar Arumugam, Utku Kose, Sachin Sharma, Jerald Nirmal Kumar S.
Description: Hershey PA : Medical Information Science Reference, [2023] | Includes bibliographical references and index. | Summary: "The book discusses the role of people behavioral activity in the evolution of the traditional medical system to an intelligent system. It is based on the development of technical improvements considered in the process of intelligent systems by using cognitive techniques, swarm Intelligence deep learning, and machine learning techniques. These techniques will be used for multimodal biomedical data processing and non-invasive interpretation which efficiently improves the patient interpretation quality. Moreover, it objects to highlight the challenges of developing and proposing new ideas regarding the out-of hospital dedicated systems directions. Solicits contributions of this book include theory, applications, and design schemes of intelligent systems, vision techniques, and biomedical applications, as well as the methodologies behind them. This book also focuses on the economic, social, and environmental impact of swarm Intelligence smart healthcare systems. It aims to provide a detailed understanding of swarm Intelligence analysis supported applications while engaging premium smart computing methods and improved intelligent algorithms in the field of computer science. Further, the detailed assessment of IoT sensors, actuators, communication, and computing technology, and standards has been taken into considerations. Emphasis is also laid on the challenges associated with these smart healthcare systems. It includes connectivity, sensing, computation, complexity, and security issues. Therefore, this book designed for new innovations to overcome such challenges and to explore the dynamics of swarm Intelligence health analysis for the future generation. We hope to strengthen the link between the Swarm Intelligence analysis sector and mental health research in this book chapter. Various works in the digital health arena shown how real-time monitoring of mood disorders improved the overall quality of life of patients and citizens"-- Provided by publisher.
Identifiers: LCCN 2022055346 (print) | LCCN 2022055347 (ebook) | ISBN 9781668468944 (hardcover) | ISBN 9781668468951 (ebook)
Subjects: MESH: Health Information Systems | Artificial Intelligence | Data Analysis | Machine Learning | Medical Informatics Computing--trends
Classification: LCC R859 (print) | LCC R859 (ebook) | NLM W 26.55.A7 | DDC 362.10285--dc23/eng/20230207
LC record available at https://lccn.loc.gov/2022055346
LC ebook record available at https://lccn.loc.gov/2022055347

This book is published in the IGI Global book series Advances in Healthcare Information Systems and Administration (AHISA) (ISSN: 2328-1243; eISSN: 2328-126X)
British Cataloguing in Publication Data
A Cataloguing in Publication record for this book is available from the British Library.

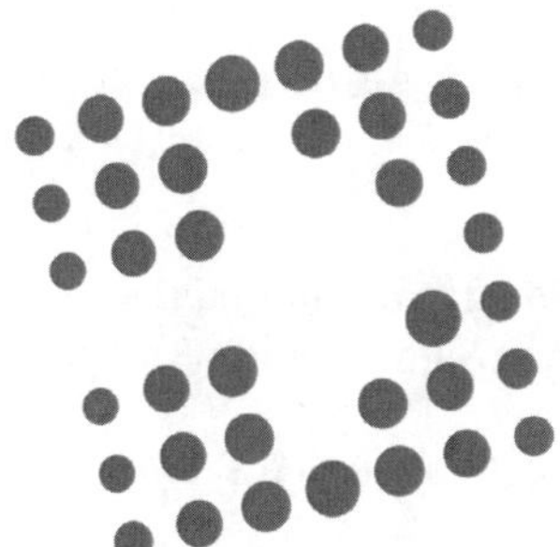

Advances in Healthcare Information Systems and Administration (AHISA) Book Series

ISSN:2328-1243
EISSN:2328-126X

Editor-in-Chief: Anastasius Moumtzoglou, Hellenic Society for Quality & Safety in Healthcare and P. & A. Kyriakou Children's Hospital, Greece

MISSION

The **Advances in Healthcare Information Systems and Administration (AHISA) Book Series** aims to provide a channel for international researchers to progress the field of study on technology and its implications on healthcare and health information systems. With the growing focus on healthcare and the importance of enhancing this industry to tend to the expanding population, the book series seeks to accelerate the awareness of technological advancements of health information systems and expand awareness and implementation.

Driven by advancing technologies and their clinical applications, the emerging field of health information systems and informatics is still searching for coherent directing frameworks to advance health care and clinical practices and research. Conducting research in these areas is both promising and challenging due to a host of factors, including rapidly evolving technologies and their application complexity. At the same time, organizational issues, including technology adoption, diffusion and acceptance as well as cost benefits and cost effectiveness of advancing health information systems and informatics applications as innovative forms of investment in healthcare are gaining attention as well. **AHISA** addresses these concepts and critical issues.

COVERAGE

- Nursing Expert Systems
- IT Applications in Physical Therapeutic Treatments
- Measurements and Impact of HISA on Public and Social Policy
- Medical Informatics
- Pharmaceutical and Home Healthcare Informatics
- IT security and privacy issues
- IT Applications in Health Organizations and Practices
- Clinical Decision Support Design, Development and Implementation
- Management of Emerging Health Care Technologies
- Decision Support Systems

IGI Global is currently accepting manuscripts for publication within this series. To submit a proposal for a volume in this series, please contact our Acquisition Editors at Acquisitions@igi-global.com or visit: http://www.igi-global.com/publish/.

The Advances in Healthcare Information Systems and Administration (AHISA) Book Series (ISSN 2328-1243) is published by IGI Global, 701 E. Chocolate Avenue, Hershey, PA 17033-1240, USA, www.igi-global.com. This series is composed of titles available for purchase individually; each title is edited to be contextually exclusive from any other title within the series. For pricing and ordering information please visit http://www.igi-global.com/book-series/advances-healthcare-information-systems-administration/37156. Postmaster: Send all address changes to above address.

Titles in this Series

For a list of additional titles in this series, please visit:
http://www.igi-global.com/book-series/advances-healthcare-information-systems-administration/37156

Contemporary Applications of Data Fusion for Advanced Healthcare Informatics
G.S. Karthick (PSG College of Arts and Science, India) and Sathishkumar Karupusamy (Gobi Arts and Science College, India)
Medical Information Science Reference • copyright 2023 • 300pp • H/C (ISBN: 9781668489130) • US $325.00 (our price)

Revolutionizing Healthcare Through Artificial Intelligence and Internet of Things Applications
Keshav Kaushik (University of Petroleum and Energy Studies, India) Susheela Dahiya (Graphic Era Hill University, Dehradun, India) Shilpi Aggarwal (State University of New York, USA) and Ashutosh Dhar Dwivedi (Copenhagen Business School, Denmark)
Medical Information Science Reference • copyright 2023 • 277pp • H/C (ISBN: 9781668454220) • US $345.00 (our price)

Global Perspectives on Probing Narratives in Healthcare
Teresa Casal (University of Lisbon, Portugal) and Maria de Jesus Cabral (University of Minho, Portugal)
Medical Information Science Reference • copyright 2023 • 349pp • H/C (ISBN: 9781668480649) • US $325.00 (our price)

Integrating Digital Health Strategies for Effective Administration
Ahmed Chemseddine Bouarar (University of Medea, Algeria) Kamel Mouloudj (University of Medea, Algeria) and Dachel Martínez Asanza (University of Medical Sciences of Havana, Cuba)
Medical Information Science Reference • copyright 2023 • 450pp • H/C (ISBN: 9781668483374) • US $325.00 (our price)

For an entire list of titles in this series, please visit:
http://www.igi-global.com/book-series/advances-healthcare-information-systems-administration/37156

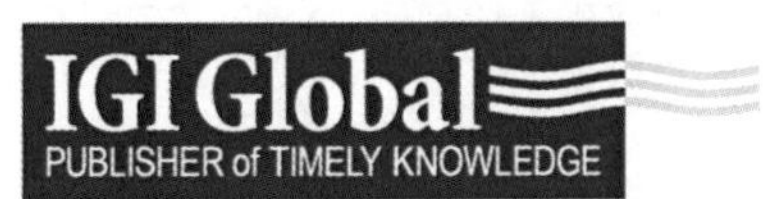

701 East Chocolate Avenue, Hershey, PA 17033, USA
Tel: 717-533-8845 x100 • Fax: 717-533-8661
E-Mail: cust@igi-global.com • www.igi-global.com

Table of Contents

Preface xv

Chapter 1
A Study on Swarm Intelligence and Its Various Clustering Algorithms in Medical Diagnosis 1
Amreen Ayesha, Presidency University, Bengaluru, India
N. Nasurudeen Ahamed, Presidency University, Bengaluru, India

Chapter 2
Healthcare Data Analytics Using Swarm Intelligence Techniques 18
K. Renuka Devi, Dr. Mahalingam College of Engineering and Technology, Pollachi, India

Chapter 3
A Generic Big Data Analytics With Particle Swarm Optimization for Clinical Machine Learning 33
Radha Subramani, Vivekanandha College of Engineering for Women, India
Aparna Chelladurai, Sengunthar Engineering College, India
Aarthi Chelladurai, Sengunthar Engineering College, India
N. Mohanapriya, Vivekanandha College of Engineering for Women, India

Chapter 4
A Modern Approach of Swarm Intelligence Analysis in Big Data: Methods, Tools, and Applications 59
Thirunavukkarasu Kannapiran, Karnavati University, India
Krishna Patel, Karnavati University, India
Thirusha T. K., CHRIST University (Deemed), India
Virendra Kumar Shrivastava, Alliance University, India
A Suresh Kumar, Jain University, India

Chapter 5
Swarm Intelligence and Evolutionary Machine Learning Algorithms for COVID-19: Pandemic and Epidemic Review..83
C. V. Suresh Babu, Hindustan Institute of Technolgy and Science, India
Sam Praveen, Hindustan University, India

Chapter 6
Swarm Intelligence Analysis of Healthcare Prediction Techniques Based on Social Media Data: Basics of Swarm Intelligence, Scope of Swarm Intelligence, Swarm Intelligence in Healthcare 104
Manivel Kandasamy, Karnavati University, India
Raju Shanmugam, Karnavati University, India
Tanya Valji Chhabhadiya, Karnavati University, India
Harshvi Kamlesh Adesara, Karnavati University, India
Pujita Sunnapu, Karnavati University, India

Chapter 7
The AI-Based COVID-19 Personal Protective Equipment Is Smarty and Secure...125
Mohd Asif Shah, Chandigarh University, India
Ramesh Sekaran, Jain University (Deemed), India

Chapter 8
Internet of Things-Integrated Remote Patient Monitoring System: Healthcare Application...137
Sampath Boopathi, Muthayammal Engineering College, India

Chapter 9
An IoMT and Machine Learning Model Aimed at the Development of a Personalized Lifestyle Recommendation System Facilitating Improved Health162
Guru Prasad, Graphic Era University (Deemed), India
A. Suresh Kumar, Jain University (Deemed), India
Sakshi Srivastava, Graphic Era University (Deemed), India
Ananya Srivastava, Graphic Era University (Deemed), India
Aditi Srivastava, Graphic Era University (Deemed), India

Chapter 10
Securing Healthcare Systems Integrated With IoT: Fundamentals, Applications, and Future Trends...186
S. Boopathi, Muthayammal Engineering College, India

Chapter 11
A Blockchain IoT Hybrid Framework for Security and Privacy in a Healthcare Database Network 210
Puneeta Singh, KIET Group of Institutions, India
Pritish Sinha, Galgotias University, India
Abhinav Raghav, Chandigarh University, India

Chapter 12
Categorical Data Clustering Using Meta Heuristic Link-Based Ensemble Method: Data Clustering Using Soft Computing Techniques 226
Kousik Nalliyanna Goundar Veerappan, Arden University, UK
Yuvaraj Natarajan, Sri Shakthi Institute of Engineering and Technology, Coimbatore, India
Arshath Raja, B.S. Abdur Rahman Crescent Institute of Science and Technology, Chennai, India
Jeyaprabhavathi Perumal, Arden University, UK
S Jerald Nirmal Kumar, Sharda University, India

Compilation of References 239

About the Contributors 268

Index 272

Detailed Table of Contents

Swarm intelligence is a manner the usage of the knowledge of collective objects (human beings, bugs, etc.) collectively to attain the optimized solution for a given hassle. "Swarm" is a set of objects (people, bugs, and so on.). In different phrases, permits say we supply a troubling statement to a single person and tell her or him to undergo this hassle after which provide the solution, then because of this we will keep in mind the solution of that specific character only; however, the problem is that the answer given with the aid of that man or woman might not be the best solution or maybe that solution is not proper for others. So, to keep away from that, what we do is we give that hassle to a certain quantity of humans together (swarm) and ask them to attain the first-class answer feasible for that problem and then compute all the responses together to reach the high-quality solution possible.

The healthcare domain plays a significant role. Healthcare information contains heterogeneous data where it has been utilized to mine data in order to provide accurate and optimized results to the user. Hence, the data mining can open up a world of possibilities in terms of diagnosis, prognosis, and therapy. It holds an important place in the medicinal field for the purpose of analyzing huge volumes of data for extracting the salient parts for evaluating the patients' reports. The swarm intelligence (SI) technique has also been utilized for disease diagnosis and treatment.

This chapter explains the importance of swarm intelligence technique under data mining in healthcare. It also focused on explaining different algorithms of SI such as particle swarm optimization (PSO) and ant colony optimization (ACO). It also explains its performance and accuracy in delivering the optimized results to the users/patients.

Chapter 3
A Generic Big Data Analytics With Particle Swarm Optimization for Clinical Machine Learning 33
Radha Subramani, Vivekanandha College of Engineering for Women, India
Aparna Chelladurai, Sengunthar Engineering College, India
Aarthi Chelladurai, Sengunthar Engineering College, India
N. Mohanapriya, Vivekanandha College of Engineering for Women, India

In the past two decades, researchers are facing challenges in analyzing biomedical data. It is a fast growing and new promising field due to vast growing information. Data analytics and machine learning are possible on huge volume of biomedical data. The primary goal of the biomedical data analysis by using swarm intelligence will help you to provide optimized prediction or analysis to the problem or diseases. Swarm intelligence is a special kind of information exchange across different nodes in a network with methods in machine learning. All the members of the swarm have equal rights. So there is no spider controlling the data web. Particle swarm optimization is used to fix the parameters and predicts the efficient nodes to pass on. Particle swarm optimization convolution neural networks (PSOCNN) minimizes the parameter space to a single block and evaluates the candidate CNN with a small subset of training data.

Chapter 4
A Modern Approach of Swarm Intelligence Analysis in Big Data: Methods, Tools, and Applications 59
Thirunavukkarasu Kannapiran, Karnavati University, India
Krishna Patel, Karnavati University, India
Thirusha T. K., CHRIST University (Deemed), India
Virendra Kumar Shrivastava, Alliance University, India
A Suresh Kumar, Jain University, India

Swarm intelligence is one of the most modern and less discovered artificial intelligence types. Until now it has been proven that the most comprehensive method to solve complex problems is using behaviours of swarms. Big data analysis plays a beneficial role in decision making, education domain, innovations, and healthcare in this digitally growing world. To synchronize and make decisions by analysing such

a big amount of data may not be possible by the traditional methods. Traditional model-based methods may fail because of problem varieties such as volume, dynamic changes, noise, and so forth. Because of the above varieties, the traditional data processing approach will become inefficient. On the basis of the combination of swarm intelligence and data mining techniques, we can have better understanding of big data analytics, so utilizing swarm intelligence to analyse big data will give massive results. By utilizing existing information about this domain, more efficient algorithm can be designed to solve real-life problems.

Healthcare delivery makes use of cutting-edge technology like AI, IoT, big data, and machine learning to prevent and treat emerging diseases. In this chapter, the authors examine SI's crucial role in analysing, preventing, and combating the COVID-19 pandemic as well as other pandemics. They gathered the most recent data on AI for COVID-19 and evaluated it to determine if it may be used to treat this illness. They discovered seven crucial AI applications for the COVID-19 pandemic. Researchers have been working to create a variety of AI models to solve the difficulties associated with medical diagnosis, prediction, and forecasting of medical data in recent years, with the healthcare system at the forefront of research. AI techniques include SI and EA. These algorithms have sped up the development of data analytics methods due to the increased availability of healthcare data. When complex issues are solved computationally in distributed systems, the SI and EA are employed to analyse collective behaviour. Deploying derivative free optimization using SI is affordable, versatile, and reliable.

The healthcare industry is rapidly developing across the world. The healthcare industry generates a large volume of diverse data. It is crucial for healthcare sectors to effectively extract, collect, and exploit data. Swarm intelligence algorithms have been

Chapter 9
An IoMT and Machine Learning Model Aimed at the Development of a Personalized Lifestyle Recommendation System Facilitating Improved Health162
Guru Prasad, Graphic Era University (Deemed), India
A. Suresh Kumar, Jain University (Deemed), India
Sakshi Srivastava, Graphic Era University (Deemed), India
Ananya Srivastava, Graphic Era University (Deemed), India
Aditi Srivastava, Graphic Era University (Deemed), India

The machine learning-based internet of medical things (IoMT) has recently gained traction in the healthcare industry because of its ability to reduce costs while simultaneously improving care quality through real-time and continuous monitoring. The advent of cutting-edge technologies has sparked a surge in interest in and demand for a more sophisticated healthcare delivery system. The chapter also shows software integration designs that are extremely important for the creation of smart healthcare systems. The developed systems are discussed in terms of their contributions, working procedures, results, and comparative merits and limits, all of which are included in the explanations. Existing system flaws and new framework introduction strategies are discussed, as well as current research difficulties and potential future paths. The goal is to give readers a thorough understanding of the most current advancements in the field of smart healthcare systems.

Chapter 10
Securing Healthcare Systems Integrated With IoT: Fundamentals, Applications, and Future Trends..186
S. Boopathi, Muthayammal Engineering College, India

This chapter provides an overview of healthcare security systems integrated with IoT, discussing fundamentals, applications, benefits, challenges, and considerations for implementation. Secure data transmission, access control, authentication mechanisms, and privacy preservation techniques are needed to ensure a secure ecosystem. The chapter discusses methods for detecting and responding to security threats, such as intrusion detection systems, security information and event management systems and user training and awareness programs. It emphasizes the importance of compliance with relevant regulations and standards to ensure legal and ethical handling of patient data. The study explores future trends and emerging technologies, such as blockchain, artificial intelligence, and 5G, and their potential impact on healthcare security. By implementing the recommendations, healthcare organizations can enhance security, safeguard patient privacy, and promote trust in the healthcare ecosystem.

Chapter 11
A Blockchain IoT Hybrid Framework for Security and Privacy in a Healthcare Database Network 210
Puneeta Singh, KIET Group of Institutions, India
Pritish Sinha, Galgotias University, India
Abhinav Raghav, Chandigarh University, India

Deep concern is rising in healthcare systems regarding medical data and computing medical customary. With advancement in blockchain technology, an advanced and more secure way of medical data management, sharing, and other services can be implemented with simple innovations in IoT and blockchain. This technology relies on grouping data into block and hold sets of information that once filled are closed and linked to other blocks of data creating a chain of data. This innovation grants high fidelity and a secure way of storing data without any involvement of third-party systems. In this research, the authors harness opportunity and trends that blockchain provides in advanced healthcare systems and how integration of other technologies can lead one of most secure and automatic systems in the health sector and medicine, records serving.

Chapter 12
Categorical Data Clustering Using Meta Heuristic Link-Based Ensemble Method: Data Clustering Using Soft Computing Techniques 226
Kousik Nalliyanna Goundar Veerappan, Arden University, UK
Yuvaraj Natarajan, Sri Shakthi Institute of Engineering and Technology, Coimbatore, India
Arshath Raja, B.S. Abdur Rahman Crescent Institute of Science and Technology, Chennai, India
Jeyaprabhavathi Perumal, Arden University, UK
S Jerald Nirmal Kumar, Sharda University, India

Conventional ensemble clustering is a consensus function that fails to produce final clusters. Such poor clusters partitioning creates poor stability with reduced clustering accuracy. This motivates to improve the final clustering quality using a hybrid ensemble-based model. In this study, an optimized link-based ensemble clustering approach is proposed to refine the incomplete datasets and to refine unknown entries in categorical dataset. The proposed work uses link-based similarity measure to find the availability of unknown datasets from link network of clusters. The ensemble clustering generates a refined cluster-association matrix in the form of weighted graphs. The final cluster partitioning acquires the final clustering partitions with a

refined matrix as its input that decomposes the graph into clusters. The comparison with conventional methods is made against performance metrics to evaluate the model efficacy.

Preface

In today's world, the smart health care supports the out-of-hospital concept which transforms and offers higher care standards. This is accomplished with individual data-driven treatment schemes and high-performance optimized devices customized to act as individual requirements with the help of mood of public. Moreover, the smart health care systems generally designed to sense the individual health status data where it can be forward to the clinical for interpretation issues. This will be crucial especially in the lake of physician's number. With the benefit of cognitive algorithms, a pre-learned intelligent system can be established for improving the diagnosis process and automating it. Besides, the valuable information from the clinical database is utilized for individual health prevention and protection through emergency situations.

Nevertheless, the swarm Intelligence analysis is a valuable tool for categorizing public opinion into different sentiments and assessing the public mood in general. Swarm Intelligence analysis was created to help with these tasks, but it has yet to find widespread use in the medical field. The design and development of next generation solutions will be influenced by the integration of several disciplines and their integration into the living environment.

We hope to strengthen the link between the Swarm Intelligence analysis sector and mental health research in this book chapter. Various works in the digital health arena shown how real-time monitoring of mood disorders improved the overall quality of life of patients and citizens.

Applications of Big data analytics, Artificial and Machine Learning approaches can provide substantial improvements in all areas of healthcare from diagnostics to treatment. This book designed to explore the dynamics of Swarm Intelligence health analysis for the future generation. data analysis and managing still represent the major trend owing to a huge number of devices that connect to the server environments that generate significant medical data. Further, the security of these data represents another challenge, where the medical data is highly classified and needs to be guarded. Hence, there is a necessity for providing stable, efficient, and scalable intelligent algorithms which lead to additional sophisticated solutions and that can make operative decisions in developing of swarm Intelligence based health care systems.

The book discusses the role of people behavioural activity in the evolution of the traditional medical system to an intelligent system. This book is based on the development of technical improvements considered in the process of intelligent systems by using cognitive techniques, swarm Intelligence deep learning, and machine learning techniques. These techniques will be used for multimodal biomedical data processing and non-invasive interpretation which efficiently improves the patient interpretation quality. Moreover, it objects to highlight the challenges of developing and proposing new ideas regarding the out-of-hospital dedicated systems directions. Solicits contributions of this book include theory, applications, and design schemes of intelligent systems, vision techniques, and biomedical applications, as well as the methodologies behind them.

This book also focuses on the economic, social, and environmental impact of swarm Intelligence smart healthcare systems. It aims to provide a detailed understanding of swarm Intelligence analysis supported applications while engaging premium smart computing methods and improved intelligent algorithms in the field of computer science. Further, the detailed assessment of IoT sensors, actuators, communication, and computing technology, and standards has been taken into considerations. Emphasis is also laid on the challenges associated with these smart healthcare systems. It includes connectivity, sensing, computation, complexity, and security issues. Therefore, this book designed for new innovations to overcome such challenges and to explore the dynamics of swarm Intelligence health analysis for the future generation.

Arumugam Suresh Kumar
Jain University (Deemed), India

Utku Kose
Suleyman Demirel University, Turkey

Sachin Sharma
Graphic Era University (Deemed), India

S. Jerald Nirmal Kumar
Sharda University, India

Chapter 1
A Study on Swarm Intelligence and Its Various Clustering Algorithms in Medical Diagnosis

Amreen Ayesha
Presidency University, Bengaluru, India

N. Nasurudeen Ahamed
Presidency University, Bengaluru, India

ABSTRACT

Swarm intelligence is a manner the usage of the knowledge of collective objects (human beings, bugs, etc.) collectively to attain the optimized solution for a given hassle. "Swarm" is a set of objects (people, bugs, and so on.). In different phrases, permits say we supply a troubling statement to a single person and tell her or him to undergo this hassle after which provide the solution, then because of this we will keep in mind the solution of that specific character only; however, the problem is that the answer given with the aid of that man or woman might not be the best solution or maybe that solution is not proper for others. So, to keep away from that, what we do is we give that hassle to a certain quantity of humans together (swarm) and ask them to attain the first-class answer feasible for that problem and then compute all the responses together to reach the high-quality solution possible.

OVERVIEW OF SWARM INTELLIGENCE (SI)

Gerardo Beni (Pham et al., 2021) first proposed the concept of swarm intelligence (SI) in 1989. SI is merely the combined behavior of dispersed, organized frameworks,

DOI: 10.4018/978-1-6684-6894-4.ch001

real or fictional. The concept is applied to attack artificial awareness. SI frameworks typically consist of a population of uncomplicated experts or boids that interact locally with one another and with their environments. The inspiration typically comes from nature, especially from organic structures. The experts follow very simple rules, and despite the absence of a centralized control structure dictating how individual operators should behave, local and in some ways arbitrary, associations between such operators foster the development of "intelligent" global behavior that is hidden from the individual operators. Examples of multiplicity insight in natural structures include insect colonies, wingless animal rushing, and birds. Swarm intelligence is the collective conduct of decentralized, self-organized structures. A regular swarm intelligence device consists of a populace of simple dealers that may talk (either immediately or indirectly) domestically with each different by means of acting on their neighborhood environment. Though the agents in a swarm follow quite simple rules, the interactions between such dealers can lead to the emergence of very complex global behavior, far past the functionality of character retailers. Examples in natural structures of swarm intelligence consist of birds flocking, ant foraging, and fish education.

Figure 1. Swarm intelligence (SI) framework

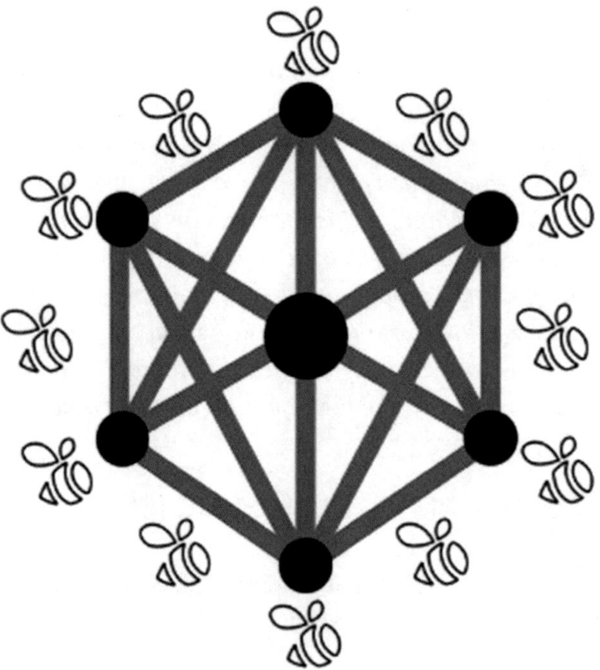

Swarm Intelligence Algorithm (SIA)

Inspired by the aid of the swarm's conduct, an algorithmic (Gong et al., 2019) class is suggested for dealing with optimization. troubles, normally below the title of swarm intelligence algorithms (SIAs). In SIAs, a swarm is made of multiple synthetic sellers. The sellers can change heuristic information within the shape of nearby interplay. Such interaction, further to sure stochastic elements, generates the conduct of adaptive search, and finally leads to global optimization. The maximum reputable and popular SIAs are particle swarm optimization (PSO) that's stimulated by using the social conduct of chook flocking or fish education, and ant colony optimization (ACO) which simulates the foraging behavior of ant colony. PSO is broadly used for real-parameter optimization whilst ACO has been efficiently carried out to clear up combinatorial optimization issues, for instance, the most famous combinatorial optimization troubles are the traveling salesman trouble (TSP) and quadratic venture hassle (QAP).

Novel SIAs with unique search mechanisms have been proposed and carried out fulfillment precise issues. Some times of novel SIAs are bacterial foraging optimization (BFO), bee set of rules, fish training search (FSS), cuckoo seek, fireworks algorithm (FWA), brain hurricane optimization (BSO), and the list is increasingly lengthier.

Here, we talk about three SI clustering algorithms (Öztürk et al., 2020), Particle Swarm Optimization (PSO), Ant Colony Optimization (ACO), and Artificial Bee Colony Optimization(ABC) for their medical diagnosis.

Particle Swarm Optimization (PSO)

Particle swarm optimization (PSO) was firstly advanced via Kennedy and Eberhart (Nasser Al-Andoli et al., 2022). In PSO every possible answer is referred to as a particle and a group of those viable answers is referred to as a populace. PSO is primarily based on how a collection of birds will randomly search for meals. Birds don't know wherein exactly the food is, in order that they follow the bird that's

Figure 2. Elements of swarm intelligence algorithm (SIA)

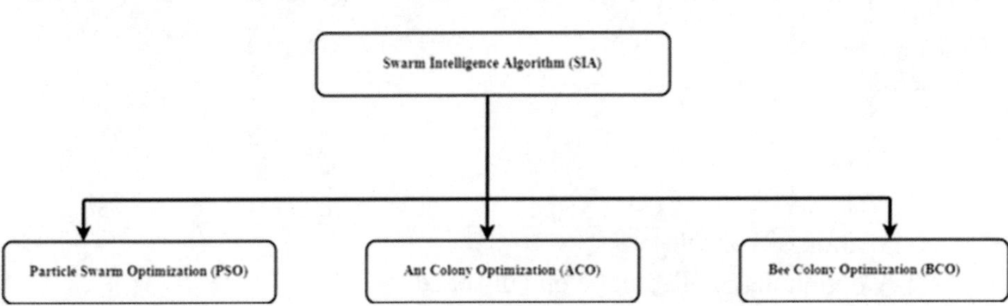

nearest to the meal. Each chicken is called a particle and each particle has its fitness feature (here it's miles a square of errors). An organization of particles is known as a swarm (Aly et al., 2019). The past two decades have visible a growing hobby in the use of particle swarm optimization (PSO) techniques, for fixing difficult numerical optimization problems, specifically the ones involving large seek spaces, discontinuous, or un-differentiable surfaces, and other troubles. PSO is beneficial because it is straightforward to apprehend and program, it does now not depend upon any assumptions approximately the underlying problem area, and it makes use of handiest a small number of parameters.

To carry out its search, the program generates a swarm of particles (Guo et al., 2011). With particular velocities, these particles continuously traverse the terrain of fitness. A particle's flight route over through the issue search space is determined by its velocity. Particles use their individual and interpersonal experiences to iteratively update their velocities as they move toward more suitable places (Li et al., 2015). PSO has been frequently used to resolve optimization issues in science and engineering due to its quick convergence time and simplicity. Band selection for hyperspectral pictures, feature selection, localization in Wireless Sensor Networks, Robotics, and Optimum Scheduling are some contemporary PSO uses.

Each particle in the standard PSO is attracted to two other particles and has a tendency to continue moving in the same direction. These three factors, therefore, control the fly trajectories of particles. The impact of these factors on a particle's flying pattern is controlled by a set of coefficients (Qasem & Shamsuddin, 2011). These coefficients have a significant impact on the particle's rate of motion, which in turn affects how quickly the algorithm converges. Numerous swarm structures have also been researched in the literature in an effort to exert greater command over the traveling pattern and speed of particles. Which particles can affect each particle depends on the swarm topology. Additionally, it controls how the swarm as a whole spreads information. A new trajectory and social behavior can result from altering the number of attractors.

The Speed and Space of the Swarm are mentioned below:

Speed: $V(T+1) = WV(T) + C1R1[X^2(T) - X(T)] + C2R2[G(T) - X(T)]$
Space: $X(T+1) = X(T) + V(T+1)$

Where,

- T – Time
- V – Velocity
- X- Position of Particle
- C1- Continuous intellectual element speed

- C2-Coefficient of speed for the social aspect
- R-Unreliable Randomness

Quantum PSO

The superposition principle of states governs the quantum system, it's neither a piecewise linear system nor a simple nonlinear system. As just a reason, this could encode more states than a piecewise- wise linear system. The approach taken by the particles in a quantum system is unexpected (Nasser Al-Andoli et al., 2022). According to the viable region, particles can appear anywhere, even at a location remote from the present site. The function of probability density. Different from the particle's current position positions might just have a fitter value then, the call to the overall desirability function of the existing particle population. Hence, using the stochastic quantum. This makes it feasible for the particles to more thoroughly search the search area and avoids local optimal convergence.

Time Variant Multi-Objective Particle Swarm Optimization (TVMOPSO)

By enabling its crucial parameters (flywheel mass and acceleration parameters) to change across iterations, TVMOPSO is adaptive by nature. This adaptability aids the algorithm's research of greater space search effectiveness. There has been a diversity parameter utilized. to ensure that the non-dominated solutions are sufficiently diverse maintaining fronts while maintaining the convergence up front on the Pareto-optimal side. The crowding distance computation technique is incorporated into the PSO algorithm (Li et al., 2015), specifically into the global best selection, the deletion procedure about an exterior library of non-dominated solutions, and the PSO parameters. The range of non-dominated responses in the exterior archive is maintained by the packing distance mechanism in conjunction with the mutation operator.

Multi-Objective Optimization (MOO)

The simultaneous optimization of numerous optimal solutions occurs in many real-world problems. These roles typically don't compare well and frequently have opposing goals. Instead of producing just one ideal solution, MOO with such competing objective functions produced a set of ideal solutions (Qasem & Shamsuddin, 2011). Numerous solutions are optimal because no one can be said to be superior to any other with regard to everyone's objective functions.

Binary Particle Swarm Optimization (BPSO)

Based on the quick pre-processing approach utilized to generate some of the data, data sets are made up of a large number of duplicate and heuristic features. The pre-treatment collected data is regarded as an input for selecting the most useful characteristics using Binary Particle Swarm Optimization (BPSO) (Guo et al., 2011).

Ant Colony Optimization (ACO)

ACO is based on how ants behave to forage for food. Ants leave behind pheromone as they move, and they follow the signal deposition to determine their path. Signal deposition density rises as ants return to the feeding source (Aly et al., 2019). The quality and variety of food brought to the source location affects the amount of pheromone deposition on the route back. The quantity of ants moving along that trail closely correlates with pheromone deposition and evaporation. Ants follow the most pheromone deposition to find the best route.

We might encounter very big graphs in some vision-based based and cognitive computing applications, and we might look for the best route between two nodes to reduce costs. Testing every conceivable path is not a viable option due to the size of the graph network. It is clear from this activity that ants are able to determine the shortest route between their source of food and their colony (Kurdi, 2022). The most crucial aspect of assisting ants in discovering this route is to emit a chemical known as a pheromone. The quickest way can become apparent over time.

Hyperbox Clustering With Ant Colony Optimization (HACO)

Unlabeled data can be categorized using a clustering technique called HACO (Hyperbox clustering with Ant Colony Optimization), which (Ramos et al., 2009) uses hyperboxes and an ant colony concept. While searching in a constrained search

Figure 3. The probability of find shortest path

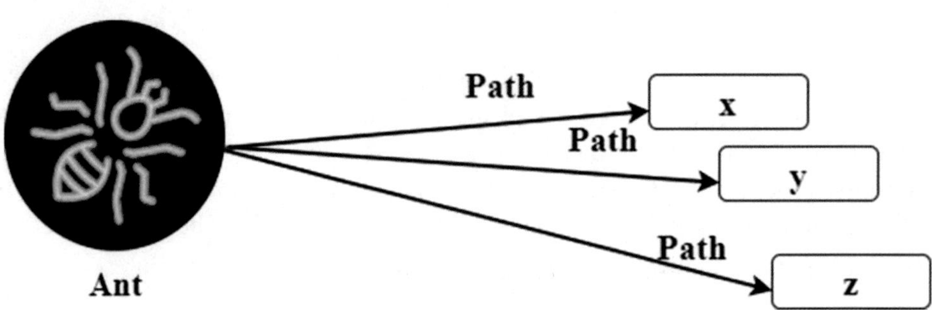

Figure 4. Classification of medical image signal processing methods

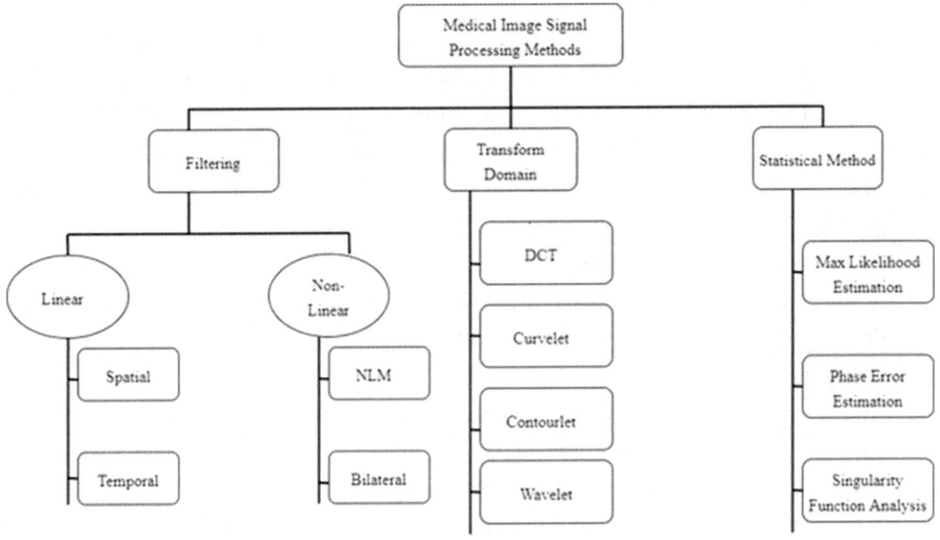

area (Miri et al., 2018), it takes into account the topological information (which is inextricably linked to categorization) included in the data, producing highly accurate results quickly. It is tested on fictitious 2D data sets before being applied to actual medical data, mechanically deriving clinical risk accounts for time-consuming tasks for medical professionals.

The ACO metaheuristic is used to insert hyperboxes in the search space, and the Closest place approach is then used to cluster them. It is typical for the number of hyperboxes to perform the search to be less than (or, in the worst-case case, equal to) the number of samples. This allows for fewer rounds of the search, which makes HACO (Ramos et al., 2009) a quick classifier. Three computer-generated 2D data sets (Miri et al., 2018) with substantial topological information are used to test the effectiveness of HACO as a classification method in order to achieve accuracy.

To search the feature space, hyperboxes to condense the space, and a local optimization technique to take into account the topological information. The HACO (Ramos et al., 2009) approach is used to identify likely risk profiles and enable early diagnosis, which is essential for averting the development of the disease into cancer. It is validated for data categorization with three computer-generated 2D data sets (Miri et al., 2018). The findings of HACO for clustering (and the simple collection of classifiers) suggested that this work should be developed further.

Ant Bee Colony (ABC)

Medical imaging, as well as how these images are interpreted, is critical for ensuring human health and tracking disorders. Technology advancements have contributed to a rise in the use of medical imaging equipment in recent years. Medical imaging technology (Aly et al., 2019) development continues to be the focus of intense study. 18.1 million new cases of cancer are anticipated in 2018, and 9.6 people are anticipated to pass away. Getting rid of many fatal diseases that endanger human life requires early detection. It is acknowledged that early diagnosis is difficult, nevertheless, given the relative scarcity of specialists compared to the global population. There aren't many experts in low-income nations. very long to be processed are medical photographs.

For example, due to their size and texture, medical photographs require more time to analyze. Fortunately, using artificial intelligence techniques in image processing has substantially enhanced automatic picture analysis. Furthermore, there are other effective techniques available exclusively for medical image (Sağ & Çunkaş, 2015) analysis. Minimizing the cost function increases the efficiency parameter. Algorithms for optimization achieve excellent success for this purpose. Optimization approaches typically result in the creation of new solution clusters. The most common swarm intelligence (SI) optimization techniques are ant colony optimization, bee colony optimization, particle swarm optimization, and whale optimization, even though that new one is added to the field practically weekly (Aly et al., 2019).

The probability distribution changes with each iteration of the ant colony optimization process, which takes an infinite amount of time to resolve. It's not too difficult to employ the particle swarm optimization technique, but its performance is greatly influenced by the initial parameters, success in problems with dispersed solutions is low, and the process is stranded at the local minimum.

In practically every industry nowadays, the ABC (Aly et al., 2019) optimization technique is preferred for artificial intelligence challenges. It is an extremely effective strategy for global optimization. This program mimics the movements of honeybee swarms and was inspired by natural phenomena. Early on, there were some issues with this algorithm's ability to solve composite and non-separable functions.

The ABC algorithm excels in resolving a wide range of problems. Due to recent changes made to its structure, it is employed in forms of instruction. According to new research, the ABC algorithm is becoming more and more popular, especially in the area of analysing clinical data. The main objective of this paper is to evaluate the ABC algorithm's approach for issues in healthcare image processing. Particularly when assessing medical images, which are essential for preserving public wellbeing (Shunmugapriya & Kanmani, 2017). The working and its variations are displayed.

The use of ABC analysis to vision based and feature extraction is closely examined in this research.

Working Principle

SI is a naturally occurring algorithm that takes inspiration from the way that insects behave and solve scientific challenges. It works with both organic and synthetic agents to strengthen the scientific solution in a number of fields, such as the analysis of medical photographs. It has a huge number of agents whose actions are coordinated via distributed control and self-organization (Shunmugapriya & Kanmani, 2017). The way these individuals communicate with one another determines how intelligent a swarm is. This insect intelligence activity improves several scientific issues in a variety of domains, such as the processing of medical photographs. Immune Algorithm, Ant Colony, Bat Algorithm etc. are a few other algorithms that draw inspiration from nature.

The honeybees have a variety of skills, including decision-making, information communication through movement, and memorization of the location (distance and direction) of food sources. They use their collective intelligence to discover food sources. These bees more dynamically assign duties and modify their roles in response to environmental changes. Honeybee life can be summed up by a food supply, bees that are working or not, bees that are foraging and bees that are employed or not (Wen et al., 2020).

Sources of food: A concerned here looks for its sources (flowers) then collects information about it, the ease with which it may be gathered, the direction and distance of the food source from the beehive, as well as the amount of nectar that is accessible. Profitability of food sources is influenced by factors like mobility, income, and simplicity of extraction. Figure 1 shows a variety of bees.

Employed and jobless working bees are yet another name for bees. A worker bee makes use of the sources of food and monitors the nectar flow. They provide information on the location, flow, and profitability of the food supply to an idle bee in the combs buzzing area. Bees that aren't making honey are actively searching for food sources to exploit and, if any are found, to share with bees that are. The unemployed bees also fall into the groups of scout bees and observer bees. In order to apply the knowledge to identify a food source, Scout bees search for a new source when the current one runs out. Spectator bees make comprise the remaining 50% of the beehive and are the only bees left. 10% of the beehive is made up of scout bees.

The hunt for food sources and nectar is the first step in the foraging process. After locating a food source, the bee begins to extract nectar and store it for 30 to 120 minutes. The amount of nectar is delivered inside the hive and is based on the hive's location and how rich the food supply is. Finally, by engaging in a

Figure 5. Classification of bee colony

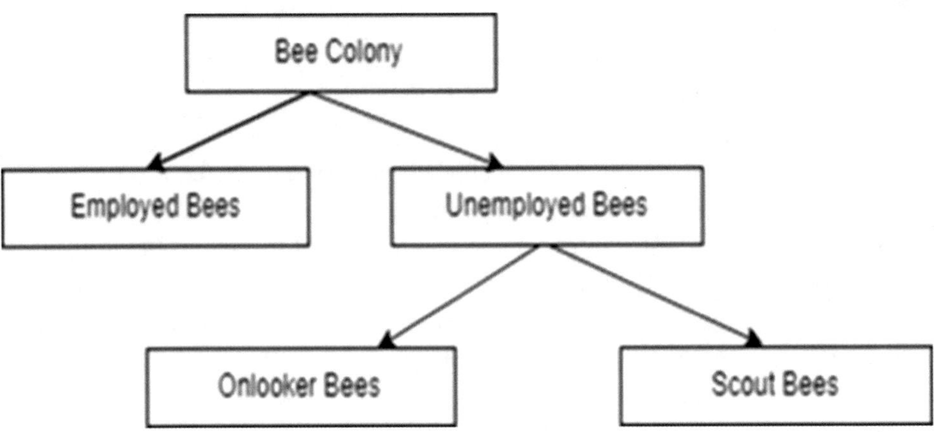

specific action known as dancing on various regions of the hive, the employed bees communicate information about the location, distance, and direction of their food supply. The orientation of the food supply in relation to the sun is indicated by the bee dance, whereas distance is indicated by several dances. The key indicator of a new food source location is the forager's body's flowery odor. The floral scent and dance language represent intercultural communication. The bee dance represents the likelihood of extracting food for decision-making. Other bees touch a dancing bee's antenna during the dance in order to sample the source's nectar (Wen et al., 2020) (Öztürk et al., 2020).

Engaged bees do a waggle, tremble, and round dance. The Round Dance is conducted if there is a close food supply to the hive. There is no mention of where the food source is located. Waggle Dance is located distant from the hive and, in relation to sunlight, points in the general vicinity of the food and water supply. The dancing becomes faster the farther away from the food source the colony is. A bee will do the Tremble Dance when it has taken a moment to drain the nectar and is dubious of the quantity and its profitability (Schranz et al., 2021).

Algorithm for Artificial Bee Colonies

Dervis Karaboga proposed the ABC algorithm in 2005. It is an inhabitants morpho algorithm inspired by the foraging behaviour of honeybees. Limit, maximum iteration size, and response number are examples of less efficient control variables (Sağ & Çunkaş, 2015). This response value represents the entire amount of food sources accessible to the population. The maximum iteration size denotes the most generations, whilst the maximum signifies the run out of food. Processes associated to the ABC include selection and population processes. Whereas, the population is a variance approach that examines the various search space areas, the selection method makes sure that earlier experiences are being used (Rostami et al., 2021). The four processes of ABC include the beginning process, engaged bees process, observant bee process, and scout bee process. The ABC's placement of the basis of food and the amount of honey it produces points to a potential solution quality (fitness).

Given that each hired bee is connected to a single food source, the number of working bees and sources of food(solutions) is equal. It depicts ABC algorithm's general algorithmic process and organizational structure. During the commencement process, scout bees commence the food source solutions, as well as the selected variables are established. New sources of food are searched out in the surrounding during the employed bees' phase, and if any are found, their fitness is evaluated using the greedy approach (Pham et al., 2021).

Inquisitive bees in the dance area talk to these worker bees about where the source of food is located. The observation bee process makes its choice of food on the basis of collective fitness information. The hired bees are turned into Scouts and its recommendations are given up during the scout process if their keys don't improve after a specific number of trials (referred to as the limit). These scouts start at random hunting for novel ideas. Pseudocode for the ABC algorithm is shown. In the sections that follow, we describe the mathematical depiction of several steps.

Establishment of the populace, the ABC process creates an initial population with a probability sampling that is uniform. Each solution in this population has a Resolution Key (RK), where a_x(x=1,2,3,...RK) represents the xth source of food in the original population and is a D-dimensional vector. Equation -1 is used to accomplish the calculation.

Based on the information about nectar fitness, the employed bee phase enhances the employed bee's current solution. This also involves the adjustment of the food source's position in the sections that follow, we describe the mathematical depiction (Equation -2) of several steps, while those with lower amounts than the previous ones are deleted (Aly et al., 2019).

The observation bee phase chooses the best course of action based on the fitness probability after assessing shared nectar quality and location information given by bees. The improved fitness probability updates the hired bees position Equation -3.

$$a_x^{\,y} = a^y_{min} + \text{rand}\,(0, 1)\,(a^y_{max} - a^y_{min}),\ \forall y = 1, 2, \ldots, D \qquad (1)$$

where a^y_{min} and a^y_{max} are bounds of a_x in y^{th} direction

$$V_{xy} = a_{xy} + \Phi_{xy}\,(a_{xy} - a_{zy}) \qquad (2)$$

where $\Phi_{xy}(a_{xy}-a_{zy})$ refers to current iteration and z ∈ {1, 2, . . ., RK}, y ∈ {1, 2, . . ., D}, are two identifiers selected at random and $\Phi_{xy} \in (-1, 1)$.

$$p_x = f_{x/(}\sum^{NS}_{y=1} f_{y)} \tag{3}$$

The fitness of the xth solution is represented by f_x in Equation-3. The scout bee phase starts searching for other sources once the current source is depleted. When a foodstuff is forcibly taken away, the aforementioned location is not revised to include the required number of sessions, this happens. The one that is linked to discarded source changes into a scout fly and starts looking for new sources nearby.

The major goal of this study is to look at how the ABC algorithm and its variations affect applications for analyzing medical images. In order to advance academics' and researchers' upcoming work in this area, the efficacy of the proposed technique and its versions for issues relating to computer vision has just been evaluated (Aly et al., 2019).

For the search for research papers, numerous electronic journal databases have been utilized. Various standard electronic journal databases were the most significant ones employed in this study

Steps to Be Followed in ABC Algorithm

1. Defining the Problem.
2. Initializing the parameters. Build a newly employed bee colony and Analyze bees fitness potential.
3. Repeat
4. Initialize N=0, z= solution near I, Φ as any random number between -1 & +1
5. Using Equation 2 to find new solutions.
6. Greedy Selection process is to be applied.
7. Using Equation 3 to find new probability values.
8. Allocate Onlooker bees, Apply the Greedy method. Check whether the ability probability w.r.t Onlooker bees is inferior to fitness probability of employed bees and replace it with Employed bees.
9. Check if the fitness (Best Onlooker) < fitness (Best), Replace it with the Best solution.
10. Say N=+1, until N reaches the number of Employed Bees.
11. Using Equation 1, ascertain the abandoned solution. Replace them if the Scout solution is superior to the one being used.

Upcoming Task in ABC

In this study, the efficiency of the ABC approach in applications involving photo processing is examined. These changes are proposed to be implemented by changing the control settings of ABC or one of its phases. By completing the fitness function and startup, adaptations aim to improve overall quality and hasten the accomplishment of outcomes. The scout bee capacity to recall food source's locations is boosted by the numerous ABC process innovations, such as the greedy selection algorithm's optimum use of watcher bees. In the bee process, repeated scout search and random search are used to improve exploration and exploitation (Aly et al., 2019).

Using local search encourages intelligent and highly qualified exploitation. As a result, it improves the bees' capacity for information transmission, The cross-cooperation mechanism improves the bee-to-bee communication paradigm. As a result, the information flow during the initial exploration phase is improved, as well as the bee-to-bee communication paradigm. The numerous parameters of the fundamental ABC algorithm were altered, and the results in terms of selecting the best threshold, bunch centers for gathering methods, resolving initial value challenges, and multi-class centers are more encouraging (Wen et al., 2020).

Today, there is a growing need for SI algorithms. Compared to photos of the natural world, people, the earth's surface, or satellites, medical images differ greatly from other types of images. Additionally, a variety of medical imaging methods produce a variety of multi-class challenges for artificial intelligence algorithms. Convolutional neural network design optimization is a prominent topic right now since it revolutionizes practically every image processing problem, including in the area of processing images (Guo et al., 2011).

ABC algorithm-based CNN structure initialization (Wen et al., 2020), backpropagation, and optimization solutions are the open rooms of medical image analysis. ABC algorithm convergence with shrink computations; effects of ABC phase parameter on convergence time and computation; examination of the method to avoid local minima for better convergence; investigation of the influence of control parameters on the performance parameters of the application algorithm. creation of an all-encompassing experimental design with a control parameter configuration; a performance analysis of the algorithm using large-scale imagery; Bee communication has improved for swift convergence and quick response (Li et al., 2015).

The ABC algorithm's utility in applications for image processing is investigated in this work. This allows for a deeper investigation of how ABC methods affect picture improvement, grouping, gathering, and separation tasks. These alternatives are put forth by changing either the ABC phases or its control parameters. The fitness function and initialization are performed as part of modifications in order to improve overall performance and speed of attaining the results. The various adjustments in the ABC stages, such as the greedy optimal use of watcher bees, improve scout bees' memory capacity for locating food sources. Better exploration and exploitation are accomplished by using the numerous scout hunt methods and random search at the employed bee process (Li et al., 2015).

Utilizing local search promotes skilled and highly fit exploitation. The ability of the bees to transmit information is thus improved, enhancing exploration during the challenging exploitation time. The multi-population cooperative mechanism is used to enhance the bee-to-bee communication paradigm. As a result, the bee-to-bee communication paradigm is enhanced, and information sharing during the initial exploratory phase is improved. In terms of choosing the best verge, group centers for grouping, fixing preliminary worth difficulties, and multi-class centers, adjustment of a number of the basic ABC algorithm's parameters yields more encouraging results.

Medical Image Diagnoses Method

PSO has been used as an MRI segmentation algorithm, and many PSO methods, including "Darwinian Particle Swarm" DPSO, have been described. Additionally, the outputs were categorized using SVM, and the overall system had reliability close to 100%. Different techniques (Li et al., 2015)(Miri et al., 2018) (Mandal et al., 2014), such as Ant colony optimization and Bee colony efficiency, look for the quickest routes. To enhance the image processing techniques based on the feature subset selection, apply ACO (ant colony optimization). As a segmentation algorithm, Artificial Bee Optimization (ABO) is used. Actually, they have used MRI scans to apply the approach (Nasser Al-Andoli et al., 2022).

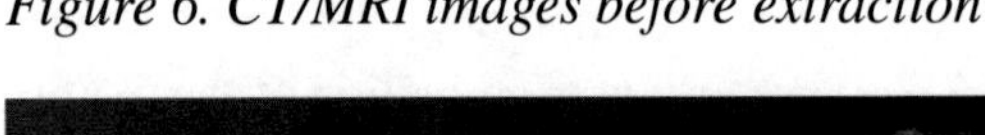

Figure 6. CT/MRI images before extraction

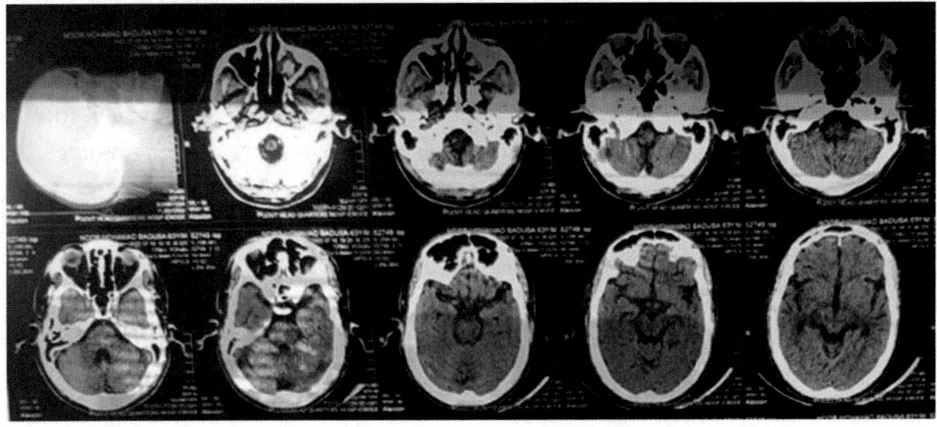

Figure 7. CT/MRI images after extraction

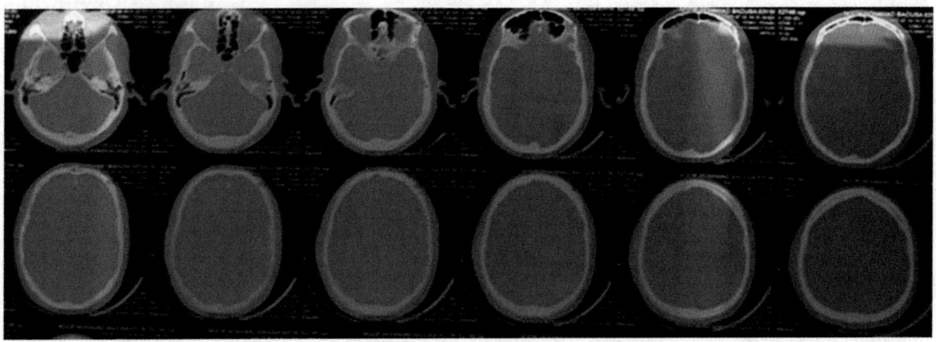

To evaluate the MRI/CT pictures (Anter et al., 2020) of the brain images, identify the different types of problems, categorize them, and forecast potential problems, we employ, integrate, and alter some of the aforementioned techniques (Wen et al., 2020).

CONCLUSION

Many of these datasets' attributes are either duplicated or unnecessary, which lowers the accuracy of the prediction model. In machine learning, and more specifically in the high-dimensional dataset, feature selection is crucial. The variables of the classification algorithm are determined by reducing the size of the medical dataset, which also lowers the computational complexity. As a result, the prediction model's accuracy will rise. Large-scale datasets have rapidly grown during the past few decades as a result of the rapid development of computer and database technologies. The features of brain MRI/CT images can be extracted in order to diagnose malignancies, and numerous approaches and algorithms have been presented. Particle swarm optimization (PSO), ant colony optimization based on trip salesman (ACO), and bee colony optimization was introduced as the three primary feature extraction strategies in this work (BCO).

REFERENCES

Al-Andoli, M. N., Tan, S. C., & Cheah, W. P. (2022). Distributed parallel deep learning with a hybrid backpropagation-particle swarm optimization for community detection in large complex networks. *Information Sciences*, *600*, 94–117. doi:10.1016/j.ins.2022.03.053

Aly, R. H. M., Rahouma, K. H., & Hamed, H. F. (2019). Brain Tumors Diagnosis and Prediction Based on Applying the Learning Metaheuristic Optimization Techniques of Particle Swarm, Ant Colony and Bee Colony. *Procedia Computer Science*, *163*, 165–179. doi:10.1016/j.procs.2019.12.098

Anter, A. M., Bhattacharyya, S., & Zhang, Z. (2020). Multi-stage fuzzy swarm intelligence for automatic hepatic lesion segmentation from CT scans. *Applied Soft Computing*, *96*, 106677. doi:10.1016/j.asoc.2020.106677

Gong, X., Liu, L., Fong, S., Xu, Q., Wen, T., & Liu, Z. (2019). Comparative research of swarm intelligence clustering algorithms for analyzing medical data. *IEEE Access : Practical Innovations, Open Solutions*, *7*, 137560–137569. doi:10.1109/ACCESS.2018.2881020

Guo, X., Wang, C., & Yan, R. (2011). An electromagnetic localization method for medical micro-devices based on adaptive particle swarm optimization with neighborhood search. *Measurement*, *44*(5), 852–858. doi:10.1016/j.measurement.2011.01.022

Kurdi, M. (2022). Ant colony optimization with a new exploratory heuristic information approach for open shop scheduling problem. *Knowledge-Based Systems*, *242*, 108323. doi:10.1016/j.knosys.2022.108323

Li, Y., Jiao, L., Shang, R., & Stolkin, R. (2015). Dynamic-context cooperative quantum-behaved particle swarm optimization based on multilevel thresholding applied to medical image segmentation. *Information Sciences*, *294*, 408–422. doi:10.1016/j.ins.2014.10.005

Mandal, D., Chatterjee, A., & Maitra, M. (2014). Robust medical image segmentation using particle swarm optimization aided level set based global fitting energy active contour approach. *Engineering Applications of Artificial Intelligence*, *35*, 199–214. doi:10.1016/j.engappai.2014.07.001

Miri, A., Sharifian, S., Rashidi, S., & Ghods, M. (2018). Medical image denoising based on 2D discrete cosine transform via ant colony optimization. *Optik (Stuttgart)*, *156*, 938–948. doi:10.1016/j.ijleo.2017.12.074

Öztürk, Ş., Ahmad, R., & Akhtar, N. (2020). Variants of Artificial Bee Colony algorithm and its applications in medical image processing. *Applied Soft Computing*, *97*, 106799. doi:10.1016/j.asoc.2020.106799

Pham, Q. V., Nguyen, D. C., Mirjalili, S., Hoang, D. T., Nguyen, D. N., Pathirana, P. N., & Hwang, W. J. (2021). Swarm intelligence for next-generation networks: Recent advances and applications. *Journal of Network and Computer Applications*, *191*, 103141. doi:10.1016/j.jnca.2021.103141

Qasem, S. N., & Shamsuddin, S. M. (2011). Radial basis function network based on time variant multi-objective particle swarm optimization for medical diseases diagnosis. *Applied Soft Computing*, *11*(1), 1427–1438. doi:10.1016/j.asoc.2010.04.014

Ramos, G. N., Hatakeyama, Y., Dong, F., & Hirota, K. (2009). Hyperbox clustering with Ant Colony Optimization (HACO) method and its application to medical risk profile recognition. *Applied Soft Computing*, *9*(2), 632–640. doi:10.1016/j.asoc.2008.09.004

Rostami, M., Berahmand, K., Nasiri, E., & Forouzandeh, S. (2021). Review of swarm intelligence-based feature selection methods. *Engineering Applications of Artificial Intelligence*, *100*, 104210. doi:10.1016/j.engappai.2021.104210

Sağ, T., & Çunkaş, M. (2015). Color image segmentation based on multiobjective artificial bee colony optimization. *Applied Soft Computing*, *34*, 389–401. doi:10.1016/j.asoc.2015.05.016

Schranz, M., Di Caro, G. A., Schmickl, T., Elmenreich, W., Arvin, F., Şekercioğlu, A., & Sende, M. (2021). Swarm intelligence and cyber-physical systems: Concepts, challenges and future trends. *Swarm and Evolutionary Computation*, *60*, 100762. doi:10.1016/j.swevo.2020.100762

Shunmugapriya, P., & Kanmani, S. (2017). A hybrid algorithm using ant and bee colony optimization for feature selection and classification (AC-ABC Hybrid). *Swarm and Evolutionary Computation*, *36*, 27–36. doi:10.1016/j.swevo.2017.04.002

Wen, T., Liu, H., Lin, L., Wang, B., Hou, J., Huang, C., Pan, T., & Du, Y. (2020). Multiswarm Artificial Bee Colony algorithm based on spark cloud computing platform for medical image registration. *Computer Methods and Programs in Biomedicine*, *192*, 105432. doi:10.1016/j.cmpb.2020.105432 PMID:32278250

Chapter 2
Healthcare Data Analytics Using Swarm Intelligence Techniques

K. Renuka Devi
Dr. Mahalingam College of Engineering and Technology, Pollachi, India

ABSTRACT

The healthcare domain plays a significant role. Healthcare information contains heterogeneous data where it has been utilized to mine data in order to provide accurate and optimized results to the user. Hence, the data mining can open up a world of possibilities in terms of diagnosis, prognosis, and therapy. It holds an important place in the medicinal field for the purpose of analyzing huge volumes of data for extracting the salient parts for evaluating the patients' reports. The swarm intelligence (SI) technique has also been utilized for disease diagnosis and treatment. This chapter explains the importance of swarm intelligence technique under data mining in healthcare. It also focused on explaining different algorithms of SI such as particle swarm optimization (PSO) and ant colony optimization (ACO). It also explains its performance and accuracy in delivering the optimized results to the users/patients.

INTRODUCTION

Data mining is one of the growing area where it has been utilized to resolve main issues and difficulties in various domains such as healthcare, commercial applications, banking areas, customer analysis (Ramzan & Ahmad, 2014). Data mining contains various algorithms to resolve those issues such as Apriori algorithm, Naïve Bayes

DOI: 10.4018/978-1-6684-6894-4.ch002

algorithm, SVM, etc., whereas the swarm intelligence plays a significant role in data mining by analyzing the result (Janardhanan & Umamaheswari, 2020) through combining the objectives of several users to obtain one of the optimized and efficient result (Suresh & Padmajavalli, 2007). From the optimized result, the user can able to obtain the efficient output (Du & Zhou, 2016) which is depicted in Figure 1.

DATA MINING

The task of uncovering valuable and intriguing patterns and correlations in large amounts of data is known as data mining (Deepa & Geetha, 2013). It is largely useful and worthy for various kinds of domains such as healthcare organizations, insurance agencies and patients etc., To classify chronic diseases and identify high-risk patients, various data mining algorithms have been explored (Costa et al., 2019). This will allow the healthcare industry to compare different symptoms, possible causes, and treatment strategies (Lakshmi & Raghunandhan, 2011). Various symptoms can be analyzed, their causes revealed, and the most effective treatment method anticipated as a result. As a result, a standard for the treatment of specific disorders can be developed (Mudimigh et al., 2009).

SWARM INTELLIGENCE

Swarm intelligence is defined as the branch of computational intelligence where it generally focused on defining how self-organizing communities of agents develop collective behavior (Kirschenbaum & Palmer, 2015). It is normally adopted by the behavior of movement of birds and fish. It is defined as the branch of self-organized

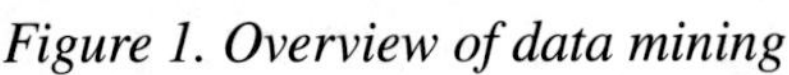
Figure 1. Overview of data mining

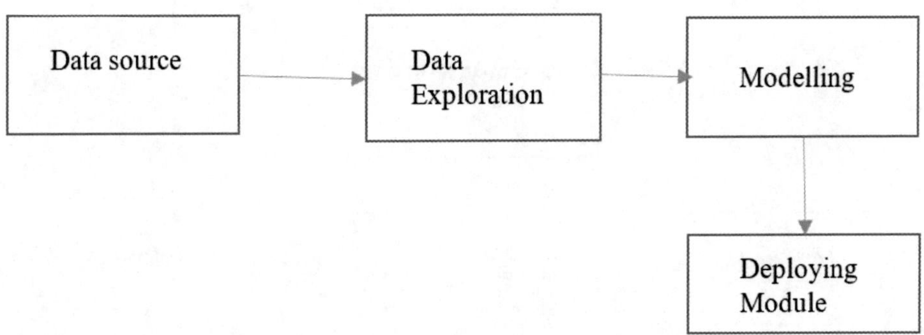

systems that tends to make its movement in a well-defined coordinated manner (Bharne & Gulhane, 2011). Swarms exist naturally in nature, and scientists have studied natural processes like ant colonization, bird flocking, and mammal herding to learn how distinct biological organisms collaborate with their surroundings to achieve a common purpose (Zhu & Tang, 2010).

The swarm intelligence holds different capabilities such as optimization, routing, clustering, scheduling (Sasa & Dongqing, 2009) which is depicted in Figure 2.

Scheduling

Scheduling is a decision-driven methodology which has been utilized in several manufacturing and service industries (Liu & Liang, 2009). This process is highly useful for allocation of resources in a short span of time and to achieve the optimized result in a more efficient manner (Deng, 2009).

Clustering

A clustering mechanism is defined as a grouping of data of comparable types (Chen & Meng, 2004). It is helpful for identifying the data of similar type and also to group the item in one similar group. The data/items in one single cluster will share the same properties which is largely helpful for the swarm intelligence technique (Khosla & Kumar, 2005).

Figure 2. Swarm intelligence: Capabilities

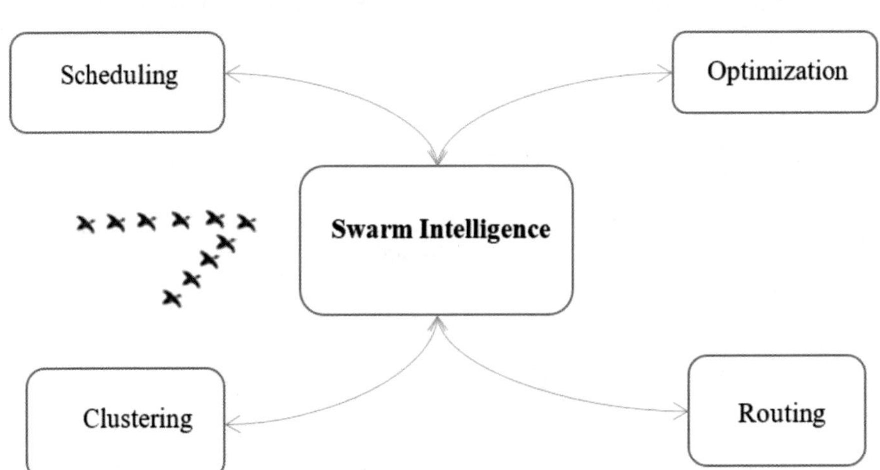

Optimization

The term "optimization" is the process of determining the optimal solution to a problem (Du & Liu, 2017). The swarm intelligence is to find the solution by collective behavior of objects. Whereas the optimization capability is highly recommended to find the best optimal solution from the result obtained. This helps to find out the best optimal result of the problem (Wei & Feifan, 2009).

Routing

Routing is based on the rule that helps to find out the optimal route from source to destination (Zhang & Gao, 2010). Swarm intelligence, on the other hand, is extremely important for ants or bees in determining the best path to goal from advanced agents (Zhang & Zhu, 2014).

SWARM INTELLIGENCE IN HEALTHCARE

The healthcare sector is growing in a rapid manner by utilizing huge amount of data (Jemal & Kechaou, 2014). This domain usually comprises of heterogeneous data and so it is highly difficult to process as well as to mine in a more effective manner. Data mining plays a significant role in analyzing the patients' records and to process the huge volume of data (Chen & Wang, 2018). The swarm intelligence has been utilized to fine tune the results obtained from mining the data. The SI is highly helpful for retrieving the most optimized result in the perspective of healthcare domain (Renuka Devi & Balasamy, 2022) which is depicted in Figure 3. For instance, if a patient is suffering from diabetes, the prediction of the patients' condition should be accurate (Fong & Deb, 2014). Hence, the SI under data mining could be highly useful for predicting the patients result in a more accurate and optimized manner.

The above figure depicts that the patients might be suffering from diabetics or any ill conditions and the data of those patients were collected and analyzed by means of data mining (Yekkala & Dixit, 2017). Data mining plays a significant role in analyzing those data in providing appropriate results to the users. Data mining utilizes swarm intelligence (SI) as a technique to process the patients' data where it tends to produce optimized and accurate results to the users by fine tuning the data in more efficient manner (Nandy & Adhikari, 2022).

Figure 3. Swarm intelligence in healthcare

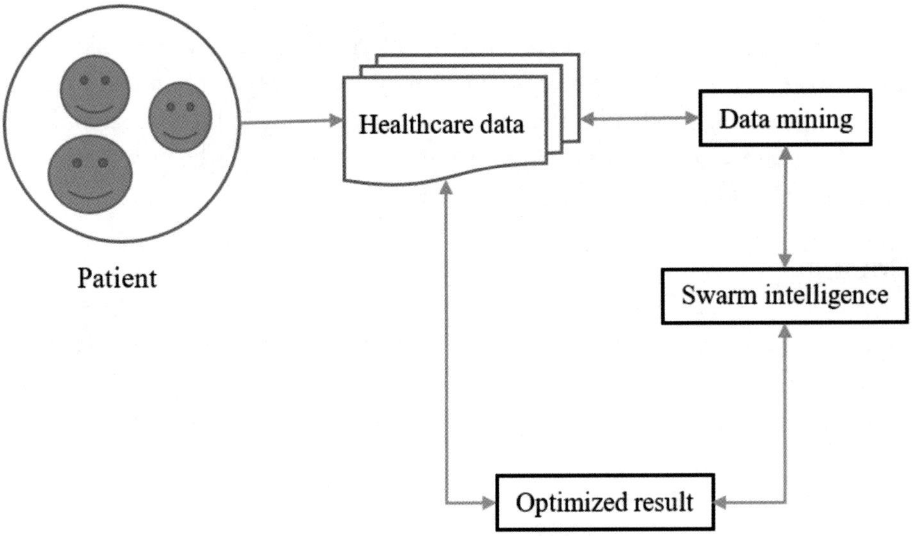

ALGORITHMS IN SI

The swarm intelligence comprises of several algorithms for data processing, analysis, data optimization (Jemal & Kechaou, 2014). The SI consists of a large number of algorithms where the important one is discussed here. Algorithms such as Particle Swarm Optimization (PSO), Ant Colony Optimization (ACO), Artificial Bee Colony (ABC), and the Firefly Algorithm (FA) which is depicted in Figure 4.

Particle Swarm Optimization (PSO)

PSO is a part of bio-inspired algorithm and tends to provide the most optimal solution to the users. It varies from generic optimization algorithm such that it requires only the objective function rather than any kind of gradient (Shen et al., 2018). It is considered to be the efficient meta- heuristic optimization technique where it gets inspired by bird or fish flocking. It was originally inspired by the inspiration of bird flocks. Technically, this algorithm explains that for any given data or measured quality, it processes those data and provide us the optimal results (Yitong & Mengyin, 2007) which is given through equation 1.

Benefits:

When compared to mathematical algorithms and other heuristic optimization techniques, the PSO algorithm has the following primary benefits:

Figure 4. Swarm intelligence algorithms

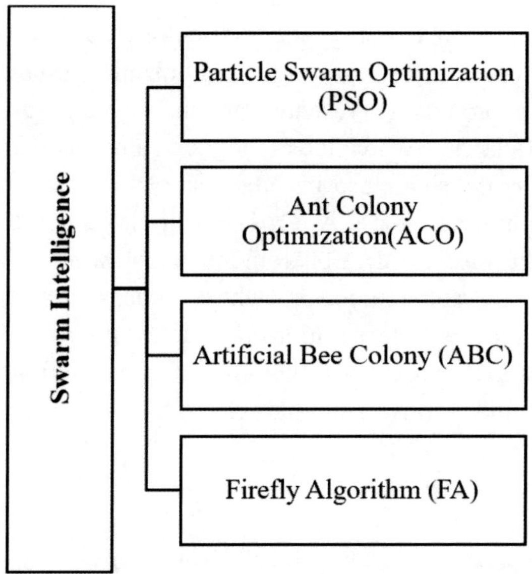

- A straightforward concept,
- Straightforward implementation,
- Robustness to control parameters, and
- Computational efficiency.

$$x_i(k+1) = x_i(k) + v_i(k+1) \tag{1}$$

Where,

i = particle index

k = discrete time index

v_i = velocity of ith particle

x_i = position of ith particle

Ant Colony Optimization (ACO):

A population-based metaheuristic called ant colony optimization (ACO) can be utilized to approximately solve challenging optimization issues.

An optimization problem is presented, and in ACO, a group of software agents referred to as artificial ants which looks for good solutions (Jangra & Kait, 2017). The optimization issue is changed into the task of locating the optimum path on a weighted graph in order to use ACO. The artificial ants move about the graph to develop solutions piecemeal. A pheromone model, which referred to as a set of parameters linked to graph components whose values are changed at any runtime by the ants, biases the stochastic solution construction process (G. Ping, X. Chunbo, 2014) has been given through equation 2. In ACO, the solution to the optimization problem will be found by traversing through the fully connected graph.

Benefits:

Benefits of Ant Colony Optimization includes:

- Positive feedback explains how quick answers are found.
- Effective for the "Traveling Salesman Problem" and related issues.
- Suitable for dynamic applications.

$$T_{i,j}=\left(1-\rho\right)T_{i,j}+\Delta T_{i,j} \qquad (2)$$

Where,

$T_{i,j}$ denotes the amount of pheromone,
A indicates the amount of pheromone evaporated,
$\Delta T_{i,j}$ indicates the amount of pheromone deposited.

Artificial Bee Colony (ABC)

The ABC algorithm is a kind of swarm-based metaheuristic model which is utilized for analyzing and to optimize those numerical problems. It was influenced by how honeybees used intelligence in their foraging (Bing & Youwei, 2021). The algorithm is especially formulated on the design for honeybee colony feeding behavior. Foraging bees that are working and not working, as well as food sources, make up the model. The first two elements, working and unemployed foraging bees of a kind, look for abundant food sources nearby their hive, which is the third element.

The model also identifies two key behaviors that must occur for self-organization and collective intelligence: Foragers must be drawn to abundant food sources, which produces favorable feedback, and they must be driven away from poor sources, which results in negative feedback.

In ABC, a colony of synthetic forager bees looks for plentiful synthetic food sources. For utilizing Artificial Bee Colony, the optimization problem under consideration is first transformed into a problem of determining the optimum parameter vector that tends to reduce a target function (Zhang & Zhang, 2021). The artificial bees then use a neighbor search technique to move towards better solutions while discarding inferior ones to iteratively increase the population of the initial solution vectors that they have randomly discovered which is explained through equation 3.

Benefits:

- ABC has few control parameters.
- Rapid convergence.
- Utilized for both exploration and exploitation strategies.

$$v_{ij}=x_{ij}+\varphi_{ij}(x_{ij}-x_{kj}) \tag{3}$$

Where,
k & j is a randomly selected parameter index,
x_{kj} is a randomly selected food source.

Firefly Algorithm (FA)

The physiological and social features of actual fireflies serve as the basis for the Firefly Algorithm (FA) which is also a metaheuristic. It could deal with multimodal combinational and numerical optimization problems more effectively and naturally (X. Qi, S. Zhu, 2017). It was used in a variety of fields, including in-line spring-mass systems and the codebook for vector quantization, because to its few adjustable parameters and ease of comprehension, realization, and computation.

The flashing behavior of fireflies serves as the basis for the Firefly algorithm. The basic foundation of FA is idealized by the three following rules: Since every firefly is gender neutral, they will all attract one another regardless of their gender. Attractiveness is inversely correlated with brightness, which declines as a firefly's distance from another firefly increases (S. K. Sarangi, R. Panda, 2016) which is given through equation 4.

Benefits:

- Efficient for non-linear, multimodal problems.
- Doesn't use velocities.
- High convergence speed.
- Doesn't require initial solution to begin its iteration.

$$x_{ik} = x_{ik} + \beta_{\circ}.e^{-\gamma.r_{ij^2}}.\left(x_{ik} - x_{jk}\right) + \propto .S_k.\left(rand_{ik} - \frac{1}{2}\right) \tag{4}$$

Where,
$\propto$ and S_k denotes the scaling parameters,
$rand_{ik}$ denotes the random integer between 0 and 1.

EXPERIMENT

The experiment was carried out by utilizing diabetes dataset from UCI machine learning repository. The dataset contains attributes such as age, gender, location, glucose level of each patient. The experiment was carried out by utilizing Windows 8.1 operating system by programming in Java using netbeans 8.1 with varying CPU and RAM capacity.

EXPERIMENTAL RESULTS

Figure 5 depicts the performance of particle Swarm Optimization algorithm. The result shows that the speed in detecting results increases with the increase in number of attributes. In the perspective of accuracy, the percentage gets higher with the number of attributes. This shows that the user/patient gets accurate results in a more efficient manner.

Figure 6 depicts the performance of Ant Colony Optimization algorithm. The result shows that the speed in detecting results decreases with the increase in number of attributes. In the perspective of accuracy, the percentage moderately decreases with the number of attributes. This shows that the detecting results and providing more accurate results will be lesser for ACO algorithm.

Figure 7 depicts that the comparison of Particle Swarm Optimization (PSO) algorithm and Ant Colony Optimization (ACO) algorithm in terms of performance analysis. From the figure, it is inferred that PSO performs better than ACO, since the accuracy and speed of PSO is higher when compared with ACO. The PSO performs

Figure 5. PSO algorithm: Performance

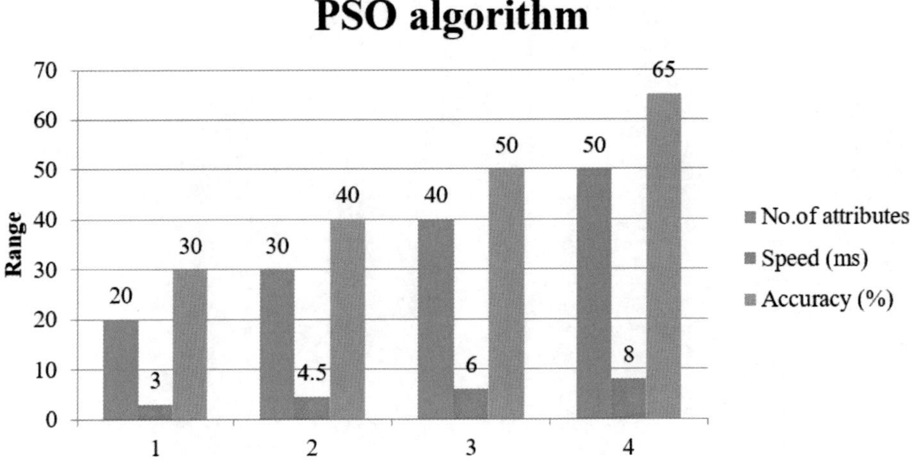

Figure 6. ACO algorithm

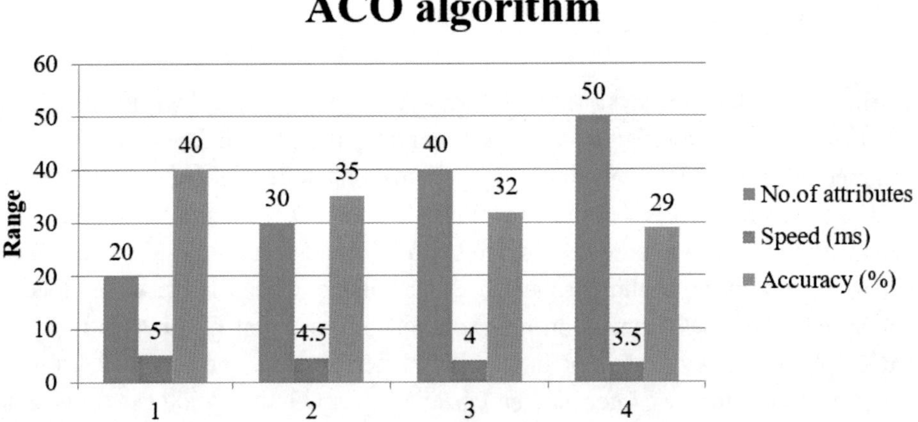

better when the number of attributes increases. When the number of attributes is 20, PSO performance would be 45% whereas ACO would be 33%. When the number of attributes is 30, PSO performance would be 53% whereas ACO would be 42%. But, when the number of attributes is 40, PSO performance would be 74% whereas ACO would be 61%. Likewise, when the number of attributes is 50, PSO performance would be 85% whereas ACO would be 70%.

Figure 7. Comparison: PSO and ACO

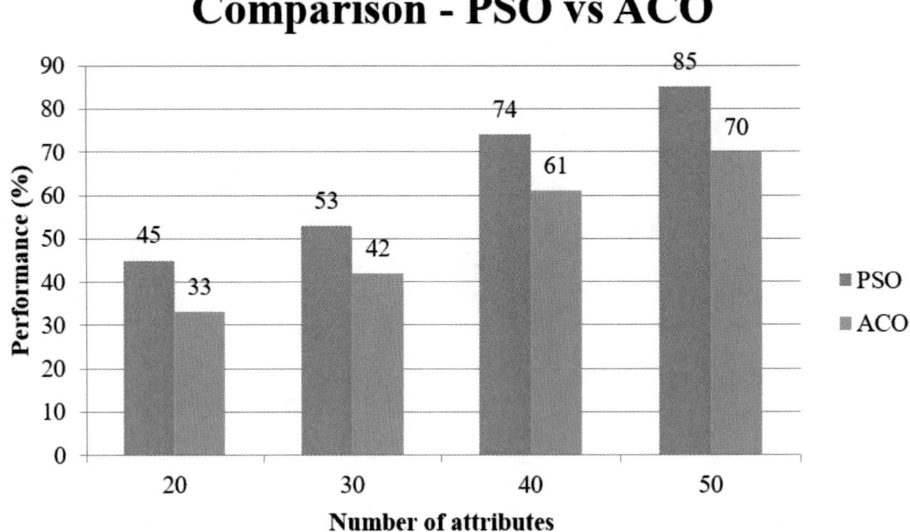

CONCLUSION

The healthcare domain plays one of the most significant and vital roles in today's world. The medicinal field consists of a huge amount of sensitive data. Several technologies and methods prevail for analyzing those patients' data for providing efficient results. One of the techniques is that the swarm intelligence under data mining which aims in analyzing the data in order to provide optimized and accurate results to the users/ patients. Various algorithms under SI are available whereas this paper focused on Particle Swarm Optimization (PSO) algorithm and Ant Colony Optimization (ACO) algorithms by explaining in terms of its performance and accuracy. From the experimental results, we infer that the Particle Swarm Optimization performs better than Ant Colony Optimization. Since, the result computing speed and accuracy tends to increase as the number of attributes increases. Hence, it can be able to provide more optimized and accurate results to the user/patients in healthcare domain.

REFERENCES

Bharne, P. K., Gulhane, V. S., & Yewale, S. K. (2011). Data clustering algorithms based on Swarm Intelligence. *2011 3rd International Conference on Electronics Computer Technology*, 407-411. 10.1109/ICECTECH.2011.5941931

Bing, X., Youwei, Z., Xueyan, Z., & Xuekai, S. (2021). An Improved Artificial Bee Colony Algorithm Based on Faster Convergence. *2021 IEEE International Conference on Artificial Intelligence and Computer Applications (ICAICA),* 776-779. 10.1109/ICAICA52286.2021.9498254

Chen, Y., Wang, Y., Cao, L., & Jin, Q. (2018). An Effective Feature Selection Scheme for Healthcare Data Classification Using Binary Particle Swarm Optimization. *2018 9th International Conference on Information Technology in Medicine and Education (ITME),* 703-707. 10.1109/ITME.2018.00160

Chen, Z., & Meng, Q.-C. (2004). An incremental clustering algorithm based on swarm intelligence theory. *Proceedings of 2004 International Conference on Machine Learning and Cybernetics, 3*, 1768-1772. 10.1109/ICMLC.2004.1382062

Costa & Santos. (2019). An Overview of Data Mining Representation Techniques. *2019 7th International Conference on Future Internet of Things and Cloud Workshops (FiCloudW),* 90-95. 10.1109/FiCloudW.2019.00029

Deepa, V. K., & Geetha, J. R. R. (2013). Rapid development of applications in data mining. *2013 International Conference on Green High Performance Computing (ICGHPC),* 1-4. 10.1109/ICGHPC.2013.6533916

Deng, X. (2009). System Identification Based on Particle Swarm Optimization Algorithm. *2009 International Conference on Computational Intelligence and Security,* 259-263. 10.1109/CIS.2009.167

Du, J., Zhou, J., Li, C., & Yang, L. (2016). An overview of dynamic data mining. *2016 3rd International Conference on Informative and Cybernetics for Computational Social Systems (ICCSS),* 331-335. 10.1109/ICCSS.2016.7586476

Du, S.-Y., & Liu, Z.-G. (2017). Diversity based hybrid particle swarm algorithm. *2017 International Symposium on Intelligent Signal Processing and Communication Systems (ISPACS)*, 444-449. 10.1109/ISPACS.2017.8266520

Fong, S., Deb, S., Yang, X.-S., & Li, J. (2014, July-August). Feature Selection in Life Science Classification: Metaheuristic Swarm Search. *IT Professional, 16*(4), 24–29. doi:10.1109/MITP.2014.50

Janardhanan, J., & Umamaheswari, S. (2020). Data Analytic Tools an Overview. *2020 International Conference on Smart Innovations in Design, Environment, Management, Planning and Computing (ICSIDEMPC),* 46-50. 10.1109/ICSIDEMPC49020.2020.9299645

Jangra, R., & Kait, R. (2017). Analysis and comparison among Ant System; Ant Colony System and Max-Min Ant System with different parameters setting. *2017 3rd International Conference on Computational Intelligence & Communication Technology (CICT),* 1-4. 10.1109/CIACT.2017.7977376

Jemal, H., Kechaou, Z., & Ben Ayed, M. (2014). Swarm intelligence and multi agent system in healthcare. *2014 6th International Conference of Soft Computing and Pattern Recognition (SoCPaR),* 423-427. 10.1109/SOCPAR.2014.7008044

Khosla & Aggarwal. (2005). A Framework for Identification of Fuzzy Models through Particle Swarm Optimization Algorithm. *2005 Annual IEEE India Conference - Indicon*, 388-391. 10.1109/INDCON.2005.1590196

Kirschenbaum, M., & Palmer, D. W. (2015). *Perceptualization of particle swarm optimization. In 2015 Swarm/Human Blended Intelligence Workshop*. SHBI. doi:10.1109/SHBI.2015.7321681

Lakshmi, N., & Raghunandhan, G. H. (2011). A conceptual overview of data mining. *2011 National Conference on Innovations in Emerging Technology,* 27-32. 10.1109/NCOIET.2011.5738828

Liu, Y., & Liang, F. (2009). An Adaptive Hybrid Particle Swarm Optimization. *2009 Second International Symposium on Computational Intelligence and Design*, 87-90. 10.1109/ISCID.2009.29

Mudimigh, F. S., & Ullah, Z. (2009). Efficient implementation of data mining: Improve customer's behaviour. *2009 IEEE/ACS International Conference on Computer Systems and Applications*, 7-10. 10.1109/AICCSA.2009.5069289

Nandy, S., Adhikari, M., Khan, M. A., Menon, V. G., & Verma, S. (2022, May). An Intrusion Detection Mechanism for Secured IoMT Framework Based on Swarm-Neural Network. *IEEE Journal of Biomedical and Health Informatics*, *26*(5), 1969–1976. doi:10.1109/JBHI.2021.3101686 PMID:34357873

Ping, G., Chunbo, X., Yi, C., Jing, L., & Yanqing, L. (2014). Adaptive ant colony optimization algorithm. *2014 International Conference on Mechatronics and Control (ICMC),* 95-98. 10.1109/ICMC.2014.7231524

Qi, X., Zhu, S., & Zhang, H. (2017). A hybrid firefly algorithm. *2017 IEEE 2nd Advanced Information Technology, Electronic and Automation Control Conference (IAEAC),* 287-291. 10.1109/IAEAC.2017.8054023

Ramzan, M., & Ahmad, M. (2014). Evolution of data mining: An overview. *2014 Conference on IT in Business, Industry and Government (CSIBIG),* 1-4. 10.1109/CSIBIG.2014.7056947

Renuka Devi, K., & Balasamy, K. (2022). Securing Clinical Information Through Multimedia Watermarking Techniques. In D. Samanta & D. Singh (Eds.), *Handbook of Research on Mathematical Modeling for Smart Healthcare Systems* (pp. 86–109). IGI Global. doi:10.4018/978-1-6684-4580-8.ch005

Sarangi, S. K., Panda, R., Priyadarshini, S., & Sarangi, A. (2016). A new modified firefly algorithm for function optimization. *2016 International Conference on Electrical, Electronics, and Optimization Techniques (ICEEOT),* 2944-2949. 10.1109/ICEEOT.2016.7755239

Sasa, M., Dongqing, L., Jia, X., & Xingqiao, F. (2009). Research on Continuous Function Optimization Algorithm Based on Swarm-Intelligence. *2009 Fifth International Conference on Natural Computation,* 61-65. 10.1109/ICNC.2009.9

Shen, Y. (2018). Research on Swarm Size of Multi-swarm Particle Swarm Optimization Algorithm. *2018 IEEE 4th International Conference on Computer and Communications (ICCC),* 2243-2247. 10.1109/CompComm.2018.8781013

Suresh, R. M., & Padmajavalli, R. (2007). An Overview of Data Preprocessing in Data and Web Usage Mining. *2006 1st International Conference on Digital Information Management*, 193-198. 10.1109/ICDIM.2007.369352

Wei, X., & Feifan, Y. (2009). Swarm Intelligence in Modeling Adaptive Behavior of the Industry Cluster. *2009 WRI Global Congress on Intelligent Systems*, 213-217. 10.1109/GCIS.2009.50

Yekkala, S. D., & Jabbar, M. A. (2017). Prediction of heart disease using ensemble learning and Particle Swarm Optimization. *2017 International Conference On Smart Technologies For Smart Nation (SmartTechCon),* 691-698. 10.1109/SmartTechCon.2017.8358460

Yitong, L., Mengyin, F., & Hongbin, G. (2007). A Modified Particle Swarm Optimization Algorithm. *2007 Chinese Control Conference*, 479-483. 10.1109/CHICC.2006.4347362

Zhang, H., Gao, M., & Zhang, X. (2010). Improved hybrid particle swarm optimization algorithm. *2010 Sixth International Conference on Natural Computation*, 2642-2646. 10.1109/ICNC.2010.5583000

Zhang, J., Zhu, X., Wang, W., & Yao, J. (2014). A fast restarting particle swarm optimizer. *2014 IEEE Congress on Evolutionary Computation (CEC),* 1351-1358. 10.1109/CEC.2014.6900427

Zhang, Z. Z., & Lin, X. (2021). An Improved Artificial Bee Colony with Self-Adaptive Strategies and Application. *2021 International Conference on Computer Network, Electronic and Automation (ICCNEA),* 101-104. 10.1109/ICCNEA53019.2021.00032

Zhu, Y., & Tang, X. (2010). Overview of swarm intelligence. *2010 International Conference on Computer Application and System Modeling (ICCASM 2010),* 400-403. 10.1109/ICCASM.2010.5623005

Chapter 3
A Generic Big Data Analytics With Particle Swarm Optimization for Clinical Machine Learning

Radha Subramani
Vivekanandha College of Engineering for Women, India

Aparna Chelladurai
Sengunthar Engineering College, India

Aarthi Chelladurai
Sengunthar Engineering College, India

N. Mohanapriya
Vivekanandha College of Engineering for Women, India

ABSTRACT

In the past two decades, researchers are facing challenges in analyzing biomedical data. It is a fast growing and new promising field due to vast growing information. Data analytics and machine learning are possible on huge volume of biomedical data. The primary goal of the biomedical data analysis by using swarm intelligence will help you to provide optimized prediction or analysis to the problem or diseases. Swarm intelligence is a special kind of information exchange across different nodes in a network with methods in machine learning. All the members of the swarm have equal rights. So there is no spider controlling the data web. Particle swarm optimization is used to fix the parameters and predicts the efficient nodes to pass on. Particle swarm optimization convolution neural networks (PSOCNN) minimizes the parameter space to a single block and evaluates the candidate CNN with a small subset of training data.

DOI: 10.4018/978-1-6684-6894-4.ch003

INTRODUCTION

Huge opportunities exist in data science, which has recently received a lot of attention. Data analytics, which results in the data extraction of a required knowledge base from large volumes of data, is the basic component of data science. The primary focus of traditional methods is on preprocessing the gathered data and fitting it to some predetermined mathematical models. However, when faced with issues like volume, dynamic changes, noise, and so forth, these models might not be effective. The prevalence of the aforementioned issues makes using conventional data analysis methods ineffective or inefficient. Due to the aforementioned challenges, new and effective techniques should be created to handle data analysis. Now the methods for analysis are migrating from model-driven to innovative data-driven paradigms and concentrating on the variety of data to be analyzed.

Any model or system that has "the five V" issues can benefit from using big data analytics techniques to increase its capacity for making decisions (variety, volume, velocity, validity, and volatility). A significant portion of the healthcare industry analyzes the data and processing of vast volume of patient data. The hurdles with variety, veracity, and validity are frequently used to describe them. Big data and machine learning are primarily used for diagnostic purposes in medicine, which entails using classification or regression algorithms to predict and analyze various diseases. Huge volume of data or Big and deep data has the potential to produce significant results when merged with soft computing techniques like neural networks, machine learning, data mining, and swarm intelligence and fuzzy logic.

Most of the applications in data analytics might be transformed to make the complex problems into optimal solutions. So, it expects the methodologies to be able to explore the solution space and forage the optimal result (Ahmadi et al., 2007). Conventional model-driven techniques have complex problems that can be coded and follow the form of discriminable procedures. However, while handling huge volume of massive data and complex process, it is challenging to find the solutions. Two groups of methodologies are used from the most powerful algorithms in neural and soft computing. The most required classes of algorithms (i.e., to be self-learned by inducing proficiency present in the training labels and data) are available in Artificial Neural Networks (ANNs). They are influenced by the architecture and operation of the nervous system. By devising basic parts, the democracy-based meta-heuristic analysis methods are very much efficient by solving those complex tasks, which the conventional model driven methods cannot be able to do and is a challenging to find a optimal solution (Shi, 2011). SI is a kind of meta-heuristic analysis algorithm is fascinating much concentration, also manifested to be sufficient to solve the large and multi-dimensional problems in training data.

As in the approaches of SI stated in Figure 1, when using SI algorithms in data science, there are primarily two types of approaches (Kennedy & Eberhart, 1995). Data extraction technologies such as supervised/unsupervised learning, deep learning, statistics, and others may be used in the first approach as a method for parameter tuning and optimization. The second type applies SI algorithms to data organization such as moving the data multi-objects to a 2-dimensional extracted feature solution space to obtain an appropriate grouping or decreases the various dimensions of the big data.

SI is a group of natural search and optimized analysis and prediction methods that examines a group behavior in a growth of low complexity individuals with complex problems (Li & Yao, 2012). The relationship of SI in Data Science among single groups or multiple groups, which involve various kinds of tackling and cooperating along with the training data, are the inspiration for the SI algorithms (Shi, 2011). SI algorithms search in a domain using a population of people. Every person represents the ability for giving answers to the issue being optimized. When conducting a self-guided search, Intelligence algorithms keep track of and enhance a pool of best findings until a predetermined stopping criterion is satisfied, i.e., the outcome is satisfactory, or the predetermined count of repetitions is determined (Abualigah et al., 2018).

SWARM INTELLIGENCE

Basic Method of SI Algorithm

A group of specific intelligent methods called SI Algorithms were inspired by the macro and micro-level behaviors of biological swarms. They typically have decentralized, self-organizing paradigms that are scalable, adaptable, robust, and simple on an individual level. In SI based algorithm, Growth of specific parameters

Figure 1. Two approaches of swarm intelligence for data science

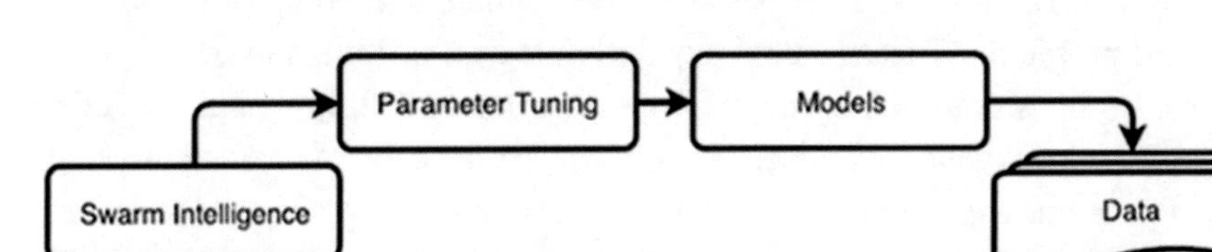

that represents efficient candidate solutions cooperates with one another and statistically improves over iterations to finally find satisfactory solutions (Kennedy & Eberhart, 1995). Numerous swarm intelligence methods have been put forth in recent years. These methods employ a variety of operations and draw their inspiration from various sources. Generally speaking, these various operations aim to balance the exploration as well as exploitation, or the concurrence of the search process.

Algorithm summarizes the common process of swarm intelligence algorithms. Swarm algorithms can finally find the optimized findings from the digitization of a growth of specifics in feature space, preceded by the relevant task and generating solutions. As more resources related to computation in time or space are provided, the expected fitness value of a complex solution may increase as a general rule.

Algorithm 1. General procedure of swarm intelligence algorithms

1. Population Initialization: Generate random solutions for an optimized problem, repair solutions if solutions violate any of the constraints;
2. Evaluate all initialized individuals;
3. **While** *not terminated* **do**
4. Reproduce individuals to form a new population;
5. Evaluate the fitness of each solution;
6. Select solutions with better fitness values;
7. Update solutions in the archive;

Result: Relatively good solution(s)

The quality of the solution should improve monotonically over iterations, i.e., the fitness value of the solution at time $t + 1$ should be no worse than the fitness at time t.

Development of Swarm Intelligence

There have been many SI algorithms developed over the past 30 years. They draw ideas from various phenomena and develop new operations for generating solutions in a way that balances the swarm's convergence and diversity. It is becoming increasingly difficult to find the best solutions dynamically due to the prevalence of NP-hard problems. These issues frequently have an infinite number of potential solutions. In this situation, coming up with a workable solution quickly is crucial. Almost all areas of science, engineering, and industry have found use for SI algorithms in solving nonlinear problems, including data mining, computational intelligence, optimization, bioinformatics, business planning, and industrial applications. These scientific and engineering issues are somewhat related to data, since we are in the era of cloud and big data. Numerous successful applications of swarm intelligence in relation to data exist. In the meantime, there are still a lot of opportunities as well as the challenges while applying the swarm intelligence algorithm with data science due to the growth of noises, and complexity of tasks.

THEORETICAL APPLICATIONS

Data Preprocessing

As soon as we receive the Electronic Health Record of each patient (EHR) from the various health data sources, data preprocessing is necessary. Data preprocessing comes first, followed by normalization to deal with missing and erroneous values (Nguyen & Shirai, 2013). Unwanted words, spaces, or symbols could be present in the featured data. Stop-word elimination methods are used to get rid of those components. To enhance the accuracy of the analytical models, the data set's noise needs to be eliminated. The majority of the data that is available in the healthcare industry is unstructured. The healthcare data is varied, making it difficult to aggregate or integrate them. By synchronizing and combining their formats, we integrated the data. Our efforts eventually yielded a number of CSV files with a 1 GB maximum training data size. To handle the interpreted or missing or erroneous values, they calculated missing data with the value of median of the remaining data for the set of variables.

Dataset Collection, Feature Extraction, and Feature Selection

First Experiment

The author obtained the datasets Framingham and Hungarian for the first experiment from the Kaggle website (Abualigah et al., 2018). They retained the 13 variables that Khan and Algarni (Li & Yao, 2012) chose from the 76 available attributes: Age (Middle, Old, Young) (Young, Medium, Old), Gender(M, F), chest pain (Non-Anginal pain, Atypica, Angina, Asymptomatic), Serum cholesterol, resting blood pressure (High, Medium, Low) Fasting Blood [Yes/No (120 mg=dl)], electrocardiogram at rest (Medium, abnormality, Left ventricular), heart rate (High, Medium, Low), Whether regular exercise causes the case angina, Exercise-induced pressure in comparison to a test (Low, Risk, Terrible), Exercises for the ST segment's slope of the peak include major vessels (0–3), fixed defects, and reversible defects on a thalium scan. This dataset's target variable was a variable such as (Disease: Yes 1/No 0).

Second Experiment

They used the health training Dataset from the Health website of USA (Alexander et al., 2011), which contains information from the countries. The training dataset has an enormous number of features. For feature selection, a wide range of techniques are available (Chen & Huang, 2017; Shi, 2011). Using the modified crow search algorithm (MCSA), created by Guptaet.al. (Ahmadi et al., 2007), an evolutionary optimization algorithm which is nature-inspired, we chose the features. Each crow in MCSA forages for food and stores it in their nests or places. Each crow silently follows the other group of crows to learn where they hide the food. Each crow stores the top solution in its memory (referred to as mem in the following), which is used to store the hiding places. A fitness function assesses the solution's goodness. There are only two variables that control CSA: flight length and probability of awareness (by awaking a crow that is silently preceded by another flock of crows, noted as Ap). MCSA depicts an improved method for choosing a destination and a procedure for adjusting the flying duration. The location of the i-th crow is noted by l_i and shows an optimal result in the solution feature space. For the use of the above algorithm in feature extraction and selection the solution space of all the feasible combination of knowledge features. A d-dimensional cube can be used to represent the solution space for this purpose, and any point within its volume is mapped to a computable result by ceiling each direction to the nearest number (1 - insert, 0 -delete) before finding a solution by means of a function called fitness. The function for a selection of features and extraction may be any classifier, normally a classifier which incurs possibly low extraction cost, like the k-nearest neighbor. The following steps are to be followed in feature selection and extraction by applying the MCSA method.

1. There are n data files for patients' health records. First split the health data into simple clusters or portions.
2. Two constraints may occur: the crow might be conscious or unconscious of being followed. Otherwise, if the crow knows, the new location is created randomly.
3. The storage has the location of the crow is to be modified randomly. The value of the present location of the crow is calculated by fitness method. If the calculated value is greater than the present value and change is reverted back in the memory.
4. Repeat until a maximum iteration is to be repeated or an adequately stable optimal value is found.

The primary factors ultimately taken into account in their research were Year, Age, Diseases, Symptoms, Death ratio and Treatment. Disease Names was the pickout variable, and it could be any of the following: Alzheimer's disease, anemia, asthma, diabetes, fibroids, gastroenteritis, hepatitis, kidney disease, nephropathy, Parkinson's disease, and heart disease. Noteworthy linguistic variables include Symptoms and Treatment. Only the prescription's type was indicated by the treatment (Lotion, spray, suspension, Ointment, tablets, injections, or powder).

In the area of Computer Technology statistics, data analysis has been a famous research topic for many years. The SI algorithm is employed in data analytics tasks, as previously mentioned, either as a parameter tuning algorithm or as a data organizing algorithm. Dimensionality reduction, classification, prediction, clustering, and machine learning are common applications.

Dimensionality Reduction

The task of diminishing the variables in a dataset under deliberation is known as dimensionality reduction. It is essential for preprocessing data in data mining. The two operations that make up dimensionality reduction are typically feature selection and extraction of possible features. The process of choosing the best subset of pertinent features to use when building a model is known as feature selection. While extracting the features of projected features data in a three-dimensional space onto a lesser data dimension. Rather than using all the features present in a vast amount of data, carefully chosen/projected features will improve the accuracy of a model. SI algorithms are discovered as a promising solution to the possible kinds of complex problem depending on feature selection.

Recent years have seen the rise of many related works, including some of the following: Based on variant PSO known as Competitive based Swarm Optimizer, Gu et al. proposed for high dimensional classification (Jordan, 2007). An FA based method for feature data selection and extraction that can delay convergence was created by Abualigah et al. (2018). For selection of features, Pourpanah et al. combine the BSO algorithm and the Fuzzy ARTMAP (FAM) model Ari et al. (2019) contains a more review on SI powered feature selection.

Classification and Clustering

Data science must include classification and clustering. Over the years, they have received extensive research in the fields of fuzzy neural networks, statistics, supervised/ unsupervised machine learning, and knowledge management systems. Classification involves predicting the target class using the training dataset, whereas clustering involves grouping similar types of targets by taking the most favorable condition into account.

Automated Machine Learning

Deep or Convolutional Networks (DNNs) Chakraborty and Datta (2017) have made significant advancements in a wide range of application fields, and machine learning research and applications have both grown rapidly in the last decade. Too many design choices, however, can significantly affect how well some machine learning techniques perform. In specific, designing the architecture of DNNs is extremely difficult and heavily depends on the experience of the experts. Numerous SI-based methods for designing DNNs automatically have been proposed as solutions to this issue Cui et al. (2005).

Using Wang et.al. efficient PSO (EPSOCNN) method, convolutional neural network architectures can be generated automatically Shi (2011). (CNNs). In order to reduce the computational cost, the hyper parameter of EPSOCNN is minimized. Using a small set of the training dataset, CNNs are condensed into a single block and evaluated. Based on the classifiers computed accuracy and the PSO computational cost, Shi, Y. et al. (2011) proposed a multi-objective CNNs (MOCNN) to find the non-dominant CNN architectures. It introduces a preliminary encoding method for CNNs and employs OMOPSO, a multi-objective PSO method, to empower the potential CNN architectures.

PARTICLE SWARM OPTIMIZATION

PSO is one of the eminent algorithms and it is a basic algorithm to search for finding an optimal outcome in the solution and feature space. It may vary from other algorithms by using the objective function and it is independent of the any differential part of the objective.

Particle Swarms

Kennedy et al. introduced the concept of swarm optimization in 1995. According to the concept, socio-biologists think that a bunch of fish or a flock of birds that moves together "can materialize from the expertise of all other members". All of the birds in the group can exchange their findings and aid in the best compatible hunt when a bird is flying and searching randomly for food, for example.

While simulating the displacement of a group of birds, they also considered the possibility of each bird is meant to assist in the search for the best answer in a high-dimensional problem space, and that the flock's best find is the best solution in the space.

Example Optimization Problem

Finding the low and high of optimization function based on a multi-dimensional space is the adoptable application for PSO. Applying PSO requires that the function f(X) which generates a possible value from X (such as the coordinates (x,y) in a plane) and X can take any value in the feature space. For instance, f(X) may be the altitude point on plane. The PSO algorithm give output as parameter X that it discovered to produce the lowest value of f(X).

As from the plot, this function produces a graph that looks like a curved egg carton. It is not a convex function and therefore it is very complex to analyze its minimum because a local minimum found is not necessarily the global minimum.

They determined this function's minimum point by conducting thorough research using the value of f(x,y) for each point on the plane. If they believed that it would be too expensive to search every point, we can also randomly select a few points on the plane and find which one plots the lowest value on f(x,y). However, they also noticed from the shape of f(x,y) that it is simpler to find smaller value close to a point where f(x,y) has been found to be smaller.

It starts with a set of random points on the plot plane (let's call them particles) and makes them search for the lower point in random directions, much like a flock of birds searching for food. Every particle should search around the lowest plot it has ever located at each iteration, as well as the lowest plot of the entire swarm of

Figure 2. f(x,y)

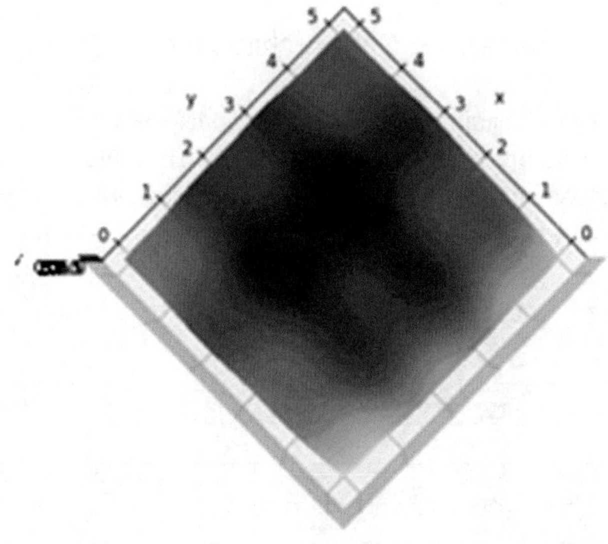

particles has ever discovered. By doing a certain number of steps, they believed that this swarm of particles has never gone further than the minimum point of the function.

As can be depicted from the aforementioned paragraph, deep or machine learning networks have produced superior outcomes with fewer adjustments to parameter fixings. Deep Convolutional Neural Networks are used frequently because of their elasticity in data-driven methodology (single dimensional Convolutional node for signal data) and model based methodology(data transformed to a two dimensional image). The use of multiple layers and careful parameter initialization are required for improved model performance. This calls for in-depth knowledge of both the dataset and the CNN architecture.

To analyze and find the optimum CNN without the interruption of a human, a meta heuristic algorithm PSO may be used which is quite easy to construct and adopt with lower cost.

Parameter Settings for PSO

The PSO algorithm's behavior is controlled by the parameters used in this category. It has three parameters: iterations, swarm size, and (Cg), which emphasizes the likelihood of choosing a particular layer from the top-performing layer when calculating the velocities of individual particles. The actual number of repetitions that the ideal technique will execute before PSO optimization is finished. After the final particle is optimized, the efficient CNN architecture with the highest accuracy is achieved. The PSO algorithm's size of the swarm gives the count of particles. Each particle in this case is a complete CNN architecture, and the algorithm will evaluate its performance.

Parameters for initializing CNN Architecture

The second category's parameter initialization regulates how the particles move at first. There are eight parameters involved, which are listed in Table 2. An initial population of CNN-based swarms is present in this step. Particles with CNN architectures selected randomly according to the attributes make up this initial population. The

Table 1. Initialization of parameters

Description	Value
Iterations	10
Size of Swarm	20
Cg	0.5

lowest and highest number of outcomes from a convolution layer must be specified in order to restrict the number of feature or solution maps produced. The kernel size is selected between the kernel's starting and ending sizes. These attributes only affect the basic architecture; following initialization, the architecture is updated in accordance with the design requirements.

Convolutional Neural Network: Parameter Settings for Training

The attributes denote training given to the data set of every particle. It insists four attributes to set and controls the process of updating during the training of each particle dataset. The count of epoch denotes the count of training repetition of the particle using full dataset. The drop out attribute is applied in the particle to prevent overfitting. The model incorporates group normalization among the convolutional layers to prevent it while training.

PSO is a growth dependent stochastic algorithm that is enhanced by the characteristics of animal swarms, such as swarms of different kinds of insects or ants, or schools of fish Cui et al. (2005). It is additionally classified as a meta-heuristic algorithm in the article. Swarm is a common term used to describe the population. Although there are some similarities between them in terms of their

Table 2. CNN initialization

Description	Value
Min.of outputs from a convolution layer	3
Max of outputs on convolution layer	256
Min. neurons in a FC layer	1
Min. layers	3
Max. layers	20
Min. size of Kernel	3
Max. size of kernel	7

Table 3. Convolutional neural network training

Description	Value
Epochs - particle	100
Epochs - global	256
Dropout rate	0.5
Batch normalizer of a particle	yes

inner workings, these kinds of methodologies are being referred to as inspired, as negation to evolutionary dependent techniques such as evolutionary computing like genetic algorithms. Artificial Intelligence is a related research area. Even though PSO's predecessor was the study and modelling of behavior of an animal, it enhanced as an optimizer, but well-defined information. The term and algorithm were first proposed in 1995 Abraham et al. (2006). PSO and swarm intelligence are inextricably linked by definition.

Swarm optimization processes are appealing for a variety of reasons. Biological swarms come in a variety of forms, so it is secure to deduce that they represent a prominent source of ideas, resources, and methods. Swarms exhibit fluid and elegant coordination in their behavior, which makes their cooperative activities and decision-making methodologies but not strictly effective. Additionally, humans are able to see and understand how a biological swarm behaves. As a result, we have a brief introduction and better understanding of the motivations, objectives, communication, and utilization for a natural phenomenon, is abstract and make it difficult to develop a method or model that is well-structured.

Numerous PSO variants have been introduced since the method was first introduced. In order to adapt to particular problems, many algorithms are developed and are still being introduced with certain parameters and packages. Due to the extensive use and examination of these numerous variations, PSO has developed into a very potent method. The swarm and its behavior are described in more general terms in the subsection that follows, while the sequel provides in-depth explanations of particular algorithms.

The biological swarm has three distinct characteristics, according to Clerc and Kennedy (2002). First, cohesiveness: Because everyone in the group is related to everyone else and belongs to the same group, there is a certain amount of "sticking together" going on. The members actively work to avoid colliding with one another and migrate with some respect for the standard separation between the members. Alignment is the next process, in which every member of the population actively works to move in the same direction. This is the target of food in biology, the solution to the problem in optimization. The swarm is not compelled to have separation because particles are intended to lack mass and volume. All particles come to an end at or very close to the precise position denoting the solution when they converge to it. However, particle "collision" does not have shape or any form prevent particles from moving apart as a principle. Due to the fact that each particle is created with unique characteristics (such as initial positions, personal bests, clan leaders, and more, depending on the algorithm), they are somewhat independent of one another even though they search in union based on the swarm.

Basic Methodology of Swarm Intelligence

We provide an understandable list of SI principles in reference to Millonas' classification to provide clarity to establish the connection between PSO and Swarm Intelligence.

Principle of Proximity. The group's members can grasp and perform simple space complexity and time calculations.

Principle of Quality. It cannot respond to time and space features, but also verifies for quality parameters, e.g., safety.

Diverse Response. It should not give response to its surroundings in an absolutely ordered manner.

Stability Principle. It should not reorganize its behavior into a completely different mode every time an update happens.

Adaptability Principle. However, it should also be able to interchange its behavioral pattern, provided this modification in a positive.

Kennedy et al. confirmed that the PSO algorithm has designated to function the particles stabilize their location and velocity and need the ability to reconsider surrounding time and space stimuli in the case to upgrade them. When performing the abovesaid updates, the swarm responds to the best value g along with other QoS factors, upholding the quality principle. As a result of the swarm's avoidance of acting in an overly restricted way, the aforementioned quality factors do not avoid the diverse reaction. The diversity and noise that exist in the swarm promote this. Finally, the swarm exhibits adaptability without jeopardizing its stability because it bases behavioral changes on a clear set of criteria (which includes the global best position g). When a behavior is advantageous and practical, it changes.

The PSO Algorithm

The PSO algorithm carries out all the methodologies, principles and characteristics mentioned so far. By default, an optimizer is considered by the way the model works, but there exist methods to efficiently use an algorithm in order to find minima as well.

The flock's activities were influenced by Heppner's simulation, known as a cornfield vector, and was based on it. Heppner aimed to replicate the movements of a group of birds as they are in search of food and shelter, specifically at the time simulation's "cornfield." The way that birds react in the real world strategies suggests that they possess what we call common sense or knowledge, which is the capacity for flock members to impart knowledge acquired from their group without any experience of it. It provides a cognitive process as well as a communication tool.

This phenomenon occurs frequently; flocks of birds can quickly become accustomed to a new feeder in its area by spending a few minutes exploring it. As time goes on, an increasing number of birds will systematically begin visiting the feeder. In the simulation, where the birds were allotted with different categories of memory, this behavior was modeled. They were given global best g for the flocks of birds' memory of food sources, and for its allotted memory, they stored information about the best location they had ever visited x. Additional controls were added to modify the degree to which each memory location affected the behavior and movement.

Kennedy et al. (2002) designed the PSO algorithm to utilize these specified observations. So, in the PSO algorithm, the model is as follows.

- When particles identify the best optimal solution to the complex problem, this idea is transferred to full swarm.
- Each particle can be attractive towards best solutions, but not in an abstract.
- all particles have own memory spot for their value $x*$
- The particles migrate with respect to Newton's theory of motion.

Shi et al. (2002) proposed the constraints such as how to optimize the attributes of the PSO algorithm. Eventually, they proposed to use the inertia mechanism and the same may be applied to the particles' migration. Usually, the inertia is reduced as a linear sequence while the occurrences of the algorithm run, and it gets modified once per iteration i.

Algorithm

By denoting the model, a fixed algorithm can be established for the computational intelligence implementation. The algorithm is depicted in Figure 3.

Regarding the certain parameters, usually a size of 20 to 30 for N is identified, but these numbers may change depending on the optimization problem. The bigger the swarm, take much more evaluations of the function f are made during each iteration, thus due to the complex computations, the algorithm takes more time to find optimal solution.

MACHINE LEARNING

The adage "experiments and experience make the man perfect" holds true for machines as well in today's advanced world of internet technologies (IT). The development of "Machine Learning" is a result of experiments and experience producing creative and productive machines. Machine learning enables sensor-equipped machines to

Figure 3. PSO pseudocode

Algorithm 1: Particle Swarm Optimization (PSO)

Input: N, $\mathbf{x}_l$, $\mathbf{x}_u$, c_1, c_2, $i_{\max}$, f
Output: A swarm S of size N (N position vectors)
Initialize S, randomly generate the position $\mathbf{x}$ of each particle w.r.t. the bounds $\mathbf{x}_l$, $\mathbf{x}_u$ of the objective function;
Initialize all velocities $\mathbf{u}$ to zero;
Initialize best positions $\mathbf{x}^*$ (and respective values) for individual particles and find $\mathbf{g}^*$;
Choose randomly two values in $[0, 1]$ for r_1 and r_2;
Iteration $i = 0$;
Initialize $\theta_{\min}, \theta_{\max}$;
while $i < i_{\max}$ **do**
Calculate inertia: $\theta = \theta_{\max} - \frac{\theta_{\max} - \theta_{\min}}{i_{\max}} i$;
For each particle in S, the values for iteration i are:

1. Update velocity: $\mathbf{u}_i = \theta\, \mathbf{u}_{i-1} + c_1 r_1 [\mathbf{x}^* - \mathbf{x}_{i-1}] + c_2 r_2 [\mathbf{g}^* - \mathbf{x}(i-1)]$;
2. Update position: $\mathbf{x}_i = \mathbf{x}_{i-1} + \mathbf{u}_i$;
3. Compute the value of the new position according to f;
4. Check/Update: $\mathbf{x}^*, \mathbf{g}^*$

(Optional) Check for convergence;
Upgrade iteration: $i = i + 1$;
end
return S;

attempt to replace people. Machine learning is based on an analytics engine that processes experience and learns from it, much like a human brain does.

Machine learning, which is essentially having specialized algorithms that aid system in self-learning A programmed algorithm known as machine learning takes data as input and analyzes it to find the output values that occurs within a predetermined range. When new data is fed into algorithms, they will automatically learn it and optimize their activities by means of increasing performance, gradually gaining "intelligence."

Few Applications of Machine Learning:

Speech recognition (Tang et al., 2018).
Classifying the Text Documents (He et al., 2014).
Autonomous vehicles (Pretz, 2013).
Healthcare (Hepp et al., 2007).
Computation based biological application (Guinard et al., 2010).
Computer vision such as image processing and face recognition J(oshi & Kim, 2008).

Recommendation and information extraction systems (Lim et al., 2018).
Collaborative filtering (Aceto et al., 2020).
Web page ranking system (Balaji et al., 2019).

To classify the Machine learning algorithms based on its operation, there are four types namely,

1. Supervised
2. Semi-supervised
3. Unsupervised
4. Reinforcement Learning

Supervised Learning

The machine will be well trained in the case of supervised methodology. The operator will use an existing dataset to train the machine learning algorithm, which will then analyze the dataset to produce the desired output. The algorithm is trained to recognize patterns in data using the training dataset, which the trainer uses to know the precise solutions to the problem. The algorithm then trained from observations and makes classification and predictions. The trainer will assess the algorithm's prediction in the training state, and the same process will continue until the algorithm reaches a high level of performance/accuracy.

Further Supervised Learning is classified as Classification, Forecasting, Regression and Prediction.

Figure 4. Supervised learning process in machine learning

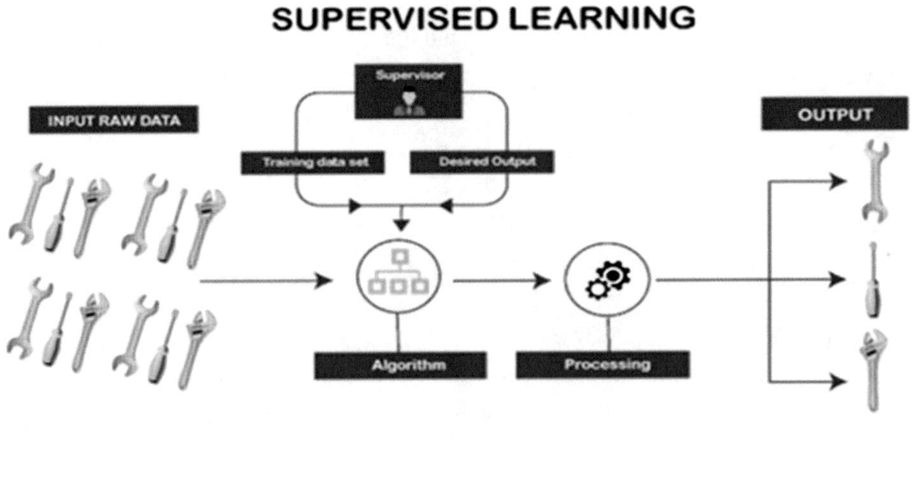

a. **Classification:** The outcome will be predicted based on the observed value and also the category which it belongs to.
b. **Regression:** In regression tasks, the relationship between the variables will be estimated. It always concentrates on base variables and with the sequence of other variables, in other words it is specifically used for predicting and finding in which the future is predicted based on statistical values.

Linear Regression:

In linear regression, inputs are multiplied with the help of constants to extract the output that produces a correlation of the dependent variable (Y) and the explanatory variable (X), using a line known as the regression line of curvature. Its implementation Bayoumi and McCaslin (2016) can be carried out using the equation for linear regression.

$$Y = a + bX$$

Where,

Y –base Variable,
X – Explanatory parameter

Support Vector Machine Regression:

Let's say that in a particular training set, X is the space of input patterns represented by (x1, y1), (xi, yi),.... The primary goal of SVM regression is to find a fitting function f(x); the data loss from the target (yi) achieved for the relevant training set should be less than. Any error less than is acceptable provided the function is rationally flat Jaidka et al. (2020).

The linear function (f) can be represented as

f (x) = (w, x) + b with, w ƀ'X, b ƀ' R (2)

Here (w, x) represents the product of X,
Rationally flat is given by w.

Semi-Supervised Learning

Semi-supervised learning stand between both labeled which is essential, meaningful tags and in turn unlabeled lacks in information.

Figure 5. Support vector machine

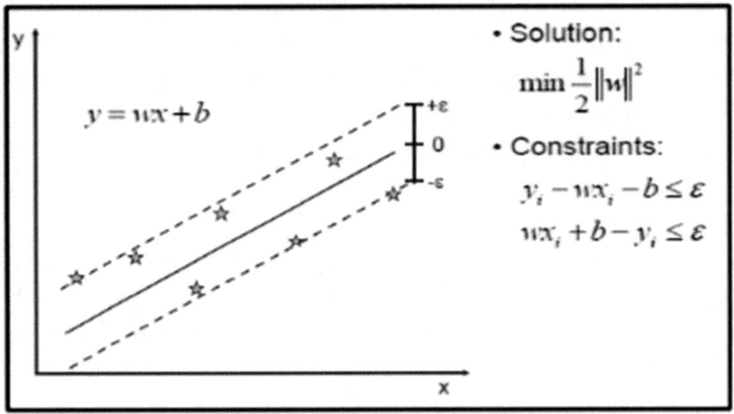

Figure 6. Semi-supervised learning process

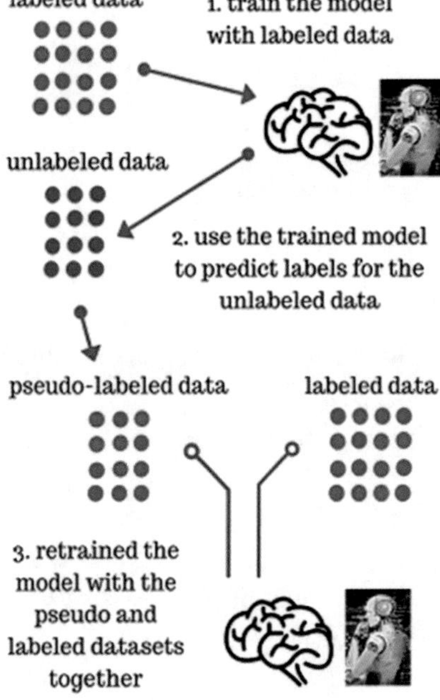

Unsupervised Learning

The analysis of the training data to find the pattern will be carried out by machine learning. In this case, there will be no human involvement and no answer key; Apart from, the machine will determine the correlation between the data and systems by looking into the data that is available. In contrast, the process relies on large training data sets and responds to that dataset appropriately. The information will be organized or grouped into clusters for forecasting. Since the prediction is based on interrupting with additional data, the effectiveness of drawing conclusions from that data becomes gradually better and more honed. It can be divided further into.

Clustering

In Clustering, collecting a set of similar data set or attributes based on stipulated condition will be processed which means partitioning a data into different groups for performing analysis of it to find the patterns. Clustering is applicable for the examination of interrelationships among few samples which is made preliminary step for assessing the sample structure of clusters. It is difficult for humans to interpret or invigilate the data in a multi-dimensional space, grouping is employed in tern it has real time challenges (Kawa, 2012). The clustering can be implemented in several ways such as centralized, Distributed and Decentralized.

Dimension Reduction

In this case the count of variables will be reduced to identify the required information which is specified.

Reinforcement Learning

It focuses mainly on systematic tasks, here a set of activities, variables and the end resultants will be provided for prediction. A set of rules will be defined in order to explore the options and possibilities, then the monitoring and evaluation process will

Figure 7. Unsupervised learning process in machine learning

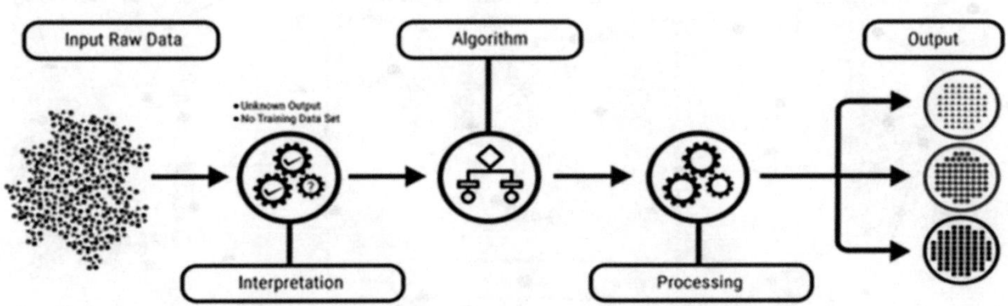

be carried out to identify the optimal solution. The reinforcement learning process is done on the machine trial and error basis, in turn the machines learn from past experiences to achieve the best possible result.

Reinforcement learning commonly used in industrial manufacturing (Kim & Tran-Dang, 2019), robotic control using AI (Leminen et al., 2020), simulations for prediction (Niranjan et al., 2017), optimization and scheduling (Radanliev et al., 2019; Xu et al., 2014), and gameplay algorithms (Deng & Li, 2013; Nguyen & Shirai, 2013).

The most familiar algorithms are

a. **Naïve Bayes (Supervised Learning - Classification):** Using the Bayes theorem, the Naive Bayes (Chen & Huang, 2017) classifier is built, and the values are classified independently of one another. It is most effective for classifying text because it encourages us to classify and predict a category based on a training data set of features that are currently available.
b. **K-Means Clustering:** It is an algorithm for unsupervised learning methodology (Kononenko, 2011), mainly used for categorizing unlabeled data, without any dedicated categories or groups.
c. **SVM (Supervised Learning - Classification):** It comes under supervised learning (Jaidka et al., 2020), which analyzes the data used for Regression, classification, and prediction analysis. It will basically filter training data set into classifiers and categories, by giving a set of testing and training samples.
d. **Linear Regression:** Linear regression (Bayoumi & McCaslin, 2016) is supervised leaning that allows us to find the correlation between two continuous or discrete variables.
e. **Logistic Regression:** In Logistic regression (Jordan, 2007), it mainly concentrates on the probability of a data based on the existing data provided. The representation will be as a binary dependent variable either 0 or 1,

Figure 8. Reinforced learning process in machine learning

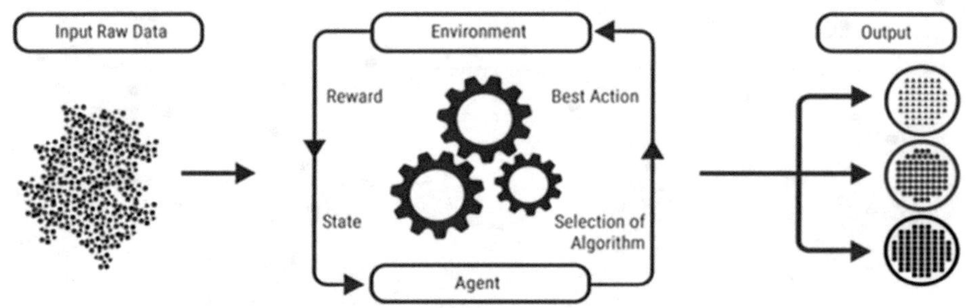

represents the outcomes. The main use of logistic regression is to deal with data classifications.

f. **ANN (Reinforcement Learning):** An Artificial Neural Network (Abraham et al., 2006); Ahmadi et al., 2007) will learn by experimentation and previous expertise which is extremely applied in constructing of non-linear relationship on high dimensional data.

g. **Decision Trees (Classification/Regression):** In this diagrammatic representation as a hierarchical like tree structure for branching, which examines every possibility of outcomes in Decision Tree (Alexander et al., 2011; Clerc & Kennedy, 2002) in machine learning persuaded from data, rendering to a top-down approach.

h. **Random Forest (Supervised Learning – Classification/Regression):** Random Forest (Cui et al., 2005) which is a more efficient and predominant algorithm in which multiple algorithms are combined to attain results for classification, analysis, prediction, regression and other tasks.

On an overall all the algorithms defined in machine language are efficient only based on the application where it is applied.

MODELLING APPROACH FOR CLINICAL MACHINE LEARNING

Challenges and Opportunities

- **Unified Swarm Intelligence**

There are a greater number of SI algorithms that have been proposed and shared the same kind of operations or methodologies for finding the solutions to the problems. There is a unified model for SI algorithms that has the responsibility and ability to implement its learning capacity that can be effective to find optimized solution for a problem at algorithms evaluation, implementation time.

- **Handling High Dimensional and Dynamical Data**

When the dimension of the data space rises, multi-dimensional training, data extraction problems experience the "curse of dimensionality." The nearest neighbor approach, for instance, is useful for categorization. The similarity search problem, however, is challenging to solve for high dimensional data because of the computational complexity brought on by the increase in dimensionality. Additionally, when issues arise in unstable or non-stationary environments., the criteria for training and testing data dynamically updated over a time, extra measurement can be taken, so that SI algorithms can be able to solve complex and dynamic problems.

- **SI Based AutoML**

Swarm intelligence algorithms, as previously notified, can be used to automatically design the model structure to optimize the hyper parameters of machine learning models. Swarm intelligence has a vast amount of potential and efficiency in this area with the development of AutoML. The specification of learning models and the process of evaluation, however, also present difficulties in addition to meta-heuristic optimization.

CONCLUSION

Swarm Intelligence ill help us to analyse the clinical data to find the diseases on a human body. This chapter reviews all the option that may be used to predict and analyse the behaviour of the disease. It has been widely used by data science applications with the rapid development of Artificial Intelligence Methodologies. By deeper involvement of patients, results in better outcomes while diagnosing the health issues. Swarm characteristics might facilitate the creation and distribution of knowledge among the particle swarms. Swarm behaviour may also be destructive. Few innovations and ideas may be hindered as they might be found as outliers and may affect to the actual behaviour. However, this negative impact and effect of swarms may also be reacted by a conscious perception and detailed study of the swarm aspect of our behaviour's amount of collected training data is increasing vastly and recommender systems are enhancing globally in parallel. These innovative tools and technologies will provide us with information that is not accessible and available until the present situation. As with many sources of input or training samples, it will be a keen to see how they will be interacted and applied by academician and industry person. This information does not need be given or processed; it lies before and between us and all we need that is to become aware of it.

REFERENCES

Abraham, A., Das, S., & Konar, A. (2006). Document clustering using differential evolution. *Proceedings of the 2006 IEEE Congress on Evolutionary Computations (CEC 2006),* 1784-1791. 10.1109/CEC.2006.1688523

Abualigah, L. M., Khader, A. T., & Hanandeh, E. S. (2018). A new feature selection method to improve the document clustering using particle swarm optimization algorithm. *Journal of Computational Science*, *25*, 456–466. doi:10.1016/j.jocs.2017.07.018

Aceto, G., Persico, V., & Pescapé, A. (2020). Industry 4.0 and health: Internet of things, big data, and cloud computing for healthcare 4.0. *Journal of Industrial Information Integration*, *18*, 100129. doi:10.1016/j.jii.2020.100129

Ahmadi, A., Karray, F., & Kamel, M. (2007). Multiple cooperating swarms for data clustering. *Proceedings of the 2007 IEEE Swarm Intelligence Symposium (SIS 2007),* 206-212. 10.1109/SIS.2007.368047

Alexander, F. J., Hoisie, A., & Szalay, A. (2011). Big data. *Computing in Science & Engineering*, *13*(6), 10–13. doi:10.1109/MCSE.2011.99

Ari, A. A. A., Gueroui, A., Titouna, C., Thiare, O., & Aliouat, Z. (2019). Resource allocation scheme for 5G C-RAN: A swarm intelligence based approach. *Computer Networks*, *165*, 106957. doi:10.1016/j.comnet.2019.106957

Balaji, S., Nathani, K., & Santhakumar, R. (2019). IoT technology, applications and challenges: A contemporary survey. *Wireless Personal Communications*, *108*(1), 363–388. doi:10.100711277-019-06407-w

Bayoumi, A., & McCaslin, R. (2016). Internet of Things – A Predictive Maintenance Tool forGeneralMachinery, Petrochemicals and Water Treatment. Sustainable Vital Technologies in Engineering &. *Informatics (MDPI).*

Bida, I., & Aouat, S. (2019). A new approach based on bat algorithm for inducing optimal decision trees classifiers. In A. Rocha & M. Serrhini (Eds.), *EMENA-ISTL 2018.SIST* (Vol. 111, pp. 631–640). Springer. doi:10.1007/978-3-030-03577-8_69

Boveiri, H. R., Khayami, R., Elhoseny, M., & Gunasekaran, M. (2019). Swarm Intelligence in Data Science: An efficient swarm intelligence approach for task scheduling in cloud-based internet of things applications. *Journal of Ambient Intelligence and Humanized Computing*, *10*(9), 3469–3479. doi:10.100712652-018-1071-1

Breivold, H. P., & Sandström, K. (2015). Internet of Things for Industrial Automation –Challenges and Technical Solutions. In *IEEE International Conference on Data Science and Data Intensive Systems.* Sydney: IEEE. 10.1109/DSDIS.2015.11

Chakraborty, T., & Datta, S. K. (2017). Application of swarm intelligence in internet of things. In *2017 IEEE International Symposium on Consumer Electronics (ISCE)* (pp. 67–68). IEEE 10.1109/ISCE.2017.8355550

Chen, H. L., Yang, B., Wang, G., Wang, S. J., Liu, J., & Liu, D. Y. (2012). Support vector machine based diagnostic system for breast cancer using swarm intelligence. *Journal of Medical Systems*, *36*(4), 2505–2519. doi:10.100710916-011-9723-0 PMID:21537848

Chen, Z., & Huang, X. (2017). End-to-end learning for lane keeping of self-driving cars. *IEEE Intelligent Vehicles Symposium (IV)*. 10.1109/IVS.2017.7995975

Cheng, S. (2017). Cloud service resource allocation with particle swarm optimization algorithm. In C. He, H. Mo, L. Pan, & Y. Zhao (Eds.), *BIC-TA 2017. CCIS* (Vol. 791, pp. 523–532). Springer. doi:10.1007/978-981-10-7179-9_41

Cheng, S., Liu, B., Shi, Y., Jin, Y., & Li, B. (2016). Evolutionary computation and bigdata: key challenges and future directions. In Y. Tan & Y. Shi (Eds.), DMBD. Academic Press.

Cheng, S., Liu, B., Ting, T., Qin, Q., Shi, Y., & Huang, K. (2016). Survey on data sciencewith population-based algorithms. *Big Data Analytics*, *1*(1), 3. doi:10.118641044-016-0003-3

Cheng, S., Shi, Y., Qin, Q., & Bai, R. (2013). Swarm intelligence in big data analytics. In *IDEAL 2013. LNCS* (Vol. 8206, pp. 417–426). Springer. doi:10.1007/978-3-642-41278-3 51

Chu, X., Wu, T., Weir, J. D., Shi, Y., Niu, B., & Li, L. (2018). Learning-interaction diversification framework for swarm intelligence optimizers: A unified perspective. *Neural Computing & Applications*, *32*(6), 1–21. doi:10.100700521-018-3657-0

Clerc, M., & Kennedy, J. (2002). The particle swarm-explosion, stability, and convergence in a multi dimensional complex space. *IEEE Transactions on Evolutionary Computation*, *6*(1), 58–73. doi:10.1109/4235.985692

Cui, X., Potok, T. E., & Palathingal, P. (2005). Document clustering using particle swarm optimization. *Proceedings of 2005 IEEE Swarm Intelligence Symposium (SIS 2005),* 185-191. 10.1109/SIS.2005.1501621

Deng, L., & Li, X. (2013). Machine Learning Paradigms for Speech Recognition: An Overview. *IEEE Transactions on Audio, Speech, and Language Processing*, *21*(5), 1060–1089. doi:10.1109/TASL.2013.2244083

Eberhart, R., & Kennedy, J. (1995). A new optimizer using particle swarm theory. *Proceedings of the Sixth International Symposium on Micro Machine and Human Science*, 39-43. 10.1109/MHS.1995.494215

Guinard, D., Trifa, V., Karnouskos, S., Spiess, P., & Savio, D. (2010). Interacting with the SOA-based internet of things: Discovery, query, selection, and on-demand provisioning of webservices. *IEEE Transactions on Services Computing*, *3*(3), 223–235. doi:10.1109/TSC.2010.3

He, W., Yan, G., & Da Xu, L. (2014). Developing vehicular data cloud services in the IoT environment. *IEEE Transactions on Industrial Informatics*, *10*(2), 1587–1595. doi:10.1109/TII.2014.2299233

Hepp, M., Siorpaes, K., & Bachlechner, D. (2007). Harvesting Wiki consensus: Using Wikipedia entries as vocabulary for knowledge management. *IEEE Internet Computing*, *11*(5), 54–65. doi:10.1109/MIC.2007.110

Honghao, C., Zuren, F., & Zhigang, R. (2013). Community detection using ant colony optimization. In *2013 IEEE Congress on Evolutionary Computation* (pp. 3072–3078). IEEE. 10.1109/CEC.2013.6557944

Jaidka, H., Sharma, N., & Singh, R. (2020). *Evolution of IoT to IIoT: Applications & Challenges.* Available at SSRN 3603739.

Jordan, M. (2007). Statistical Machine Learning and Computational Biology. *IEEE International Conference on Bioinformatics and Biomedicine (BIBM 2007).*

Joshi, G. P., & Kim, S. W. (2008). Survey, nomenclature and comparison of reader anti-collision protocols in RFID. *IETE Technical Review*, *25*(5), 234–243. doi:10.4103/0256-4602.44659

Kawa, A. (2012). *SMART logistics chain.* Intelligent Information and Database Systems. ACIIDS. doi:10.1007/978-3-642-28487-8_45

Kennedy, J., & Eberhart, R. (1995). Particle swarm optimization. *Proceedings of IEEE International Conference on Neural Networks (ICNN),* 1942-1948. 10.1109/ICNN.1995.488968

Kim, D. S., & Tran-Dang, H. (2019). An Overview on Industrial Internet of Things. In *Industrial Sensors and Controls in Communication Networks* (pp. 207–216). Springer.

Kononenko, I. (2011). Machine learning for medical diagnosis: History, state of the art and perspective. *Artificial Intelligence in Medicine*, *23*(1), 89–109. doi:10.1016/S0933-3657(01)00077-X PMID:11470218

Leminen, S., Rajahonka, M., Wendelin, R., & Westerlund, M. (2020). Industrial internet of things business models in the machine-to-machine context. *Industrial Marketing Management*, *84*, 298–311. doi:10.1016/j.indmarman.2019.08.008

Li, X., & Yao, X. (2012). Cooperatively coevolving particle swarms for large scale optimization. *IEEE Transactions on Evolutionary Computation*, *16*(2), 210–224. doi:10.1109/TEVC.2011.2112662

Lim, S., Kwon, O., & Lee, D. H. (2018). Technology convergence in the Internet of Things (IoT) start up ecosystem: A network analysis. *Telematics and Informatics*, *35*(7), 1887–1899. doi:10.1016/j.tele.2018.06.002

Nguyen, T., & Shirai, K. (2013). *Text Classification of Technical Papers Basedon Text Segmentation.* Natural Language Processing and Information Systems.

Niranjan, M., Madhukar, N., Ashwini, A., Muddsar, J., & Saish, M. (2017). IOT Based Industrial Automation. *IOSR Journal of Computer Engineering (IOSR-JCE),* 36-40.

Pourpanah, F., Shi, Y., Lim, C. P., Hao, Q., & Tan, C. J. (2019, July). Feature selection based on brain storm optimization for data classification. *Applied Soft Computing*, *80*, 761–775. doi:10.1016/j.asoc.2019.04.037

Pretz, K. (2013). *The Next Evolution of the Internet.* Retrieved 2018/3/11 from http://theinstitute.ieee.org/technology-focus/ technology-topic/the-next-evolution-of-the-internet

Radanliev, P., De Roure, D. C., Nurse, J. R., Montalvo, R. M., & Burnap, P. (2019). *The Industrial Internet of Things in the Industry 4.0 supply chains of small and medium sized enterprises*. University of Oxford.

Shi, Y. (2011). Brain storm optimization algorithm. In Advances in Swarm Intelligence, Vol. 6728, lecture notes in computer science. Springer. doi:10.1007/978-3-642-21515-5_36

Tang, C.-P., Huang, T. C.-K., & Wang, S.-T. (2018). The Impact of Internet of Things Implementation on Firm Performance. *Telematics and Informatics*, *35*(7), 2038–2053. doi:10.1016/j.tele.2018.07.007

Xu, L. D., He, W., & Li, S. (2014). Internet of Things in Industries: A Survey. *IEEE Transactions on Industrial Informatics*, *10*(4), 2233–2243. doi:10.1109/TII.2014.2300753

Chapter 4
A Modern Approach of Swarm Intelligence Analysis in Big Data:
Methods, Tools, and Applications

Thirunavukkarasu Kannapiran
https://orcid.org/0000-0001-8640-9103
Karnavati University, India

Krishna Patel
Karnavati University, India

Thirusha T. K.
CHRIST University (Deemed), India

Virendra Kumar Shrivastava
Alliance University, India

A Suresh Kumar
Jain University, India

ABSTRACT

Swarm intelligence is one of the most modern and less discovered artificial intelligence types. Until now it has been proven that the most comprehensive method to solve complex problems is using behaviours of swarms. Big data analysis plays a beneficial role in decision making, education domain, innovations, and healthcare in this digitally growing world. To synchronize and make decisions by analysing such a big amount of data may not be possible by the traditional methods. Traditional model-based methods may fail because of problem varieties such as volume, dynamic

DOI: 10.4018/978-1-6684-6894-4.ch004

changes, noise, and so forth. Because of the above varieties, the traditional data processing approach will become inefficient. On the basis of the combination of swarm intelligence and data mining techniques, we can have better understanding of big data analytics, so utilizing swarm intelligence to analyse big data will give massive results. By utilizing existing information about this domain, more efficient algorithm can be designed to solve real-life problems.

INTRODUCTION

The word swarm means a group of insects especially bees moving together. Swarm intelligence is a type of AI that works on the science of swarms. It uses the collective studies of individuals who work in a flock or group to solve any kind of problem. It`s a computational technique used to solve complex problems and a type of meta-heuristic algorithm that is currently attracting more and more attention. It has been proven to be sufficient to handle large-scale, dynamic, multi-objective problems in data analytics. SI is already playing a very important role in library materials acquisition, heating system planning, medical dataset classification, dynamic control, communications, moving objects tracking, and prediction.

A database with a large volume of data is called big data. Data analytics aims to automatic extraction of knowledge from massive data. The term big data analytics has been used since the early 1990s. Of course, it was not the first time when data analysis was used. In ancient times, different empires were used to analyse their respective empires' statistics and make decisions. However, in the last two decades, the volume and the speed of data generation have changed. The total amount of data in the world was 4.4 zettabytes (4.4 trillion gigabytes) in the year 2013. This amount increased to 44 zettabytes in 2020. This shows how the speed of data generation has increased over time. So, to analyze such a big amount of data traditional methods are not efficient. SI can play a big role to give a new dimension to industries by giving a new approach to big data analytics.

LITERATURE SURVEY

Table 1. Literature survey

Sr. no	Author	Year	Name of Paper	Technique Used	Applications
1.	G. Thippa Reddy, M. Praveen Kumar Reddy, Kuruva Lakshmanna, Rajesh Kaluri, Dharmendra Singh Rajput, Gautam Srivastava, And Thar Baker	2020	Analysis of Dimensionality Reduction Techniques on Big Data	Principle component analysis and Linear Discriminant analysis	Cardiotocography dataset
2.	Sofia Oikonomidi	2020	Impact of Big Data Analytics in Industry 4	SWOT Analysis Technique	Production data, Operational data, Supply chain data etc.
3.	Ahmed Afif Monrat, Raihan Ul Islam, Mohammad Shahadat Hossain, and Karl Andersson	2018	Challenges and Opportunities of Using Big Data for Assessing Flood Risks from Applications of Big Data Analytics Trends, Issues, and Challenges	Rule-based inference methodology using the evidential reasoning(RIMER)	human-generated data (Twitter, web traffic)
4.	Santosh Ray and Mohammed Saeed.	2018	Applications of Educational Data Mining and Learning Analytics Tools in Handling Big Data in Higher Education from Applications of Big Data Analytics Trends, Issues, and Challenges	Educational Data Mining and Learning Analytics	-
5.	Mohammed Dighriri, Gyu Myoung Lee, and Thar Baker	2018	Big Data Environment for Smart Healthcare Applications Over 5G Mobile Network from Applications of Big Data Analytics Trends, Issues, and Challenges	Data Traffic Aggregation Model	4G and 5G mobile networks data traffic
6.	Amir Mosavi, Alvaro Lopez, and Annamária R. Varkonyi-Koczy	2018	Industrial Applications of Big Data: State of the Art Survey	-	Data generated by vehicles
7.	Kan Zheng, Zhe Yang, Kuan Zhang, Periklis Chatzimisios, Kan Yang, and Wei Xiang	2016	Big Data-Driven Optimization for Mobile Networks toward 5G	Big Data-Driven (BDD) mobile network optimization	-

continued on following page

Table 1. Continued

Sr. no	Author	Year	Name of Paper	Technique Used	Applications
8.	Sindhu P Menon, Nagaratna P Hegde	2015	A Survey of Tools and Applications in Big Data	-	-
9.	Saurabh Arora and Inderveer Chana	2014	A Survey of Clustering Techniques for Big Data Analysis	DMM stream	Real-time and streaming data
10.	Chun-Wei Tsai, Bo-Chi Huang, and Ming-Chao Chiang	2014	A Novel Spiral Optimization for Clustering	Distributed spiral algorithm	Data mining
11.	R. Madhuri, M. Ramakrishna Murty, J.V.R. Murthy, P.V.G.D. Prasad Reddy, and Suresh C. Satapathy	2014	Cluster Analysis on Different Data Sets Using K-Modes and K-Prototype Algorithms	K-Modes and K-Prototype Algorithms	Numerical data, categorial data and mixed data
12.	Mahya Ameryan, Mohammad Reza Akbarzadeh Totonchi, Seyyed Javad Seyyed Mahdavi	2014	Clustering Based on Cuckoo Optimization Algorithm	Cuckoo search algorithm	Iris dataset, Wine dataset, Cancer dataset, Vowel dataset
13.	N.N.R. Ranga Suria, M. Narasimha Murty and G. Athithan	2014	A ranking-based algorithm for detection of outliers in categorical data	A novel algorithm for mining categorical outliers through ranking	Benchmark datasets
14.	Younghoon Kim, Kyuseok Shim, Min-Soeng Kim, June Sup Lee	2013	DBCURE-MR: An efficient density-based clustering algorithm for large data using MapReduce	An efficient density-based clustering algorithm	Disjoint set data structure
15.	Qing He, Xin Jin, Changying Du, Fuzhen Zhuang, Zhongzhi Shi	2012	Clustering in extreme learning machine feature space	Extreme learning machine	Synthetic control chart time series data set, Libras movement data set, NIST topic detection and tracking corpus,

METHODOLOGY FOR BIG DATA ANALYSIS

There are mainly four types of clustering algorithms. 1. Partitioning algorithm 2. Hierarchical algorithm 3. Density-based algorithm 4. Generic algorithm. There are different subtypes of each. Some algorithms are explained below for big data analysis.

Algorithm: General Procedure of swarm intelligence

Figure 1. Types of clustering algorithms for big data analysis
Source: Arora and Chana (2014)

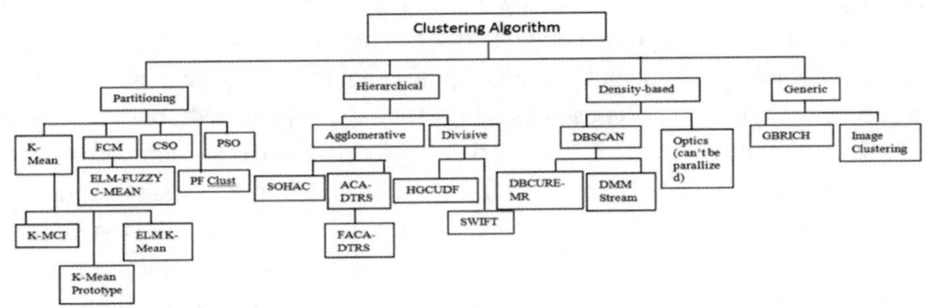

1. Population Initialization. Generate random solutions for an optimized problem, and repair solutions if solutions violate any of the constraints.
2. Evaluate all initialized individuals
3. While not terminated do
   Reproduce individuals to form a new population;
   Evaluate the fitness of each solution;
   Select solutions with better fitness values;
   Update solutions in archive;
   Result: Relatively good solution(s)

Figure 2. Types of algorithms added in chapter

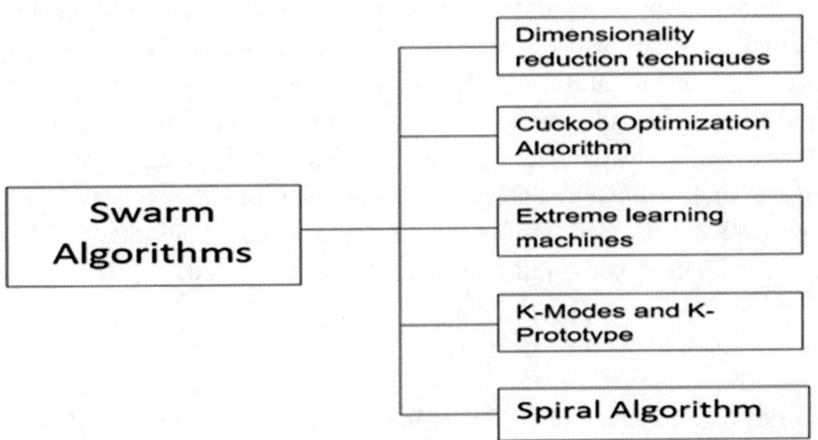

Spiral Algorithm

The main idea of spiral optimization is that all the points (individuals) rotate about the centre (i.e., the elitist or optimal solution) to search the solution space, and the population converges to the best solution in the end. In the spiral model, all the points attracted by the centre move to their next positions using the rotation operator, the only SO operator. Although SO outperforms the traditional single-solution-based algorithms for continuous optimization problems, the centre of SO is still easy to fall into a local minimum.

The SDO algorithm for an n-dimensional system is explained, along with the idea of origin. By creating both conventional and hypotrochoid spiral trajectories, the impact of changing the spiral's radius and angle is examined for both two- and three-dimensional systems. The focus is also on the present applications of SDO and its variations. To comprehend spiral behaviours, various spiral kinds, XY-plane coordinates, and trajectories are constructed. Furthermore, a thorough presentation of the developments of numerous unique optimization techniques using these spirals is provided. Therefore, by using SDO and its derivatives to address a variety of engineering challenges, this review paper aids in directing several scholars who are already working on the subject or who wish to (Tsai et al., 2014).

K-Modes and K-Prototype Algorithms

k-Modes is an algorithm based on the k-Means algorithm paradigm and is used for clustering categorical data. k-modes define clusters based on matching categories between the data points. The k-Prototype algorithm is an extension to the k-Modes algorithm that combines the k-modes and k-means algorithms and can cluster mixed numerical and categorical variables.

Large data sets can be efficiently clustered using the K-means algorithm; however, it can only handle numerical data types. However, the physical world is made up of a variety of data-typed objects. If we use a modified k-modes algorithm to expand the K-means algorithm to categorical domains and the K-prototypes method to domains with mixed category and numerical data. By using three measures—"using a simple matching dissimilarity measure for categorical data," "replacing means of clusters by modes," and "using a frequency-based method to find the modes of a problem used by the K-means algorithm"—the Modified K-modes algorithm will replace the means with the modes of the clusters (Madhuri et al., 2014).

Extreme Learning Machines

Extreme learning machines are feedforward neural networks for regression, classification, clustering, compression, sparse approximation, and feature learning with a single layer

Figure 3. Cuckoo optimization algorithm

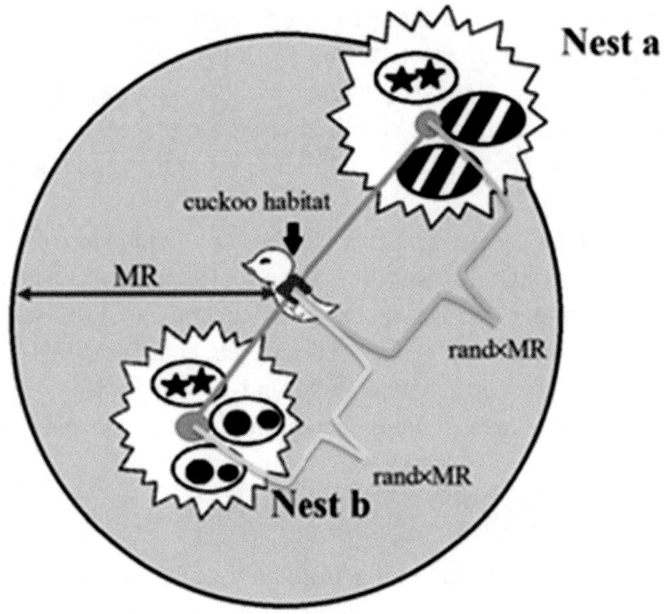

or multiple layers of hidden nodes, where the parameters of hidden nodes need not be tuned. These hidden nodes can be randomly assigned and never updated or can be inherited from their ancestors without being changed. In most cases, the output weights of hidden nodes are usually learned in a single step, which essentially amounts to learning a linear model. These models can produce good generalization performance and learn thousands of times faster than networks trained using backpropagation. In literature, also shows that these models can outperform support vector machines in both classification and regression applications. Most of the time, ELM is used as a single hidden layer feedforward network (SLFN) including but not limited to sigmoid networks, RBF networks, threshold networks, fuzzy inference networks, complex neural networks, wavelet networks, Fourier transform, Laplacian transform, etc. A hidden node in ELM is a computational element, which need not be considered a classical neuron. A hidden node in ELM can be classical artificial neurons, basis functions, or a subnetwork formed by some hidden nodes (He et al., 2012).

Cuckoo Optimization Algorithm

Cuckoo birds, known for their brood parasite habit, have recently caught the interest of research organizations. The aggressive egg-laying and migration patterns of cuckoo birds served as the inspiration for Rajabioun's Cuckoo Optimization Algorithm (COA). COA requires fewer iterations to obtain global optimums. Additionally, COA can accurately estimate global optima in cases where GA and PSO are unable to arrive at a viable solution. Because of this, COA is employed to resolve clustering datasets. Then, to improve stability and enrich the initial population, the chaotic Arnold's Cat function is used. Each initial cuckoo represents a solution obtained by using the K-means algorithm on a dataset to bring the initial population closer to the overall solution.

Groups of cuckoos coexist. Existing cuckoos are divided into a certain number of groups using K-means. In the wild, cuckoo birds migrate to more favourable locations. Each group's average fitness is calculated in COA. As a destination point, the best point of the best group is chosen. Cuckoos fly in this direction while taking the interval distance, deviation angle, and current position into account. The algorithm iterate until the termination condition is met (Ameryan, 2014).

Dimensionality Reduction Techniques

In this section, the two popular dimensionality reduction techniques, Principal Component Analysis and Linear Discriminant Analysis are discussed.

1) Assessment of Principal Components

A statistical technique called PCA makes use of an orthogonal transformation. A group of correlated variables is transformed into a group of uncorrelated variables using PCA. For exploratory data analysis, PCA is employed. PCA can also be used to examine the connections between a collection of variables. Therefore, it can be applied to reduce dimensions.

2) LDA (Linear Discriminant Analysis)

Another well-liked method for dimensionality reduction in pre-processing for data mining and machine learning applications is LDA. LDA's major objective is to map a dataset with a lot of features onto a space with fewer dimensions and good class separability. By doing so, computational costs. LDA and PCA use methods that are quite similar to one another. LDA maximizes multiple class separation in addition to maximizing data variance (PCA). The goal of Linear Discriminant Analysis is to project a dimension space onto a lesser subspace i (where i £ x – 1) without disturbing the class information (Reddy et al., 2020).

Table 2. Methods for big data analysis

No.	Technique	Issue Addressed	Merits	Demerits
1.	ELM K-means and ELM NMF (He et al., 2012)	Solve the clustering problem by using ELM feature on K-means and Fuzzy C-means.	ELM features are easy to implement and ELM Kmeans produce better results than Mercer -kernel based methods.	Number of nodes should be greater than 300 else performance is not optimal.
2.	K-modes and K-Prototype algorithm (Madhuri et al., 2014)	K-means clustering algorithm is modified as k-modes and k-prototype.	K-prototype and k-mode produce better result as compared to k-mean. Also reduces function cost.	Quality of cluster is not very good.
3.	Ranking Based Algorithm (Ranga Suria et al., 2014)	The ranking based algorithm is given to deal with the issue of outliers. It works on two methods value frequency and inherent clustering.	The algorithm is effective to found different numbers of outliers and computational complexity is not affected by outliers.	The limitation of this algorithm is that it can be applied to categorical datasets only.
4.	A clustering approach to constrained Binary Matrix Factorization (Arora & Chana, 2014)	This approach deals with reduction in dimensionality of high dimension data.	The solution obtained is accurate and provided in better time.	Very difficult to implement.
5.	Clustering based on Cuckoo Search Optimization (Arora & Chana, 2014)	It is a metaheuristic approach which avoids problem of k-means.	It is easy to implement and has good computational efficiency. It also improves method to detect best values.	Quality of clusters obtain is not very high.
6.	Dimensionally reduction techniques (Reddy et al., 2020)	Solves the clustering problem using assessment of principal components and LDA	Helps in data compression, and hence reduced storage space.	gv to some amount of data lose.
7.	Spiral algorithm (Tsai et al., 2014)	Multi-objective optimization and truss optimization problems	A high amount of risk analysis hence, avoidance of risk is enhanced and also good for large and mission-critical projects.	Project's success is highly dependent on the risk analysis phase
8.	Parallel Annealing Particle Clustering Algorithm (Arora & Chana, 2014)	It resolves issue of large-scale computation problem by paralleling particle swarm optimization.	Computation time is reduced and clustering quality is also improved.	Does not provide the best global optimization solution.
9.	DBCURE-MR (Kim et al., 2013)	It deals with issue of clustering big data problems. It finds clusters with varying densities and is parallelized with MapReduce.	It is easy to parallelize. Cluster with varying densities are found accurately. It not sensitive to cluster with varying densities.	Its drawback is that it is inapplicable to boundary regions.
10.	ACA-DTRS and FACA-DTRS (Yu et al., 2013)	Extension of DTRS to automatically determine the number of clusters	Without a human interface, it accurately counts clusters without sacrificing the functionality and expedite execution as well.	This algorithm is proposed for tick data only.

TOOLS FOR SWARM INTELLIGENCE

Hadoop

At the beginning of the 2000s, companies like Google and Yahoo had to handle thousands of terabytes and petabytes of data. To deal with Google initiated a distributive computing framework. This was the starting point of Hadoop. After some time Yahoo contributed to this project. Then big data-related projects were developed under the Apache foundation. According to them,

Hadoop is "An open-source framework for processing, storing, and analysing massive amounts of distributed unstructured data. It is designed to handle petabytes and exabytes of data distributed over multiple nodes in parallel."

It is open source which means anyone can use this technology without paying a single penny. Hadoop handles unstructured data. It means that Hadoop can handle databases like text, and images which traditional database systems fail to handle. Hadoop handles huge quantities of data which means Hadoop handles exabytes and petabytes of data which is more expensive than using traditional database systems. Hadoop runs on multiple nodes in parallel. It means that Hadoop runs on a cluster of machines than a single machine.

Features

The big advantage of Hadoop is the easy computation of large-scale data. Ex. It Changes the economics and dynamics of large-scale computing very easily. Some key features make Hadoop reliable for the industry in current times. These features play a major part to make Hadoop the most powerful tool for big data analysis.

Hadoop is an open-source platform which means it is free to use for everybody. Its source code is available online for understanding and to modify in the future. It is largely scalable. A large amount of data can be divided into different inexpensive machines. New machines also can be added easily as per the requirement. Hadoop is highly fault tolerant. Because it uses machines that are easily available, and Hadoop makes different replicas of data. Because of this, lost data can be recovered in the situation of machine failure and it reallocates new machines in the case of hardware. It is flexible to work with both structured and unstructured types of data.

Workflow

Need and demand play a major role in handling. Known for handling unstructured/semi-structured data.

Figure 4. Master node diagram

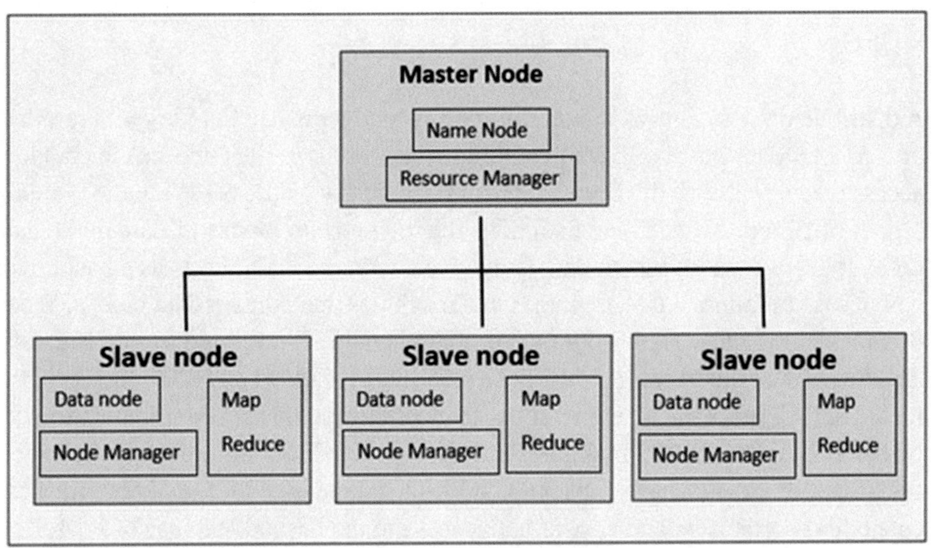

The first client loads data into Hadoop clusters and HDFS breaks this data into parts and then loads it into multiple clusters (Some of the data is replicated multiple times so that data has a backup source). This loaded data will be analysed by the map-reduce framework. The client writes a map-reduce job which is handled by the job tracker. It will be transferred to different nodes in the cluster. This job will be executed on different machines. After the map reduction is completed, the client accesses these results (Sindhu, 2015).

Hadoop Architecture

Hadoop cluster is a master-slave architecture. It consists of five deamonsas namely Name Node (NN), Data Node (DN), Secondary Name Node (SNN), Job tracker (JT), and Task Tracker (TT). A master is like metadata and a slave is an individual machine that executes the split job simultaneously. Name Node, Secondary Name Node, and Job Tracker are the parts of the master node whereas Data Node is and Task Tracker Are in every slave machine which is part of the Hadoop cluster. Name Node, Secondary Name Node, and Data Node are associated with the file handling and are also linked to HDFS whereas Job Tracker and Task Tracker are associated with Map reduce components and are job-related daemons.

Hadoop Ecosystem

HDFS

A distributed file system to run on commodity hardware. It splits files with raw data into 64 MB data blocks. It is intended for reading large files and not for random access reads. Name Node, Data Node, and Secondary Name Node are the building blocks of HDFS. Name Node maintains the reference to blocks of data in the data node. It keeps track of which data is in which data node. SNN acts as a backup for NN in case of failures. DN are individual machines that contain data blocks. When it comes to big data, HDFS components can handle all the three V's of Big data. The function of the Slave (i.e., the Data Node) is to read/ write HDFS blocks in the local HDD of the slave machine. It executes orders from NN - communicates with NN and other DN. HDFS maintains a replica of data blocks in different machines. Each data block will have a backup. Built-in redundancy and failover, Big Data capability, Portability, and cost-effectiveness are the best advantages of HDFS.

Map Reduce

A programming skeleton or language on which Hadoop systems are based. It also has a master-slave component. Map tasks take the input file, then process, create the intermediate files, and send it to the reducer. It takes input from different mappers and aggregates the results.

HBase

HBase is for structured data. It is an Apache open-source project whose objective is to provide storage for Hadoop clusters. HBase sits on top of HDFS as an additional layer. HBase consists of Master and Region.

There are some main differences between HDFS and HBase. The writing pattern of HDFS is appended whereas HBase follows random write and bulk incremental writing patterns. HDFS scans the full table at once while reading but HBase scans randomly. HDFS handles both structured and unstructured data whereas HBase handles only structured data. HDFS does not allow data updates and HBase allows it to do regularly.

There are also some differences between RDBMS and HBase. The data layout of RDBMS is oriented but the layout in HBase is column oriented. The data size in RDBMS is Terabytes whereas it is parabytes in HBase. The query language for RDBMS is SQL and for HBase is get/put/scan etc.

Figure 5. Map reduce

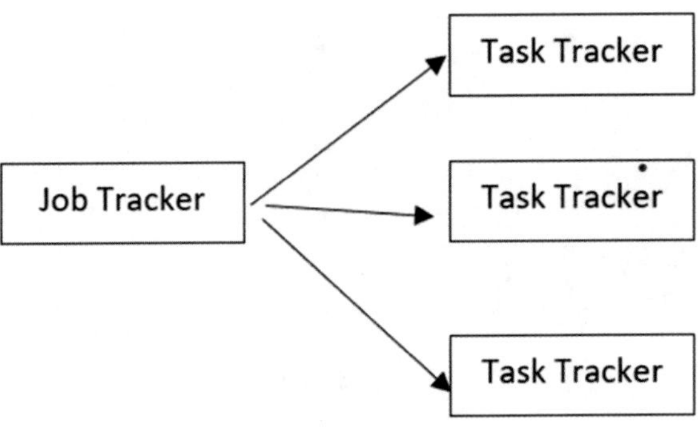

On the right is the HDFS layout and in the Middle is the data nodes or region node which contains the data. On the left is the master component. We have a zookeeper which is a component of the Hadoop ecosystem that looks into the coordination and management aspect of the slave node. Region servers would reside inside HDFS. This is the general HBase architecture to showcase the different components of HBase (Katal, 2013).

APPLICATION

Figure 6. Apache Hadoop ecosystem
Source: Hadoop ecosystem components and its architecture from ProjectPro (n.d.)

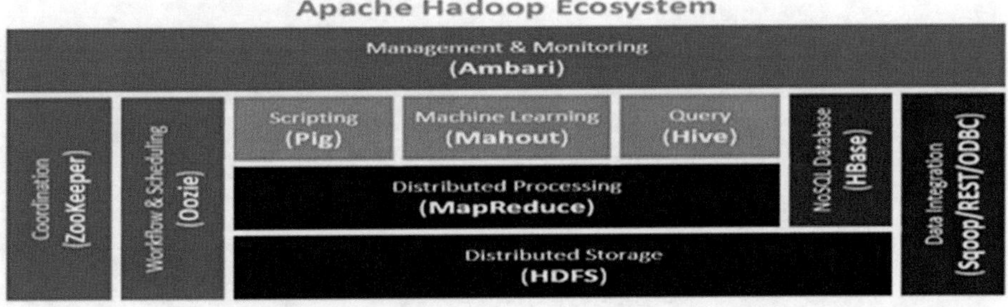

Applications of Big Data Analytics

Big data analytics is being used to examine large datasets containing a variety of data types to uncover hidden patterns, unknown correlations, market trends, customer

Figure 7. Google trends indicator of swarm intelligence algorithms from 2004 to 2022

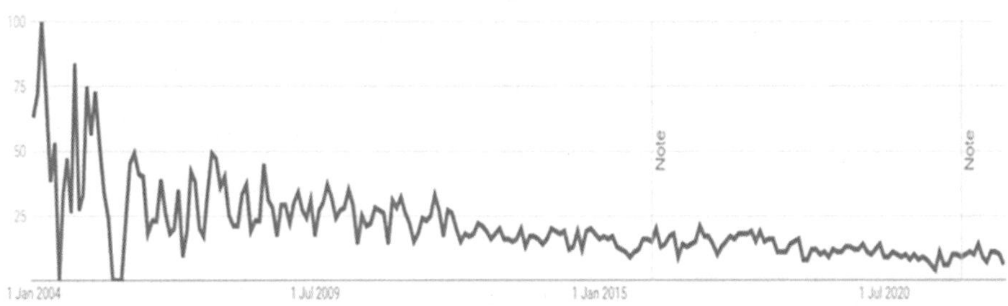

Figure 8. Various applications of swarm intelligence algorithms in different field.

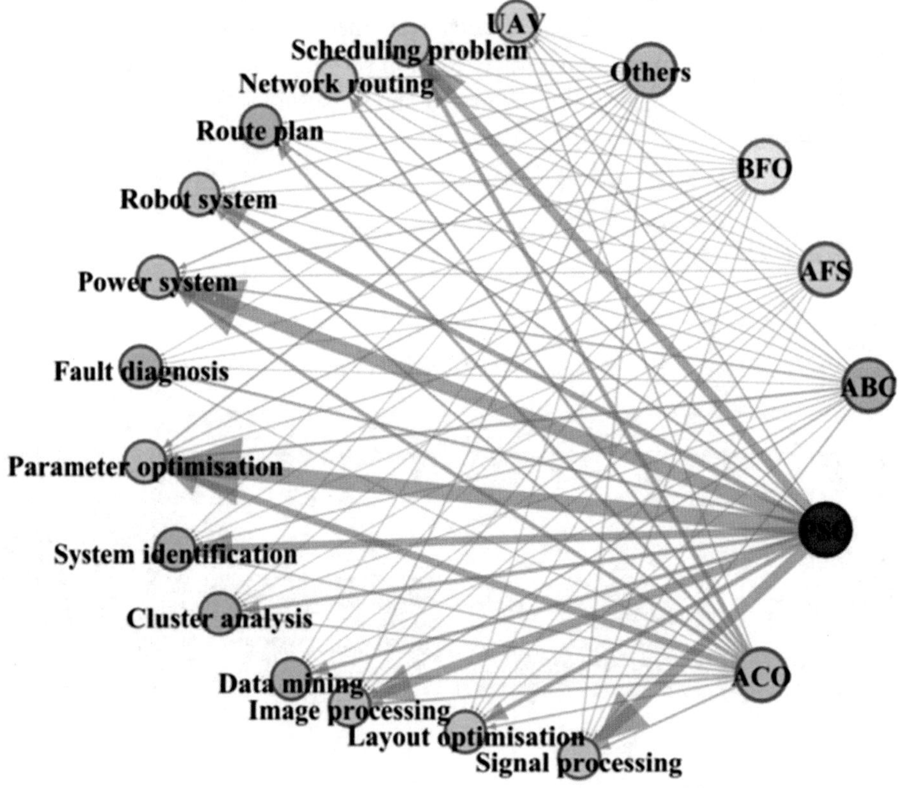

preferences, and other useful business information. Although big data analytics has been widely used in business environments to predict future trends and consumer behaviours, it has been surprisingly underutilized in the educational environment in general. The six stakeholders in education are learners, educators, educational researchers, course developers, learning institutions, and education administrators.

Flood Management

Therefore, determining the risk of flooding before it happens is essential. This allows precautionary measures to be taken by warning the people living in flood-prone areas. Eventually, the people will be able to arm themselves with the necessary tools to combat local flooding risks. Due to its ability to efficiently display, analyse, and predict risks, big data in this context could play a significant role in supporting the evaluation of flood risks. Its analytical methods are so robust that it can handle extremely large data chunks and is capable of processing complex mathematical computations to reveal patterns, trends, and associations to extract the values from the dataset to facilitate assessment or prediction more accurately.

Big Data has so much to promise in disaster management that is associated with floods. Big Data can deal with enormous volumes of data that are coming from different sources in various formats. Unlike the traditional data processing approach, Big Data has the computing resources to process large and complex data to make better decisions and provide valuable insight by assessing the patterns, trends, and association of data. Crisis response teams from different countries have turned their interest in Big Data to use its potential to come up with better prediction models for a disaster like earthquakes, wildfires, storms, or floods. The reason behind that is data are coming from different sources such as humans, organizations, and machines while dealing with a natural disaster. By evaluating the data coming from social media (Facebook or Twitter), sensors, satellite images, and disaster management organizations through API, many crises can be predicted before they occur which will give adequate time for the evacuation of people and other crucial preparations. Furthermore, Big Data is renowned for transforming disorganized collections of data into something extensive and significant.

Big Data can increase social resilience to natural disasters by providing functionalities such as monitoring hazards, predicting exposure and vulnerabilities, managing disaster response, assessing the pliability of natural systems, as well as engaging communities throughout the disaster cycle. Satellites, seismographs, and drones provide consistently enhancing remote-sensing abilities. Data that are coming from smartphones and Twitter feeds create significant opportunities for monitoring hazards like floods or earthquakes. Using satellite imagery, experts can pinpoint geographical and infrastructure concerns. Social media can be monitored to study the behaviour and movement of people after a natural calamity for guiding disaster

2 Challenges and Opportunities of Using Big Data for Assessing Flood Risks 35 response accordingly (Monrat et al., 2018).

Big Data in Higher Education

Big data can provide students with information about what they have understood well and what is otherwise. Similar to this, students can learn from the strategies used by high-performing students and adapt their learning to the system. Using big data, educators can analyse the overall performance of the class at the macroscopic level, therefore helping them to prepare general strategies for the class. Also, they can analyse the performance of an individual student at the microscopic level to find the strengths and weaknesses of that specific student. Accordingly, educators can focus on the weak points to improve the overall performance of the students. Educational researchers can use a large amount of learner data to propose new learning theories and practices and to test the effectiveness of the proposed theories and models. The course developers can take advantage of the instant availability of a large number of online users and their feedback to design new course contents or modify existing course contents. The learning institutions can use big data to reach potential students for recruiting or to establish and maintain relations with their alumni. Also, academic administrators can analyse the performance of students from all courses with less effort. They can use these data to measure the effectiveness of new initiatives taken by them to improve the performances of the learners as well as instructors. Accordingly, they can frame policies, implement programs, and adapt the policies and programs to improve teaching, learning, and retention rates. These benefits of big data analytics have generated interest among all the stakeholders in using big data analytics in the learning, administration, and analysis process in institutions.

Educating Students Using Big Data The twenty-first century has witnessed the integration of ICT into teaching and learning. Educators are using several online and offline tools to create quality and easily understandable content for learners. Web-based learning management systems were one of the ICT tools that higher education institutions utilized most throughout the first decade of this century (LMS). LMSs such as Blackboard and Moodle are helping educators in bringing together learning content and resources besides other administrative jobs such as assessment of students' work, etc. Web-based learning management systems were one of the ICT tools that higher education institutions utilized most throughout the first decade of this century (LMS). Therefore, the second decade of this century is witnessing the emergence of distributed heterogeneous tools used by all stakeholders in the learning process. These systems are embedding data mining techniques to collect the required data, analyse them, and suggest the appropriate actions. Big data can help in tracking the time taken by the students to learn a particular concept. This will be an indicator of the level of difficulty of the concept provided in the study material, or it can help to determine the learning ability of the students (Ray & Saeed, 2018).

Big Data in Mobile Networks

Applying big data in mobile networks is possible in two scenarios. Therefore, it is crucial to reduce expenses during the manufacturing process. The second scenario is to apply big data analysis for optimizing the mobile network design. Big data analysis provides three capabilities for fifth generation (5G) design (Dighriri et al., 2018). The first is full intelligence of the current network status, the second is predicting user's behaviour, and the third is related to the dynamic response association to the network parameters. The 5G technology will allow users to have high-speed Internet access consequently new applications and services will emerge (Zheng et al., 2016).

Big Data in Industry

Big data analytics has become an important tool for the progress and success of a wide range of businesses and industries. Its diversity and flexibility offer a steadily increasing scope for several applications to stay competitive in the market. For that, the big data approach provides several advantages such as advanced analytics, intelligent optimization, informed decision making, large-scale modelling, and accurate predictions. It has been especially possible to find more precise and workable solutions for contemporary engineering difficulties because of the many advantages. As a result, big-data analytics is having a greater than ever impact on the field of engineering and its applications (Mosavi et al., 2018).

Nowadays, several applications, services, and products are offered by different sectors and people are demanding access to these services or trying to obtain new products according to their preferences and tendency. An industry's responsibility is to find better solutions for a specific problem taking into account the aspects mentioned above and achieve a fault-free and cost-efficient process within the company. Solving problems in engineering fields is a demanding decision-making process and should be considered from different perspectives. Although for enterprises finding a solution for a given problem is important, they are also identifying how to increase their revenue and processes optimization. Therefore, decreasing costs during the manufacturing process is imperative. Therefore, big data analysis plays an important role during the fourth industrial revolution as it helps to find a low-cost strategy for companies to be more competitive (Al-Abassi et al., n.d.).

Big Data in Industry 4.0

According to, in 2050 about 70% of the world population will live in cities. Consequently, new challenges will appear for different sectors. Companies, that provide water supply, electricity, transportation, and health, should deal with the city's overcrowding population. Furthermore, governments want better control of natural resources and are looking for better living conditions for their citizens. All these areas can be addressed by an important technology that will help to optimize all the processes within a city. This technology is called the Internet of Things (IoT). It allows connecting multiple devices within a common network. Consequently, it is possible to have integrated management of them, but the most fascinating advantage is that all this management can be possible through the Internet. Likewise, traffic optimization network and traffic forecast can be accomplished, and it will help in decision making. On the other hand, there are advantages related to air pollution. Through big data analysis, it is possible to create a suitable traffic model which helps to reduce the fuel consumption in vehicles. The IoT is also related to Industry 4.0, where it supports factories with rapid product development, flexible production, and a complex environment. The age of smart factories is coming, and intelligent and customized products can be manufactured in a shorter period in real-time considering the customer's preferences. Such an automation process is generating big datasets. It is worth analyzing these datasets to find new strategies for the supply chain processes to increase profitability. The big amount of data generated by all these devices connecting to the Internet will generate a big amount of structured and unstructured data. This sharp increase converges once again in big data analysis. Nevertheless, the data gathered by IoT have different features compared to traditional big data because of data generation, data interoperability, and data quality. Interpretation of big datasets from IoT is a challenge because the data sources are ubiquitous the transmitted data is noisy, heterogeneous, and spatiotemporal dependent (Oikonomidi, 2020).

Big Data in Mechanical Engineering

Over the last decade, the automobile industry has developed important solutions for car driving, and all the mechanical and electronic systems within Electronic Vehicles (EV). These developments allowed the manufacturing of autonomous vehicles.

State of the Art Survey 229 which is equipped with advanced sensing, navigation devices, communication capabilities, and computer vision. Thus, these entire new characteristics in vehicles are potential support for all the users and transportation systems since they can avoid crashes, reduce travel time, assisting traffic flows, among other benefits. There are several sensors installed in vehicles, which help in different vehicle functions and, at the same time, provide a large amount of data for research purposes. By the analysis of data collected from vehicles, it is possible to improve all the systems inside. Using Big Data techniques, all the functions in the vehicle can be substantially improved. Regarding the range estimation for EV, there are several parameters to analyse and this big amount of data has different levels of accuracy, relevance, and unstructured ways. Big Data analysis provides a much better estimation of vehicle driving range. To give an optimum solution for this particular problem, the data acquisition, e.g., state of charge of the battery, battery manufacturer model, driving history, the model of the vehicle, GPS location, weather conditions, traffic report, etc. are collected and categorized according to their properties within three groups. The first is standard data, this category includes data such as GPS position, weather conditions, and estimation of the driving time to the destination. The second is historical data, within this group, there are parameters like a mile per gallon, and the data from other people who did the same trip are collected. The third is real-time data, which includes data collected when an event occurs unexpectedly, for instance, a traffic jam due to an accident (Hadoop ecosystem components and its architecture from ProjectPro, n.d.).

Applications of Swarm Intelligence

Swarm Intelligence in Robotics

Swarm intelligence serves as the model for swarm robotics, a rapidly growing subject. Animal communities serve as excellent models for the potential outcomes of robotic swarms in the future, but they are in no way constrained by biological plausibility. The creation of such systems should include possible criteria such as cost, cost-effectiveness, flexibility, and efficiency.

Foraging: This scenario has numerous applications and calls for a number of essential abilities from a group of robots, including cooperative exploration, efficient work distribution, and shortest path finding. It also includes the sub-task for transportation, which addresses the significant problem of collective transportation. Toxic waste clean-up, search and rescue (SAR), and the collection of landscape samples are a few examples of uses for foraging scenarios.

Dangerous Tasks: Because the creators of a swarm-robotic system are expendable, the system is appropriate for domains with dangerous tasks. A swarm of robots, for instance, can demine at a low cost.

Exploration and Mapping: New scenarios are now conceivable because to design innovations that significantly reduce the size and cost of robotic units. Swarms of robots can be used to inspect various types of designed structures, a process that is typically time- and money-consuming. Despite the limited sensory capabilities of the robots in a swarm, the swarm's collective awareness can be leveraged to generate global knowledge (e.g. construct a map of the area) (Jevtic & Andina, n.d.).

CHALLENGES

Unified Swarm Intelligence

This expanding field is governed by any universal principles. There aren't any essential elements to a successful swarm intelligence algorithm. Numerous SI algorithms

Table 3. Applications of big data

Sr no.	Domain	Application
1.	Flood management (Monrat et al., 2018)	• It can deal with enormous volumes of data that are coming from different sources in various formats. • It has the computing resources to process large and complex data to make better decisions and provide valuable insight by assessing the patterns, trends, and association of data. • Response teams from different countries have turned their interest in Big Data to use its potential to come up with better prediction models for a disaster like earthquakes, wildfires, storms, or floods.
2.	Higher education (Ray & Saeed, 2018)	• Can provide students with information about what they have understood well • Educators can analyse the overall performance of the class at the macroscopic level • Educational researchers can use a large amount of learner data to propose new learning theories and practices.
3.	Mobile networks (Dighriri et al., 2018)	• Provides three capabilities for fifth-generation (5G) design 1. It is full intelligence of the current network status 2. It predicts user's behaviour 3. It is related to the dynamic response association to the network parameters
4.	Industry (Mosavi et al., 2018)	• It is an important tool for the progress and success of a wide range of businesses and industries. • The big data approach provides several advantages such as advanced analytics, intelligent optimization, informed decision making, large-scale modelling, and accurate predictions.
5.	Industry 4.0 (Mosavi et al., 2018)	• It is possible to create a suitable traffic model which helps to reduce the fuel consumption in vehicles. • The big amount of data generated by all these devices connecting to the Internet will generate a big amount of structured and unstructured data. • This sharp increase converges once again in big data analysis
6.	Mechanical Engineering	• All the functions in the vehicle can be substantially improved. • It provides a much better estimation of vehicle driving range.

have been proposed thus far, all of which use the same processes to solve issues. The ability to learn and improve one's ability to solve an optimization problem that is unknown at the time an algorithm is designed or implemented is not provided by any unified framework for SI algorithms. This issue is being addressed in certain ways, but more work is necessary to make it a reality.

Handling High-Dimensional and Dynamical Data

The "curse of dimensionality" happens in high-dimensional data mining problems when the dimension of the data space increases. For instance, categorization techniques like the nearest neighbour approach are important. Due to the increased computational complexity brought on by the rise in dimensionality, it is challenging to solve the similarity search problem for large dimensional data. Furthermore, in order for swarm intelligence algorithms to continue to be able to solve adequately dynamic issues in non-stationary or uncertain situations, where the conditions of the data change over time, extra steps must be done (Yang et al., 2020).

Security Challenges in Big Data Computing

Integrity Security: The deployment of big data is significantly hampered by the filtering process and input validation. It is difficult to tell whether the data is generated from a reliable source or not because of the magnitude of the data. If the source is reliable, the information must be removed in order to prevent a risk to the entire system. Real-time security monitoring is preferred for warning institutions of assaults in their early stages. The organization appears to benefit significantly from the use of SIEM systems in spotting problems and fixing them right away.

Although data gathered through data mining can be very valuable for many different purposes, people have shown increasing concern about the flip side of the coin, which is concerned with the method poses risks to privacy. Unauthorized access to personal information, the use of personal information for non-business objectives, and the unintended revelation of embarrassing material are all threats to an individual's privacy (Sindhu, 2015). For instance, a frustrated client complained to Target that his teenage daughter received coupons for baby goods. This data was gathered via mining customer records. Analysing this situation reveals that there is tension between data mining and privacy security. PPDM, or privacy-preserving data mining, has drawn interest as a solution to problems with data mining. Its main goal is to protect personal information from unauthorized or unwanted exposure while maintaining the usefulness of the data (Sriram, n.d.).

Challenges of Big Data and SI in Education

Research: Precision education and personalised learning are gradually replacing one-size-fits-all methods of instruction in the educational system. The current concentration of AI research in education is on a particular field of intelligent computing technology. Machine-generated data should be carefully developed in terms of its structure, intent, and meaning. The widespread use of big data and AI technology has both positive and negative effects.

Policy Making: Traditional formal education systems are going through dramatic adjustments or perhaps a paradigm shift in digitally driven knowledge economy. A significant portion of instructors in training and in the classroom are not prepared to support and adopt new technology. Protections against unauthorised disclosure, economic exploitation, and other abuses of privacy and personal data are urgently needed.

Industry: There are several challenging issues with the commercialization of intelligent educational tools and systems. To preserve healthy market competition, the range of commercially and publicly available instruments must be expanded. To be current and prudent, vocational, and practical education must undergo significant modification (Sriram, n.d.).

SI-Based AutoML

Swarm intelligence algorithms can be used to automatically build the model structure as well as optimise the hyper-parameters of machine learning models. The swarm intelligence algorithm has a lot of potential in this area with the growth of AutoML (Yang et al., 2020).

REFERENCES

Al-Abassi, Karimipour, HaddadPajouh, Dehghantanha, & Parizi. (n.d.). Industrial Big Data Analytics: Challenges and Opportunities. In *Handbook of Big data Privacy*. Academic Press.

Ameryan, M. (2014). Clustering Based on Cuckoo Optimization Algorithm. Academic Press.

Arora & Chana. (2014). A Survey of Clustering Techniques for Big Data Analysis. Academic Press.

Dighriri, Lee, & Baker. (2018). Big Data Environment for Smart Healthcare Applications Over 5G Mobile Network. *Applications of Big Data Analytics Trends, Issues, and Challenges*.

Hadoop ecosystem components and its architecture from ProjectPro. (n.d.). https://www.projectpro.io/article/hadoop-ecosystem-components-and-its-architecture/114

He, Jin, Du, Zhuang, & Shi. (2012). *Clustering in extreme learning machine feature space*. Academic Press.

Indrakumari, R., Poongodi, T., Thirunavukkarasu, K., & Sreeji, S. (2020). *Algorithms for Big Data Delivery over Internet of Things. In The Internet of Things and Big Data Analytics* (1st ed.). Auerbach Publications.

Jevtic & Andina. (n.d.). *Swarm Intelligence and Its Applications in Swarm Robotics*. Academic Press.

Katal, A. (2013). *Big Data: Issues*. Challenges, Tools and Good Practices.

Khan, S., & Kannapiran, T. (2019). Indexing issues in spatial big data management. In *International Conference on Advances in Engineering Science Management and Technology (ICAESMT)*. Uttaranchal University. 10.2139srn.3387792

Kim, Shim, Kim, & Lee. (2013). *DBCURE-MR: An efficient density-based clustering algorithm for large data using MapReduce*. Academic Press.

Madhuri, R., Ramakrishna Murty, M., Murthy, J. V. R., Prasad Reddy, P. V. G. D., & Suresh, C. (2014). Cluster Analysis on Different Data Sets Using K-Modes and K-Prototype Algorithms. Academic Press.

Mangla, M., Sharma, N., Mittal, P., & Wadhwa, V. M. (Eds.). (2021). Emerging Technologies for Healthcare: Internet of Things and Deep Learning Models. Scrivener Publishing LLC.

Monrat, Islam, Hossain, & Andersson. (2018). Challenges and Opportunities of Using Big Data for Assessing Flood Risks. *Applications of Big Data Analytics Trends, Issues, and Challenges*.

Mosavi, Lopez, & Varkonyi-Koczy. (2018). *Industrial Applications of Big Data: State of the Art Survey*. Academic Press.

Oikonomidi. (2020). *Impact of Big Data Analytics in Industry 4*. Academic Press.

Ranga Suria, Narasimha Murty, & Athithan. (2014). *A ranking-based algorithm for detection of outliers in categorical data*. Academic Press.

Ray & Saeed. (2018). Applications of Educational Data Mining and Learning Analytics Tools in Handling Big Data in Higher Education. *Applications of Big Data Analytics Trends, Issues, and Challenges.*

Reddy, Kumar Reddy, Lakshmanna, Kaluri, Rajput, Srivastava, & Baker. (2020). *Analysis of Dimensionality Reduction Techniques on Big Data.* Academic Press.

Sindhu, P. (2015). A Survey of Tools and Applications in Big Data. Academic Press.

Sriram. (n.d.). *Security challenges of big data computing*. Academic Press.

Tang, Liu, & Pan. (n.d.). *A Review on Representative Swarm Intelligence Algorithms for Solving Optimization Problems: Applications and Trends.* Academic Press.

Thirunavukkarasu & Wadhawa. (n.d.). Analysis and comparison study of data mining algorithms using Rapidminer. *International Journal of Computer Science, Engineering and Applications.*

Thirunavukkarasu, K., Singh, A. S., Irfan, M., & Chowdhury, A. (2018). Prediction of Liver Disease using Classification Algorithms. *2018 4th International Conference on Computing Communication and Automation (ICCCA),* 1-3. 10.1109/CCAA.2018.8777655

Thirunavukkarasu, K., Singh, A. S., Rai, P., & Gupta, S. (2018). Classification of IRIS Dataset using Classification Based KNN Algorithm in Supervised Learning. *2018 4th International Conference on Computing Communication and Automation (ICCCA),* 1-4. 10.1109/CCAA.2018.8777643

Tsai, Huang, & Chiang. (2014). *A Novel Spiral Optimization for Clustering.* Academic Press.

Yang, J., Qu, L., Shen, Y., Shi, Y., Cheng, S., Zhao, J., & Shen, X. (2020, June 22). Swarm Intelligence in Data Science: Applications, Opportunities and Challenges. *Lecture Notes in Computer Science, 12145,* 3–14. doi:10.1007/978-3-030-53956-6_1

Yu, Liu, & Wang. (2013). *An automatic method to determine the number of clusters using decision-theoretic rough set.* Academic Press.

Zheng, Yang, Zhang, Chatzimisios, Yang, & Xiang. (2016). *Big Data-Driven Optimization for Mobile Networks toward 5G.* Academic Press.

Chapter 5
Swarm Intelligence and Evolutionary Machine Learning Algorithms for COVID-19:
Pandemic and Epidemic Review

C. V. Suresh Babu
Hindustan Institute of Technolgy and Science, India

Sam Praveen
Hindustan University, India

ABSTRACT

Healthcare delivery makes use of cutting-edge technology like AI, IoT, big data, and machine learning to prevent and treat emerging diseases. In this chapter, the authors examine SI's crucial role in analysing, preventing, and combating the COVID-19 pandemic as well as other pandemics. They gathered the most recent data on AI for COVID-19 and evaluated it to determine if it may be used to treat this illness. They discovered seven crucial AI applications for the COVID-19 pandemic. Researchers have been working to create a variety of AI models to solve the difficulties associated with medical diagnosis, prediction, and forecasting of medical data in recent years, with the healthcare system at the forefront of research. AI techniques include SI and EA. These algorithms have sped up the development of data analytics methods due to the increased availability of healthcare data. When complex issues are solved computationally in distributed systems, the SI and EA are employed to analyse collective behaviour. Deploying derivative free optimization using SI is affordable, versatile, and reliable.

DOI: 10.4018/978-1-6684-6894-4.ch005

INTRODUCTION

Problem Statement

Since COVID-19 is a recently identified infection, no known immunity exists against it in humans. Based on epidemiologic characteristics and the current situation of a surge in Covid-19 infections worldwide, it is assumed that everyone is vulnerable, albeit there may be risk factors that make people more susceptible to infection. China has made great efforts to comprehend the virus and sickness from the start of the COVID-19 pandemic. How much knowledge on a novel virus has been gathered in such a short time is astounding. Seven weeks after the outbreak started, there are still significant knowledge gaps, as with other newly emerging diseases (Cai, 2020).

Approach

Artificial intelligence (AI) can swiftly identify atypical symptoms and other "red flags," warning patients and healthcare professionals. By enabling quicker decision-making, it supports cost-effective decision-making (Guan et al., 2020). It assists in the creation of a creative diagnosis and treatment plan for COVID 19 cases through pertinent algorithms. AI can help in the diagnosis of infected patients by using medical imaging technologies like computed tomography (CT) and magnetic resonance imaging (MRI) scans of human body parts (Ruan, 2020).

COVID-19 Testing

Since SARS-CoV-2 is an RNA virus, it may be detected using any RNA detection method now in use. The viral genome needs to be reverse transcribed into a DNA complement by reverse transcriptase in order to adapt to the more frequently utilised diagnostic DNA detection formats (Verity et al., 2020). DNA amplification by PCR is currently the recommended SARS-CoV-2 diagnostic, and the real-time versions of such tests were among the first to become accessible. A PCR-based testing strategy for SARS-CoV-2 was therefore an easy choice to make, as such tests had already been established during the development of SARS-CoV and Middle East respiratory syndrome coronavirus (MERS-CoV). Additionally, identifying people who have already contracted SARS-CoV-2 and determining the efficiency of a future vaccination depend on tracking the host reaction (Yu et al., 2020).

All currently accessible technologies have been utilised over the past few months to quickly create very sensitive and highly specific detection and characterisation assays for SARS-CoV-2. We briefly touch on several test types in this section, but we won't discuss functional tests that gauge viral inactivation or the beneficial impact of cellular immune responses1. Such tests are typically only performed in extremely specialised labs, and they have little to no influence on how healthcare is now provided around the world (Kelvin & Halperin, 2020).

Diagnostic Tests Developed and Their Application

Reverse transcriptase real-time PCR (rtPCR) is the most often used direct diagnostic technique to identify active SARS-CoV-2 infections, however other molecular technologies, such as CRISPR-mediated detection or loop-mediated isothermal amplification, have also been used (Kim et al., 2020). These molecular assay's function and are applied similarly to earlier discovered tests that identify infectious pathogens.

Although other molecular technologies, such as CRISPR-mediated detection or loopmediated isothermal amplification, have also been used, reverse transcriptase real-time PCR (rtPCR) is the most common method used for direct diagnostic testing to identify active SARSCoV-2 infections (Walls et al., 2020). These molecular assays function and are used in a manner that is consistent with earlier developed tests for the detection of infectious pathogens (Wang, Qiu, Li et al, 2020).

Approximately 10 days or more after the onset of symptoms, antibody testing can play a mostly complementary role to rtPCR tests in the diagnosis of COVID-19 by evaluating prior infections and defining the dynamics of the individual humoral responses in patients individually or in patient cohorts undergoing particular treatments (Lu et al., 2020). Human IgA, IgM, and/or IgG antibodies as well as virus antigens are typically detected using immune-based techniques, such as lateral flow tests (Khailany et al., 2020). To eliminate primer and antibody mismatches and improve test quality and stability, comparative screening for genomic areas with a low mutation frequency has been used to choose the targets for the tests. Hundreds of these diagnostic tests have now been created, and technical evaluations of their performance comparisons have just lately been published (Mousavizadeh & Ghasemi, 2020).

As of September 5, 2020, information was available on more than 240 COVID-19 diagnostic tests that required an Emergency Use Authorization (EUA). The number of commercially accessible COVID-19 molecular tests and immunoassays is roughly equal. More than 250 of the more than 800 diagnostic assays being evaluated by FIND are so-called quick tests that can produce results in less than 30 minutes. The post-restriction COVID-19 control strategy does not yet include the widespread adoption of immunoassays at the point of care (POC) (Tang et al., 2020). To assist improve their medical relevance, all innovative tests urgently require useful clinical cut-off values. Due to the possibility of false-negative results, negative results from either of these test types cannot now totally rule out present or prior illnesses. The dispute over whether COVID-19 testing should be quantitative or qualitative is still going on. For the selection of a COVID-19 treatment approach, for treatment monitoring, or for the support of vaccination studies, quantitative test findings may be necessary (Cai et al., 2020).

Another critical element is surveillance, which refers to quick and ongoing efforts to identify and treat persons who are infected with the virus (van Doremalen et al., 2020). When an infection is determined to be present, typically based on a combination of clinical signs and symptoms (such as fever, sore throat, or loss of taste and smell) and a direct COVID-19 test, search and control procedures are put in place to identify anyone who has recently had direct contact with the patient and subject them to confinement and/or COVID-19 testing. Epidemiological viral typing is crucial for effective regional and worldwide surveillance and tracking. The definition of polymorphisms and the relationship between different viral strains are both determined by next-generation nucleotide sequencing. Such methods have been crucial in determining the virus's global spread and may also help identify virus variants with various biological properties (for example, ease of spread, pathogenicity and tissue tropism). Virus detection in patients or environmental materials can also be done using metagenomic next-generation nucleotide sequencing (such as wastewater).

EARLY INFECTION IDENTIFICATION AND DIAGNOSIS

Considerations for the Development, Production, and Distribution of Diagnostic COVID-19 Tests

Only the initial stages of the test development are depicted in the cursory sketch of the test design that is supplied in the preceding subsection. Initial design is followed by experimental small-scale laboratory validation, small-scale industrial scale-up, and if necessary clinical evaluation using high-quality and patient specimens. The COVID-19 test format should utilize existing platforms in addition to meeting the standard requirement that it be suitable with mass production. Any test that was quickly designed but could not be used on an existing instrument rarely makes it to the market, which is a significant drawback. Possible exclusions include the fact that tests can be coupled with any current instrument and provided in a platform-neutral format, which may be available to doctors or lab staff.

To ensure the expansion of clinical testing, tools and tests should be widely accessible on a local as well as a worldwide level. A platform's PR accessibility also permits the test's wide global distribution. If a laboratory has an installed set of instruments, additional tests in the existing format can be added to the testing repertory quickly and reliably. In these circumstances, the dissemination of the test may be a

Figure 1. Translational research

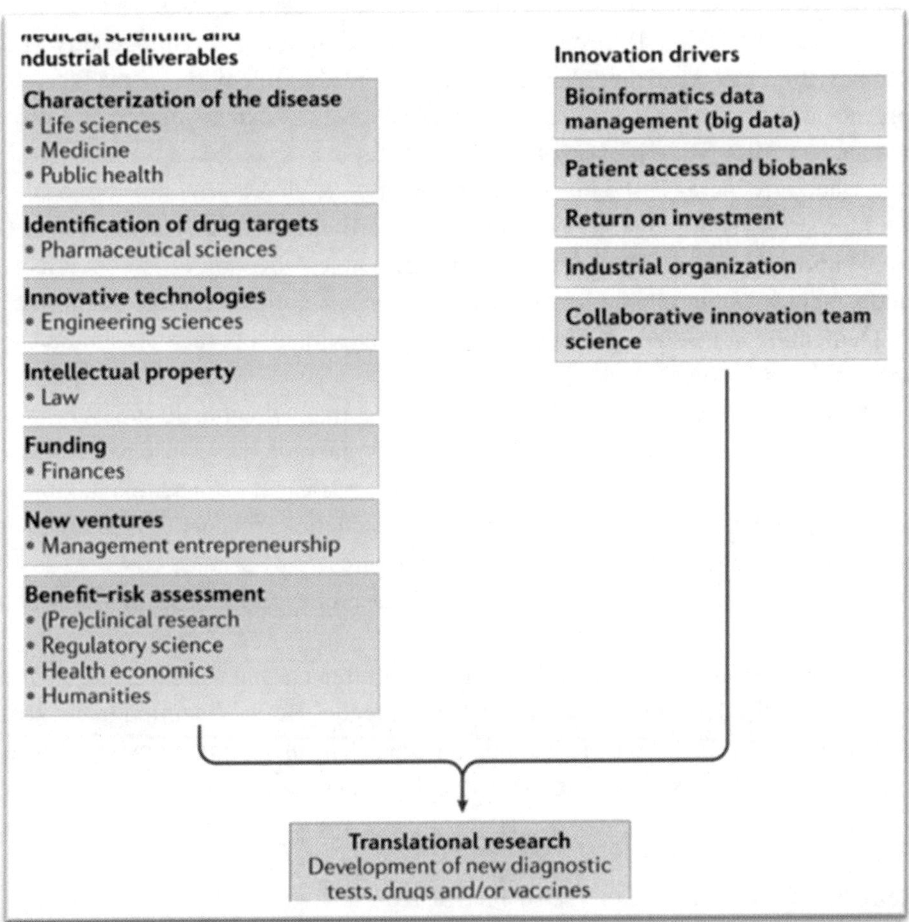

significant barrier in addition to the other challenges of assay transport and storage. The apparent ease of distribution is influenced by many factors, including the shelf life of a test, the components' resilience to temperature changes, and even seemingly unimportant details like package size and weight. Once the users have access to the instrument and assays, the use of high-throughput tests may still be constrained by human knowledge and equipment availability. The capacity of the laboratory must be balanced with the number of test requests, and problems arise when the number of requests for tests fluctuates due to changes in the priority test recommendations. It is obvious that not everyone in the world can be tested (repeatedly) at the same time, and decisions must be taken to give priority to patient groups or populations at risk of infection (for example, health-care workers). Following the identification of these groups, sampling procedures (and associated logistics) must be developed and put into practise. Other sources, such as saliva, have been suggested as alternatives specimens for COVID-19 testing. Simplicity of sampling and homogeneity of the sample itself are significant characteristics to consider. In environments where the prevalence of infection is low, testing sample pools has been advocated as a way to reduce test costs while preserving test sensitivity and specificity. Sample pooling may generally increase the burden of practical pretesting and reduce traceability; for these reasons, it may only be appropriate during reagent shortages. Due to the publication of contradicting reports, it is still unclear if pooling is cost-effective and diagnostically reliable. Additionally, it is currently accepted that prior to implementing large-scale pooling procedures, individual laboratories should carry out validation studies.

As soon as COVID-19 tests became available, many diagnostic streets or drive-through test facilities were developed, and many laboratories chose to externalise testing (using tents, dedicated buildings and separation between sample taking and actual testing). Last but not least, there is a constant need for methods of quick and accurate result dissemination. This issue is complicated by privacy concerns as well as the requirement to use test data in ways that go beyond protecting the privacy of a single patient.

Results from tests are crucial for managing outbreaks and surveillance, and they should be utilised to guide infection control strategies. Before beginning, diagnostic tests must be carefully considered and validated. This involves expensive and time-consuming processes and is frequently undervalued by scientists and the general public.

Quality Control of COVID-19 Testing

New guidelines were released for laboratories on February 29, 2020, allowing them to create and use COVID-19 molecular diagnostic tests prior to receiving EUA (see also Supplementary). The relative technical simplicity with which such diagnostic tests could be created, and the stability of the pathogen's target genetic material were contributing elements to test quality and reproducibility, leading to the development of a number of tests in a short period of time. Diagnostic testing is useless and wastes important and maybe scarce resources when there is no quality control at every stage (from design to end use).

Defining the Clinical Validation of Diagnostic Tests

According to the review, clinical validation of diagnostic tests entails evaluating the test's performance in relation to a reference test that is able to accurately determine

Figure 2. Graphical analysis of testing rate

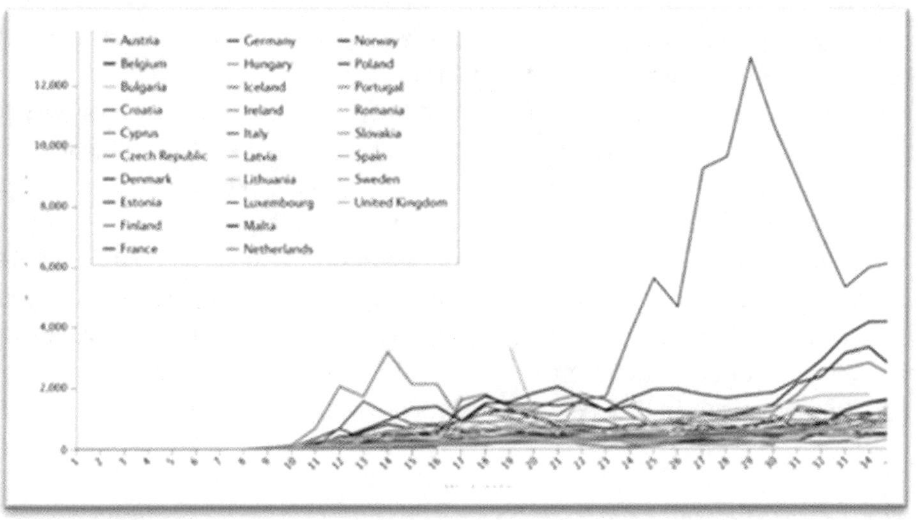

the state of the sample. To increase the likelihood of finding sources of variation and interference, the generic validation of a novel technology should be carried out on a larger scale, ideally in multiple laboratories, and should involve a much more thorough investigation of the critical parameters pertinent to the particular technology. If they are properly validated, new laboratory-developed or acquired methods that the lab uses for testing and calibration may also be competent (Chen et al., 2020). All non-standard methods and standard methods utilised outside of their intended purpose must be validated by laboratories. This includes both lab-based approaches and prediction models that make use of diagnostic data to forecast the degree of disease, for example. For amplifications and modifications to conventional procedures, it must be proven that the procedures are appropriate for the intended application by providing a carefully documented validation protocol and its consequences.

Test Sensitivity and Specificity

The ability of a molecular COVID-19 tests to exclusively identify the analyte it is intended to detect in the presence of off-target templates or interfering compounds under carefully regulated laboratory circumstances is referred to as analytical specificity. The best clinical performance will ultimately result from adequate analytical specificity and sensitivity (Hindson, 2020). The quality and relevant abundance of RNA in collected samples—which largely depend on the type and location of collection—are essential for the sensitivity of the assays in molecular COVID-19 examinations. For instance, in patients with COVID-19, the rate of rtPCR detection of SARS-CoV-2 is as high as 93% in bronchoalveolar lavage fluid, but only 72% in sputum, 63% in nasopharyngeal swabs, and only 32% in stool. A later, small hospital cohort study found that the prevalence of rtPCR positivity for SARS-CoV-2 in blood is 15-30% and in rectal swabs is 14-38% in patients with laboratory-confirmed COVID-19. In this investigation, blood samples from 23 individuals and rectal swabs from 15 patients were collected. Although a number of studies had to use target material from cultures of Vero cells or synthetic viral DNA fragments due to the regulatory inability to access samples from the early infected populations in China, the analytical sensitivity of the new molecular tests was reported to be high from the start. With clinically accessible samples from infected individuals in Europe, this validation was carried out once more.

FOLLOW-UP ON THE TREATMENT

An intelligent platform for autonomous viral monitoring and prediction may be developed using SI. To extract the visual components of this illness, a neural network might be built, which would help with adequate monitoring and treatment of those who are affected. It has the ability to offer choices for addressing the COVID-19 outbreak as well as daily updates on patients.

Artificial intelligence (AI) systems had discovered the outbreak of an unidentified type of pneumonia in the People's Republic of China (hereinafter "China") before the rest of the world was even aware of the threat posed by the coronavirus (COVID-19) (Huang et al., 2014). As the outbreak has now spread globally, policymakers, the medical community, and society at large can use AI tools and technology to support their efforts to manage the crisis and its aftermath at every stage: detection, prevention, response, recovery, and to speed up research (Figure 3) (Bénézit et al., 2020).

By quickly evaluating massive amounts of research data, AI technologies and methodologies can aid in the understanding of the COVID-19 virus and speed up research on remedies. AI text and data mining techniques can find out about the virus's origins, spread, and diagnosis, as well as on management strategies and lessons learned from other pandemics.

- Deep learning algorithms can be used to forecast potential COVID-19 therapies or medications, both new and old (Winter & Hegde, 2020). A number of institutes are utilising AI to find therapies and create vaccination prototypes. Deep learning has been employed by DeepMind and a number of

Figure 3. Accelerating research

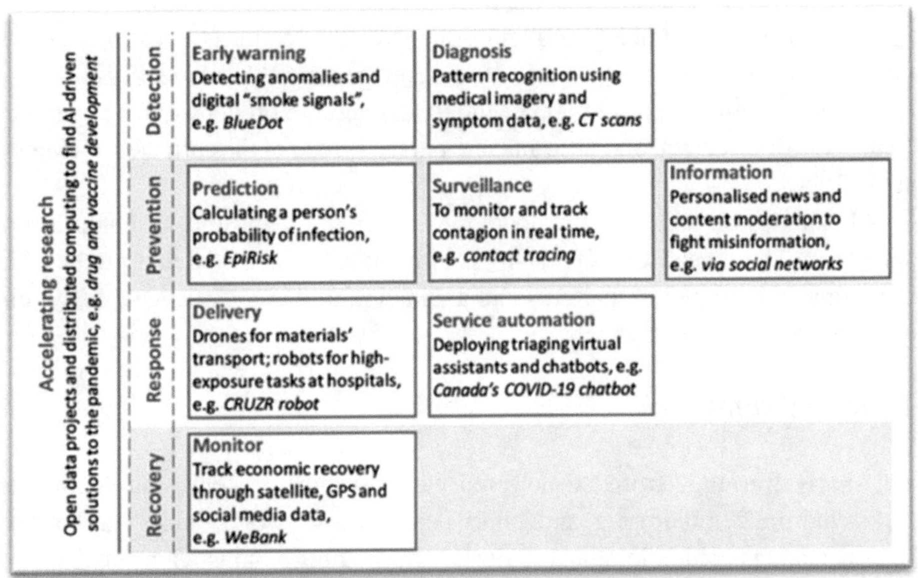

other groups to forecast the structure of proteins linked to SARS-CoV-2, the virus that causes COVID-19.

- The aggregation and exchange of diverse expertise on AI, including worldwide, is made possible by specialised platforms or fora. The US government, for instance, has started a conversation with top scientists from other countries about utilising AI to speed up examination of coronavirus material that is accessible through the Kaggle platform.
- The US government and partner organisations are making datasets in epidemiology, bioinformatics, and molecular modelling accessible, such as through the COVID-19 Open Research Dataset Challenge, which makes over 29 000 academic research publications for coronavirus and COVID-19 available.
- Technology companies like IBM, Amazon, Google, and Microsoft, as well as individuals who donate their computer processing power (such as Folding@ home), as well as public-private initiatives like the COVID-19 High Performance Computing Consortium and AI for Health, are all providing computing power for AI.
- Hackathons, open-source collaborations, and other creative strategies are advancing the quest for AI-driven remedies to the pandemic.

INDIVIDUAL CONTACT TRACING

In addition to properly tracing and monitoring individual contacts, SI can help analyse the virus's level of infection, locate clusters and "hot spots," and identify clusters. It can predict the future progression of the illness and the propensity for recurrence. Using AI to help detect, diagnose and prevent the spread of the coronavirus (Metsky et al., 2020).

AI can also be used to track down the infection, diagnose it, and stop it from spreading. The spread of COVID-19 is already being detected and predicted by algorithms that recognise patterns and anomalies, and image recognition systems are accelerating medical diagnosis.

Tracing Examples

- Early warnings from AI-powered early warning systems can supplement syndromic monitoring and other healthcare networks and data flows by detecting epidemiological patterns by mining mainstream media, web content, and other information channels in different languages (e.g. WHO Early Warning System, Bluedot).
- AI techniques can be used to track wider economic effects and track pathogen transmission chains. Numerous instances have shown that AI technologies have the ability to infer epidemiological data more quickly than traditional reporting of health data. Interactive dashboards have also been made available by organisations like Johns Hopkins University and the OECD (oecd.ai), which follow the virus' progress through real-time data on verified coronavirus cases, recoveries, and deaths.
- To prevent infection and comprehend the course of the condition, rapid diagnosis is essential. AI could assist in making a quick diagnosis of COVID-19 cases when applied to photos and symptom data. To ensure scalability and accuracy, care must be taken to collect data that is representative of the entire population.

Tracing Applications

- Several nations utilise population surveillance to track COVID-19 cases (for example, in Korea algorithms use geolocation data, surveillance-camera footage and credit card records to trace coronavirus patients). China uses mobile phone software to assign each individual a risk level (red, yellow, or green colour code) that indicates the likelihood of contagion. Search engines and social media are assisting in real-time illness tracking while machine learning models utilise travel, payment, and communications data to anticipate the location of the next outbreak and advise border checks.

- To pinpoint potential infection paths, many nations, including Austria, China, Israel, Poland, Singapore, and Korea, have established contact tracing systems. For instance, geolocation data was utilised in Israel to identify individuals coming into proximity to known virus carriers and send them text messages instructing them to immediately isolate themselves.
- In hospitals, semi-autonomous robots and drones are being used to meet urgent demands like delivering food and medications, cleaning, and sterilising, helping doctors and nurses, and making equipment deliveries.

CASE AND MORTALITY PROJECTIONS

This system can track and anticipate the features of the virus, the risks of infection, and its most likely spread using existing data, social media, and media channels. Additionally, it can predict the number of confirmed cases and fatalities in any particular area. In order to take the necessary action, AI can help identify the locations, individuals, and nations that are most vulnerable.

Figure 4. Cases A, B, C, D: Lexical analysis

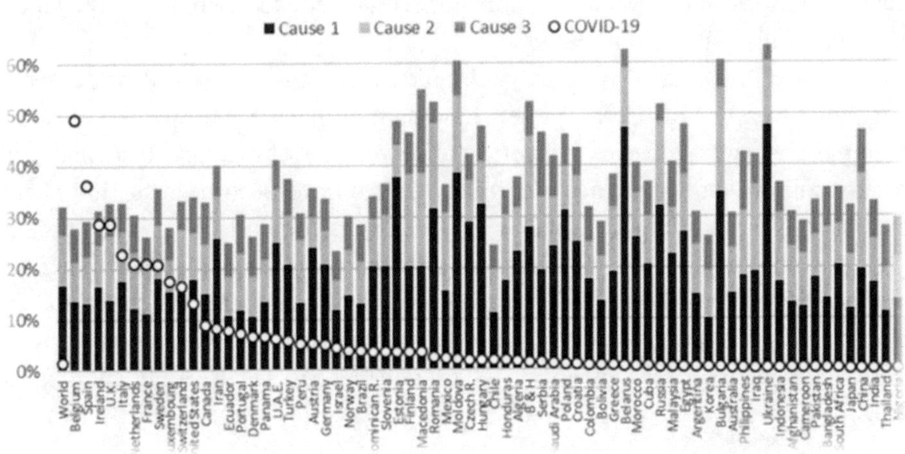

DRUG AND VACCINE DEVELOPMENT

By analysing COVID-19 data, AI is used to do drug development. Drug delivery systems can be designed and created using it. Real-time drug testing takes a lengthy time in conventional testing; therefore, this technology is utilised to speed up the process significantly (Callaway, 2020).

Drug Formulation: Application

The virtual screening of both new chemical entities and therapeutic candidates that have been repurposed is one of the most current applications of artificial intelligence for COVID19. For pharmaceuticals that have been repurposed, the objective has been to quickly forecast and leverage related biological pathways or the off-target biology of proven-safe existing therapies that can therefore be easily tested in new clinical trials. In one of the early investigations, experimentally identified 66 human proteins connected with 26 SARS-CoV-2 proteins, paving the basis for the repurposing of prospective medications. Network-based model simulation has been the primary computational strategy for examining the virus-host interactome, in addition to wet-lab methods. Peer authors discovered 30 medicines for repurposing by examining the genome sequences of the coronavirus's three primary viral family members and connecting them to the disease-based pathways in humans. Provided a combination of network-based approaches for repurposing medication combinations is an alternative strategy.

UK-based BenevolentAI leveraged its AI-derived knowledge graph, which integrates biomedical data from structured and unstructured sources. It targeted the inhibition of host protein AAK1 and identified Baricitinib, an approved drug for the treatment of rheumatoid arthritis. Similarly, The authors published an application of their DL-based drug–target interaction model that predicted commercially available antiviral drugs that may target the

SARS-COV-2-related protease and helicase. Atom-wise has also focused on targeting several SARS-CoV-2 protein binding sites that are highly conserved across multiple coronavirus species in an effort to develop new broad-spectrum antivirals.

In addition, multi-task deep learning models have been used to find current medications that can target the main viral proteins, particularly the primary protease (3CLpro) and spike protein. One outstanding example is Cyclica's development and mining of PolypharmDB, a platform of known pharmaceuticals and their projected binding to human protein targets that revealed off-target applications of 30 current treatments against, for instance, the viral protein 3CLpro and the ACE2 binding site. The open sharing of newly predicted chemical structures is one of at least two other applications of DL-based virtual screening for the SARS-CoV-2 major protease that have been published (World Health Organization, n.d.).

One of the most popular methods for virtual screening has been ML-assisted molecular docking. Typically, this procedure calls for the following: Numerous molecules have been reported to fit the binding site of various SARS-CoV-2 proteins required for viral replication and infection using the following methods: (1) Dataset of Druglike or Approved Molecules,

(2) Crystal Structure or Homology Model of the Target, (3) Molecular Docking Program, and (4) Compute. Among those examined are the host ACE2 receptor, TMPRSS2, 3CLpro, Spike

Protein, RdRP, and PLpro. For instance, the peer author developed and applied the Deep Docking (DD) network technology technique to identify at least 1000 protease inhibitors.

However, as they trained their model using the QSAR, no innovative docking score was offered (Wang, Zhang, Du et al, 2020).

It is obvious that the most frequently used target for virtual screening is 3CLpro. This is mostly due to its crucial function in viral replication and transcription as well as its clearly defined structural information. The use of viral protease inhibitors as antiviral medications has received substantial research. Furthermore, research has mostly focused on deep learning-aided techniques since they speed up discovery through automatic feature extraction. While other screened datasets include the FDA-approved LOPAC library, SWEETLEAD library, or all purchasable medications, the datasets referenced frequently make use of the ZINC database (Drugs-lib). In addition, this review examined a range of papers that made use of various computational tools.

RNA-Based

It has already been established that conserved structural components are essential to the function of coronavirus life cycles. The regulatory information stored in the viral RNA is further complicated by structural elements through direct interactions with host RNA-binding proteins and helicases. Targeted disruption of these structural elements' regulatory functions offers a mostly untested method for limiting viral loads with no negative influence on the biology of healthy cells. Despite the fact that this concept would have been unthinkable just five years ago, advancements in AI-driven computational modelling and high-throughput experimental RNA shape analysis have virtually eliminated the major obstacles.

Numerous viral families have been found to share highly conserved RNA structural components, several of which have been functionally confirmed. These stem loops, which are structural components of the 5¢UTR of SARS-CoV-2, are shared by other beta coronaviruses and are known to affect viral replication. The coding region and 3¢UTR contain a large number of structural components that are essential for functional RNA. 106 structurally conserved areas that would make good biotargets for untested antiviral medicines have been discovered. Additionally, they projected that SARS-CoV-2 contains at least 59 unstructured areas that are preserved. In target-based virtual screening, Park et al. discovered an RNA pseudoknot-binding molecule against SARS-CoV-1.

Finding new and evolved targets is also made possible by examining alterations in RNA information. Using a different strategy, the author demonstrated how a newly FDA-approved medication called Remdesivir may attach to the novel coronavirus's RNA-binding channel. By examining the proteins essential to the processes and processing of RNA, they uncovered more prospective medicines. RdRP, processed mRNA, and viral genome appear to be interesting candidates for medication repurposing.

Generative Approaches

One of the areas of drug discovery where artificial intelligence has had the largest impact over the past ten years is the production of molecules. VAE is a generator model for boosting the diversity of generated data, as was already mentioned. Together with IBM Research, we demonstrated a VAE that captures molecules in a latent space. Autoencoders train molecules into a vector that captures features such as bond order, element, and functional group. Once the desired features have been identified, modifications are performed to the original molecular vectors. These can then be reverse-engineered into fresh molecules. The structures were improved by using QED, Synthetic Accessibility, and LogP regressors to enhance the latent space variations.

By creating a novel, sophisticated deep Q-learning network with fragment-based drug design, we took a different approach and were able to resolve many of the problems with classic generative models (ADQN-FBDD). By building SARS-CoV-2 molecules one fragment at a time rather than relying on latent space adjustments, this made it possible to accelerate space exploration. A pharmacophore and descriptor filter was used to narrow the list after forming connections and rewarding compounds with the most druglike associations. They showed a reliable technique for creating brand-new, highly-binding substances tailored to the SARSCoV-2 3CLPro structure. The following is required in order to create a drug-generative network: A method of altering molecules to promote variety, a collection of druglike compounds, an in silico representation of these molecules (e.g., fingerprints, tokenizers), a way of screening and modifying the altered molecules, and so on. Insilico Medicine pursued GANrelated models and employed three of its previously validated generative chemistry methods, including crystal-derived pocket-based generation, homology modeling-based generation, and ligand-based generation, to target the major protease. The major protease has been the main focus of research for de novo drug development, similar to target-based virtual screening.

COVID-19 Vaccine Discovery

To reduce the high infection rate caused by a virus, the best targets for vaccine development must be found. A host immune system fights virus-infected cells either by T cells directly attacking the virus-infected cells or by B cells producing antibodies. MCH-I and MCHII proteins, which display epitopes as antigenic determinants, are encoded by the HLA gene.

These proteins support the binding and defence mechanisms of B-cell and T-cell antibodies. Antigens can be recognised from protein sequences using machine learning techniques, such as Random Forest (RF), Support Vector Machine (SVM), and Recursive Feature Selection (RFE).

The field of COVID-19 vaccine development has also benefited from the use of natural language processing models, particularly language modelling techniques. In the creation of a vaccine, pre-trained transformers were used to predict protein interaction and model molecular processes in carbohydrate chemistry. The application of an LSTM-based seq-2-seq model for foretelling the secondary structure of specific SARS-COV-2 proteins was explored by an author. Additionally, by foreseeing how commercially available medications might interact with SARS-COV-2 viral proteins, I employed transformers to repurpose the drugs.

Combining these studies, it is evident that spike protein has been the most frequently suggested choice for the development of a virtual vaccination. Since the SARS-COV-2 spike protein is essential for viral entry, neutralising antibodies that target Spike's receptor-binding domain can prevent viral proteins from adhering to and fusing with host proteins. This approach might deliver simulated sequences that can act as a roadmap for future COVID-19 vaccine research and perhaps novel zoonosis discovery.

Data Collection

In order to derive mathematical models, data-driven solutions rely on patterns hidden in the data. In spite of this, a data gathering campaign will encounter numerous difficulties in the case of any recently discovered virus, principally as a result of bias and imbalance in the few information available. Therefore, when trained on such datasets, even the most sophisticated modelling algorithms will be worthless. We conducted a multidimensional and thorough analysis of the current literature, datasets, and online resources to identify suitable small compounds, peptides, and epitopes in order to resolve this issue. When combined with both traditional and data-driven AI-based approaches, such features can be helpful in the process of discovering or designing innovative medications to treat COVID-19.

We decide to concentrate on both possible antiviral drugs and inhibitors of host biotargets. The information comprises the peptides and small compounds suggested by in vitro and in silico methods. The potential suppression of other respiratory tract viruses is taken into account in addition to candidate scaffolds against the structural proteins of the coronavirus in order to improve the therapeutic potential. It has been proven that antimicrobial peptides are effective antivirals that can damage either the viral membrane or another molecular mechanism of the virus. As previously mentioned, prospective immunosuppressants were also incorporated as host-targeted medicines because the cytokine storm and a heightened immune response of the host play a critical role in disease complications. In addition to potency, it is essential that a potential medication have excellent selectivity and low toxicity.

As a result, we also compiled an exhaustive toxicity dataset from other databases, such as ToxCast and Tox21. Last but not least, we obtained a large collection of epitopes that might also direct deep learning-based models for better vaccine development and epitope production.

Due to a sudden and considerable surge in patients due to the COVID-19 outbreak, healthcare professionals are overworked. In this case, artificial intelligence is being employed to lighten the load on medical staff. It provides the best training to students and professionals on this new disease and helps with early identification and treatment using digital tools and decision science. AI has the capacity to enhance patient care in the future and address more potential concerns, lessening the pressure on doctors.

RESULTS

In all, 18 out of the 80 distinct peer-reviewed and preprint records that met the requirements for inclusion in the in-depth review discussed the application of machine learning. Preferred Reporting Items for Systematic Reviews and Meta-Analyses (PRISMA) were modified as a result. One more use case not covered by peer-reviewed or preprint literature was discovered via the review of grey literature, together with supporting data for previous use cases. Overall, the in-depth analysis discovered new fields outside of managing infectious diseases, such as the consequences of a pandemic on mental health or chronic illnesses, as well as six key use cases for machine learning in pandemic preparation and response.

Colab was used to research novel model types and assess how well they performed using COVID-19 data. The proposed scheme achieves a high accuracy rate of 92.80 percent, sensitivity rate of 93.20 percent, specificity rate of 90.42 percent, precision

Figure 5. Data collection

Data provided	Discovery	Type	Mechanism of action	References
ANTIVIRAL DATA				
Total of 59,107		**Small molecules and peptides**		
50,000	*In-silico*	Small molecule	Antiviral	1
3,000	*In-silico*	Small molecule	Anti SARS2 protein	Chenthamarakshan et al., 2020
1,000	*In-silico*	Small molecule	Anti-protease	Ton et al., 2020
406	*In-vitro*	Small molecule	Inhibiting autophagy	2
802	*In-vitro*	Small molecule	Activating autophagy	2
393	*In-vitro*	Small molecule	Biotargets of coronaviruses	3
110	*In-vitro*	Peptide and small molecule	Coronavirus and respiratory disease	Pillaiyar et al., 2020
1,000	*In-silico*	Small molecule	3C protease inhibitor	Zhavoronkov et al., 2020
11	*In-silico*	Small molecule	Main protease inhibitor	Fischer et al., 2020
20	*In-vitro*	Antimicrobial peptide	Anti-SARS/MERS	Mustafa et al., 2018
7	*In-silico*	Antimicrobial peptide	Anti-MERS	Mustafa et al., 2019
277	*In-vitro*	Antimicrobial peptide	Antiviral	Wang et al., 2015
4	*In-silico*	Antimicrobial peptide	Anti-spike of sars-Cov-2	Han and Kral, 2020
379	*In-vitro*	Small molecule	Anti-respiratory syncytial virus	Plant et al., 2015
13	*In-vitro*	Small molecule	Anti-recurrent respiratory papillomatosis by HPV-6	Alkhilaiwi et al., 2019
1,280	*In-vitro*	Small molecule	Anti-respiratory syncytial virus	Rasmussen et al., 2011
16	*In-silico*	Small molecules	Anti-SARS-COV-2	Zhou Y. et al., 2020
77	*In-silico*	Small molecules	Anti-S Protein of SARS-COV-2	Smith and Smith, 2020
10	*In-silico*	Small molecules	Anti-SARS-COV2	Hu et al., 2020
25	*In-silico*	Small molecules	Anti SARS2 Proteins	Kim J. et al., 2020
10	*In-silico*	Small molecules	ACE2 and Spike inhibitors	Choudhary et al., 2020
78	*In-silico*	Small molecules	All SARS2 proteins	Wu et al., 2020
47	*In-silico*	Small molecules	3cl protease and M pro	Tang et al., 2020
16	*In-silico*	Small molecules	3cl protease inhibitor	Chen et al., 2020
36	*In-vitro*	Small molecules	Anti- Coronavirus-OC43	Shen et al., 2019
90	*In-vitro*	Small molecules	Anti- SARS-COV-2	Touret et al., 2020
ANTI-HOST PROTEINS				
Total of 677		**Small molecules and peptides**		
6	*In-vitro*	Small molecules	Anti-IL-1β and TNFα	Laufer et al., 2002
182	*In-vitro*	Peptides	Cytokine Signaling Inhibitors	4
269	*In-silico*	Small molecules	Anti-IL-6	Shukla et al., 2019
121	*In-vitro*	Small molecules	Severe acute respiratory	5
69	*In-silico*	Small molecules	Anti-protein-protein interaction of virus-host	Gordon et al., 2020
30	*In-silico*	Small molecules	Anti-host & virus interaction	Redka et al., 2020
TOXICITY DATA				
Total of 25,333		**Small molecules**		
11,800	*In-vitro*	Small molecules	Tox21 and ToxCast	Toxicology, EPA's National Center for Computational, 2018
13,533	*In-vitro*	Small molecules	Toxic for HepG2 Cell Line	Garno et al., 2010
VACCINE DATA				
Total of 517		**Epitopes and vaccines**		
182	*In-silico*	Epitopes	Anti-SARS-COV-2	Ahmed et al., 2020
174	*In-silico*	Epitope	Anti-SARS-COV-2	Prachar et al., 2020
2	*In-silico*	Epitope	Anti-SARS-COV-2	Fast and Chen, 2020
30	*In-silico*	Vaccine candidate	Anti-SARS-COV-2	Feng et al., 2020
7	*In-silico*	Epitope	Anti-SARS-COV-2	Lon et al., 2020
12	*In-silico*	Epitope	Anti-SARS-COV-2	Tilocca et al., 2020
59	*In-silico*	Epitope	Anti-SARS-COV-2	Sarkar et al., 2020
71	*In-silico*	Epitope	Anti-SARS-COV-2	Bhattacharya et al., 2020

[1] *Download CAS COVID-19 Antiviral Candidate Compounds Dataset | CAS. Available online at: https://www.cas.org/covid-19-antiviral-compounds-dataset (accessed April 27, 2020).*
[2] *Novel Coronavirus Information Center. Available online at: https://www.elsevier.com/connect/coronavirus-information-center (accessed April 27, 2020).*
[3] *https://www.elsevier.com/__data/assets/pdf_file/0004/978745/Copy-of-RMC-substances-coronovirus-targets-pX6.pdf (accessed April 27, 2020).*
[4] *Cytokines Inhibitor library|Targetmol|96-well. Available online at: https://www.targetmol.com/compound-library/Cytokines-inhibitors-Library (accessed April 27, 2020).*
[5] *https://www.elsevier.com/__data/assets/pdf_file/0007/977173/ResNet-Data_Coronavirus.pdf (accessed April 27, 2020).*

rate of 95.38 percent, recall rate of 90.24 percent, and F-measure rate of 89.78 percent when compared to existing SI schemes like SVM, logistic regression, and neural networks. It obtained a processing time of 29.12 seconds and a lower processing cost as compared to conventional methods.

CONCLUSION

The healthcare sector is expanding quickly all around the world. There has been a huge amount of mixed data produced by the healthcare industry. It has been vital for the healthcare sector to successfully complete the build-up and the data of mine. Data mining may therefore offer a great deal of flexibility in terms of crucial therapy, diagnosis, and prognosis. Data removal has played a crucial part in the medical sector, acting as both an excellent practise for additional inquiry and analysis of the patient's report and as an easier system for evaluating vast amounts of data. Swarm intelligence has typically been implemented as a population that simply interacts with its environment. Data mining is nothing more than the analysis of massive amounts of data.

REFERENCES

Bénézit, F., Turnier, P. L., & Declerck, C. (2020). Utility of hyposmia and hypogeusia for the diagnosis of COVID-19. *The Lancet. Infectious Diseases*, *20*(9), 1014–1015. doi:10.1016/S1473-3099(20)30297-8 PMID:32304632

Cai, H. (2020). Sex difference and smoking predisposition in patients with COVID-19. *The Lancet. Respiratory Medicine*, *8*(4), e20. doi:10.1016/S2213-2600(20)30117-X PMID:32171067

Cai, J., Sun, W., Huang, J., Gamber, M., Wu, J., & He, G. (2020). Indirect virus transmission in cluster of COVID-19 cases, Wenzhou, China, 2020. *Emerging Infectious Diseases*, *26*(6), 1343–1345. doi:10.3201/eid2606.200412 PMID:32163030

Callaway, E. (2020). The race for coronavirus vaccines: A graphical guide. *Nature*, *580*(7805), 576–577. doi:10.1038/d41586-020-01221-y PMID:32346146

Chen, Y., Chen, L., Deng, Q., Zhang, G., Wu, K., Ni, L., Yang, Y., Liu, B., Wang, W., Wei, C., Yang, J., Ye, G., & Cheng, Z. (2020). The presence of SARS-CoV-2 RNA in feces of COVID19 patients. *Journal of Medical Virology*, *92*(7), 833–840. doi:10.1002/jmv.25825 PMID:32243607

ClinicalTrials.gov. (n.d.). *COVID-19 | Recruiting Studies*. https://clinicaltrials.gov/ct2/results?term=COVID-19&Search=Apply&recrs=a&age_v=&gndr=&type=&rslt=

Guan, W., Ni, Z., Hu, Y., Liang, W., Ou, C., He, J., Liu, L., Shan, H., Lei, C., Hui, D. S. C., Du, B., Li, L., Zeng, G., Yuen, K.-Y., Chen, R., Tang, C., Wang, T., Chen, P., Xiang, J., ... Zhong, N. (2020). Clinical characteristics of coronavirus disease 2019 in China. *The New England Journal of Medicine*, *382*(18), 1708–1720. doi:10.1056/NEJMoa2002032 PMID:32109013

Hindson, J. (2020). COVID-19: Faecal-oral transmission? *Nature Reviews. Gastroenterology & Hepatology*, *17*(5), 259–259. doi:10.103841575-020-0295-7 PMID:32214231

Huang, C. T., Lin, H. H., Ruan, S. Y., Lee, M.-S., Tsai, Y.-J., & Yu, C.-J. (2014). Efficacy and adverse events of high-frequency oscillatory ventilation in adult patients with acute respiratory distress syndrome: A metaanalysis. *Critical Care (London, England)*, *18*(3), R102. doi:10.1186/cc13880 PMID:24886674

Imran, A., Posokhova, I., Qureshi, H. N., Masood, U., Riaz, M. S., Ali, K., John, C. N., Hussain, M. D. I., & Nabeel, M. (2020). AI4COVID-19: AI enabled preliminary diagnosis for COVID-19 from cough samples via an app. *Informatics in Medicine Unlocked*, *100378*, 1–31. doi:10.1016/j.imu.2020.100378 PMID:32839734

Kelvin, A. A., & Halperin, S. (2020). COVID-19 in children: The link in the transmission chain. *The Lancet. Infectious Diseases*, *20*(6), 633–634. doi:10.1016/S1473-3099(20)30236-X PMID:32220651

Khailany, R. A., Safdar, M., & Ozaslan, M. (2020). Genomic characterization of a novel SARS-CoV-2. *Gene Reports*, *100682*, 1–6. PMID:32300673

Kim, J.-M., Chung, Y.-S., Jo, H. J., Lee, N.-J., Kim, M. S., Woo, S. H., Park, S., Kim, J. W., Kim, H. M., & Han, M.-G. (2020). Identification of coronavirus isolated from a patient in Korea with COVID-19. *Osong Public Health and Research Perspectives*, *11*(1), 3–7. doi:10.24171/j.phrp.2020.11.1.02 PMID:32149036

Lu, R., Zhao, X., Li, J., Niu, P., Yang, B., Wu, H., Wang, W., Song, H., Huang, B., Zhu, N., Bi, Y., Ma, X., Zhan, F., Wang, L., Hu, T., Zhou, H., Hu, Z., Zhou, W., Zhao, L., ... Tan, W. (2020). Genomic characterisation and epidemiology of 2019 novel coronavirus: Implications for virus origins and receptor binding. *Lancet*, *395*(10224), 565–574. doi:10.1016/S0140-6736(20)30251-8 PMID:32007145

MaghdidH. S.GhafoorK. Z.SadiqA. S.CurranK.RabieK. (2020). A novel AI-enabled framework to diagnose coronavirus covid 19 using smartphone embedded sensors: design study. doi:10.1109/IRI49571.2020.00033

MetskyH. C.FreijeC. A.Kosoko-ThoroddsenT. S.SabetiP. C.MyhrvoldC. (2020). *CRISPRbased COVID-19 surveillance using a genomically-comprehensive machine learning approach.* doi:10.1101/2020.02.26.967026

Mousavizadeh, L., & Ghasemi, S. (2020). Genotype and phenotype of COVID-19: their roles in pathogenesis. *J. Microbiol. Immunol. Infect.* doi:10.1016/j.jmii.2020.03.022

Rahmatizadeh, S., Valizadeh-Haghi, S., & Dabbagh, A. (2020). The role of artificial intelligence in management of critical COVID-19 patients. *J. Cell. Mol. Anes.*, *5*(1), 16–22.

Ruan, S. (2020). Likelihood of survival of coronavirus disease 2019. *The Lancet. Infectious Diseases*, *20*(6), 630–631. doi:10.1016/S1473-3099(20)30257-7 PMID:32240633

Santosh, K. C. (2020). AI-driven tools for coronavirus outbreak: Need of active learning and cross-population train/test models on multitudinal/multimodal data. *Journal of Medical Systems*, *44*(5), 1–5. doi:10.100710916-020-01562-1 PMID:32189081

Tang, B., Bragazzi, N. L., Li, Q., Tang, S., Xiao, Y., & Wu, J. (2020). An updated estimation of the risk of transmission of the novel coronavirus (2019-nCov). *Infectious Disease Modelling*, *5*, 248–255. doi:10.1016/j.idm.2020.02.001 PMID:32099934

van Doremalen, N., Bushmaker, T., Morris, D. H., Holbrook, M. G., Gamble, A., Williamson, B. N., Tamin, A., Harcourt, J. L., Thornburg, N. J., Gerber, S. I., Lloyd-Smith, J. O., de Wit, E., & Munster, V. J. (2020). Aerosol and surface stability of SARS-CoV-2 as compared with SARS-CoV-1. *The New England Journal of Medicine*, *382*(16), 1564–1567. doi:10.1056/NEJMc2004973 PMID:32182409

Verity, R., Okell, L. C., Dorigatti, I., Winskill, P., Whittaker, C., Imai, N., Cuomo-Dannenburg, G., Thompson, H., Walker, P. G. T., Fu, H., Dighe, A., Griffin, J. T., Baguelin, M., Bhatia, S., Boonyasiri, A., Cori, A., Cucunubá, Z., FitzJohn, R., Gaythorpe, K., ... Ferguson, N. M. (2020). Estimates of the severity of coronavirus disease 2019: A model-based analysis. *The Lancet. Infectious Diseases*, *20*(6), 669–677. doi:10.1016/S1473-3099(20)30243-7 PMID:32240634

Walls, A. C., Park, Y. J., Tortorici, M. A., Wall, A., McGuire, A. T., & Veesler, D. (2020). Structure, function and antigenicity of the SARS-CoV-2 spike glycoprotein. *Cell*, *18*(2), 281–292. doi:10.1016/j.cell.2020.02.058 PMID:32155444

Wang, Q., Qiu, Y., Li, J. Y., Zhou, Z. J., Liao, C. H., & Ge, X. Y. (2020). A unique protease cleavage site predicted in the spike protein of the novel pneumonia coronavirus (2019-nCoV) potentially related to viral transmissibility. *Virologica Sinica*, *20*(3), 1–3. doi:10.100712250-020-00212-7 PMID:32198713

Wang, Y., Zhang, D., Du, G., Du, R., Zhao, J., Jin, Y., Fu, S., Gao, L., Cheng, Z., Lu, Q., Hu, Y., Luo, G., Wang, K., Lu, Y., Li, H., Wang, S., Ruan, S., Yang, C., Mei, C., ... Wang, C. (2020). Remdesivir in adults with severe COVID-19: A randomised, double-blind, placebo-controlled, multicentre trial. *Lancet*, *395*(10236), 1569–1578. doi:10.1016/S0140-6736(20)31022-9 PMID:32423584

Winter, A. K., & Hegde, S. T. (2020). The important role of serology for COVID-19 control. *The Lancet. Infectious Diseases*, *20*(7), 758–759. doi:10.1016/S1473-3099(20)30322-4 PMID:32330441

World Health Organization. (2020). *Coronavirus disease 2019 (COVID-19): Situation report*. www.who.int/docs/default-source/coronaviruse/situation-reports/20200624

World Health Organization. (n.d.). *Draft landscape of COVID-19 candidate vaccines*. www.who.int/publications/m/item/draft-landscape-of-covid-19-candidate

Yu, N., Li, W., Kang, Q., Xiong, Z., Wang, S., Lin, X., Liu, Y., Xiao, J., Liu, H., Deng, D., Chen, S., Zeng, W., Feng, L., & Wu, J. (2020). Clinical features and obstetric and neonatal outcomes of pregnant patients with COVID-19 in Wuhan, China: A retrospective, single-centre, descriptive study. *The Lancet. Infectious Diseases*, *20*(5), 559–564. doi:10.1016/S1473-3099(20)30176-6 PMID:32220284

Chapter 6
Swarm Intelligence Analysis of Healthcare Prediction Techniques Based on Social Media Data:
Basics of Swarm Intelligence, Scope of Swarm Intelligence, Swarm Intelligence in Healthcare

Manivel Kandasamy
Karnavati University, India

Raju Shanmugam
Karnavati University, India

Tanya Valji Chhabhadiya
Karnavati University, India

Harshvi Kamlesh Adesara
Karnavati University, India

Pujita Sunnapu
Karnavati University, India

ABSTRACT

The healthcare industry is rapidly developing across the world. The healthcare industry generates a large volume of diverse data. It is crucial for healthcare sectors to effectively extract, collect, and exploit data. Swarm intelligence algorithms have been

DOI: 10.4018/978-1-6684-6894-4.ch006

applied on the data in detecting cancer, heart disease, malignancies, and cardiology prognosis. Disease diagnosis and treatment have benefited from swarm intelligence techniques. In terms of techniques and outcomes, this chapter examines several uses of swarm intelligence with data prediction techniques using social media data in healthcare. The chapter will cover different areas where prediction techniques will be applied to the data collected by different social media platforms, like data mining, risk scoring of illnesses, and early recognition of patients' condition deterioration using data detection that will use algorithms based on swarm intelligence.

INTRODUCTION

Intelligence has made a crucial and foremost part in the fields of healthcare ever since the expansion and rise of complexity in healthcare data with different data available that involves numeric-reports, categorical-medical results, text-results and conclusions, speech-conversations (doctors, technicians, and patients), signals-ECG and EMG, image- x-rays and video-CT, MRI and Ultrasound output. Data challenges in healthcare will inevitably arise from attempting to keep up with the sheer volume of information generated by images, telehealth, electronic medical records, and other sources of data.

According to research by the International Data Corporation, the healthcare sector is predicted to generate more data than any other economic sector through 2025. Conclusions and optimized decision making is the key output of every healthcare treatment and diagnosis. The effect of a collective decision from multiple intelligent sources will be much more exact and optimized. Intelligence altogether will help healthcare industries to effectively acquire, process, and analyze the data. In the field of artificial intelligence (AI), machines imitate human intelligence and knowledge.

The healthcare sector does not only involve patients' wellbeing and treatment but is an amalgam of various different groups that make the healthcare system work efficiently. It basically includes equipment services and pharmaceuticals and biotechnology services that are further divided into various departments such as equipment supply, providers and services and technology in the first and biotechnology, life science tools and services and pharmaceuticals in the latter. The challenges that these sectors face are rising due to data growth. Using AI and ML these problems can be assisted well.

The Data Challenge

The world of data has begun to sprung after the rise of the internet and IT technology. The main growth of data happened when the world began using social media.

Several social media sites like Six Degrees, MySpace and Facebook were the very early social media sites that were launched 2-3 decades before. These sites were responsible for the birth of the new term in the field of data that is "Big Data". The modern business environment has just undergone a change because of big data. Big data is a collection of information that organizations can use for business reasons through machine learning, predictive modeling, and other sophisticated data analytics applications. It consists of a mixture of structured, semi structured, and unstructured data. To deal with all such data intelligence and technology must be well combined and used effectively for better data insights.

Data in healthcare brings various problems and challenges to be assisted that include data fragmentation, altering and transforming data, data security and privacy and data expectations. Patients today expect the same experience from health care providers, payers and pharmaceutical companies as they get from retailers and banks: they want to be more involved in their care. They expect all relevant parties, like providers, payers and pharma to collaborate and recommend the best treatment options.

Data fragmentation in healthcare is the ever challenging area that has popularized with social media data. Health care data is available in a dizzying array of types and sources, including structured data, paper, digital, images, videos, multimedia, and more. The networks that collect and aggregate data are equally dispersed, which makes it challenging to retrieve and aggregate information. Data is gathered by providers such as physicians, doctors and clinics, consumers, experts in public health employers, social network communities, and patients, but no effort is made to aggregate and consolidate the data. There is no single source of truth, and there is data deviation and redundancy. Because of this, health care user records are erroneous and deficient in details on a patient's journey to wellness and their continuously shifting connections with providers, collectors, pharmacists, friends, and family. Low compliance and high relapse risks are caused by a lack of awareness, supervision, and assistance.

The ever changing data is also one of the challenges that healthcare sectors face. Like everyone else, patients and doctors relocate, alter identities and occupations, resign, and come to an end. Additionally, provider companies could relocate, open new branches, or go through a variety of acquisitions and acquisitions. Additionally, it is challenging to keep precise, comprehensive, and up-to-date health care data due to changes in service delivery, drug development, and individualized care strategies. Data lag and obsolete information have a serious influence on both the inclusion support and the sustainability of the suppliers' operations. As a result, new treatment approaches are adopted more reluctantly, healthcare programmes need to be filled with responses, and involvement and satisfaction are poor (Phillips, 2021).

Another major concern while delivering insights from patients' data is privacy and security. Building an effective health care ecosystem depends on maintaining patient trust. Since patient privacy depends on adherence and the secure adoption of electronic health records, data security has become of the utmost significance to the healthcare sector. Additionally, it might be difficult to maintain compliance with data sets and engagements owing to the constantly changing regulatory standards. Organizations are unable to comply with new regulatory standards due to poor data integrity and strategy, which also raises the cost of examinations and monitoring. It will be difficult to improve the general public's health until data security and compliance issues are fully addressed.

The Solution

The use of emerging technologies and intelligence systems can be considered as one the solutions to all the major problems that are faced by the healthcare providers. Technologies like data mining, machine learning and artificial intelligence have paved the way in solving various problems. A part of artificial intelligence that is swarm intelligence is an optimized solution for all the challenges and provides better results (Datta et al., 2019).

Optimized solutions through the much available data can be achieved by effectively studying the patterns in the data and applying intelligence into it. A developing technology called swarm intelligence (SI) was created as a result of social behavior found in biological systems like ants, bees, birds, fish, and monkeys. Swarm intelligence will nevertheless combine the intelligent thinking of creatures into algorithms for better data driven decision making. Swarming actions of groups of organisms are the source of swarm intelligence. Organisms that live in groups can work through issues that are challenging or impossible for individuals to overcome alone. In order to establish a global emerging pattern, swarm intelligence promises to be able to control intricate networks of interdependent individuals with little communication with anybody outside of their immediate neighborhood.

Basics of Swarm Intelligence

Due to the efficiency with which social insects can solve complicated issues, such as determining the quickest route between their nest and a food source or organizing their nests, biologists and natural scientists have been investigating social insect behavior. This collective intelligence is thus termed as swarm intelligence. Swarm intelligence (SI), which was first observed in nature, is now also possible in artificial systems. Swarm intelligence is indeed a subset of the exploratory calculations that are employed in a wide range of commercial, engineering, and industrial fields because of its flexibility, efficiency, and ability to attain the absolute optimal.

There is no centralized control mechanism to anticipate the activity of individual agents also where individuals follow straightforward principles. An "intelligent" behavior that is therefore unknown to individual agents is produced by a certain degree of stochastic recurrence between the agents. There are several algorithms designed inspired from nature. These techniques are ant colony optimiser, particle swarm optimiser, artificial bee colony algorithm, glow worm algorithm, firefly algorithm, cuckoo search algorithm, bat algorithm, hunting search algorithm and many more.

Swarm intelligence is an emerging technological term that has a boost for research in the next coming years and is therefore divided into basic 3 categories that include biological, engineering and artificial intelligence. Ever since the emergence of the term swarm intelligence the researchers have been involved in studying how the study of the grouping of animal patterns can help solving many algorithmic problems and biological research.

The biological investigation of self-organized behaviors in social insects is the basis of swarm intelligence. The collective actions of these creatures have influenced many of the fundamental studies in this young field of research, from the routing of traffic in telecommunication networks to the design of control algorithms for groups of autonomous robots. The foundations of sophisticated collective actions of social insects are described in biological research, which starts with a few reminders about the fragmented character of such systems and moves on to the idea that self-organization occurs in biological systems and the concept of stigmergy (Zhu & Tang, 2010).

Kazadi designated swarm engineering to be a recognised topic of study in 2000. Swarm engineering, according to him, is a "two-step" process. The creation of a swarm condition is the first phase, followed by the creation of behaviors that can fulfill the swarm condition.

Swarm engineering's objective is to create a general condition or combination of circumstances that may be utilized to generate a variety of swarm designs, any of which can accomplish the overall objective.

Swarm Principles

1. Proximity: The fundamental elements of a swarm should be able to respond to environmental variation brought on by interactions between agents. However, several essential behaviors, like the search for live resources and nest-building, are common.

2. Quality: A swarm should be capable of adapting to quality elements like identifying a location's safety.
3. Diverse response: Resources shouldn't be gathered in a small area. The arrangement should indeed be constructed in such a way that each component will be as shielded from environmental changes as possible.
4. Stability: Every time the environment changes, the population shouldn't adjust its behavior.
5. Adaptability: The swarm is sensitive to environmental changes, which enable it to behave differently (Garnier, 2007).

Swarm Capabilities and Benefits

The capabilities of swarm intelligence are categorized into four major parts according to which the further algorithms are generated. Based on different behavior patterns found within the swarms the output of each differs and is therefore used to develop algorithms that fit into the four categories that include clustering, optimization, load balancing (scheduling) and routing.

A cluster is a group of agents that both resemble and differ from the agents in other clusters like formation of clusters of corpses to clean up the ants' nests. Finding the Best Solution or Minimal Cost Solution from all the Viable Solutions is the definition of an optimization problem that can be well observed in ants who are known to find the shortest path from their colony to a food source. Routing is based on the idea that advancing ants use the information they learn along the way to get to their destination to help the backward ants, for example the AntHocNet routing algorithm for MANETs (mobile ad hoc networks). In load balancing and scheduling the emphasis is placed on the job's relative position rather than its immediate predecessor or immediate successor in the schedule, and the global pheromone evaluation rule is adhered to just like Ant Colony Load Balancing – AntZ.

The overall benefits of swarm intelligence include various factors that are responsible for the emergence of swarm intelligence in every field. Below are some of the benefits that swarm intelligence incorporates within it.

1) Flexible: The colony reacts to both internal and external perturbations.
2) Robust: Even if several agents fail, tasks are still finished.
3) Scalable: From a few to millions of agents
4) Decentralized: The colony lacks a centralized administration.
5) Self-organized: Rather than being predetermined, the answers emerge.
6) Adaptation: The swarm system is capable of adapting to both previously known stimuli and novel ones.
7) Speed: Network changes can spread very quickly.

8) Modularity: Agents interact with different network layers independently.
9) Parallelism: Agents operate in parallel by nature.

Basic Algorithms

Particle Swarm Optimization

The social foraging behavior of some animals, such as the flocking behavior of birds and the schooling behavior of fish, served as the inspiration for particle swarm optimization. The algorithm's objective is to have all the particles locate the optima in a multidimensional space. They are initially given random positions and speeds, and they are supposed to advance gradually toward the local optima by using exploration and exploitation of advantageous, well-known positions in space. Rules that PSO follows are distancing yourself from fellow flock members, each person lines up their own heading with that of their neighbors' on average, aim to go toward your neighbors' median position and the necessity for roosting or swarming per bird, which increases if a clearly defined roosting location is approachable.

Figure 1. Benefits of swarm intelligence

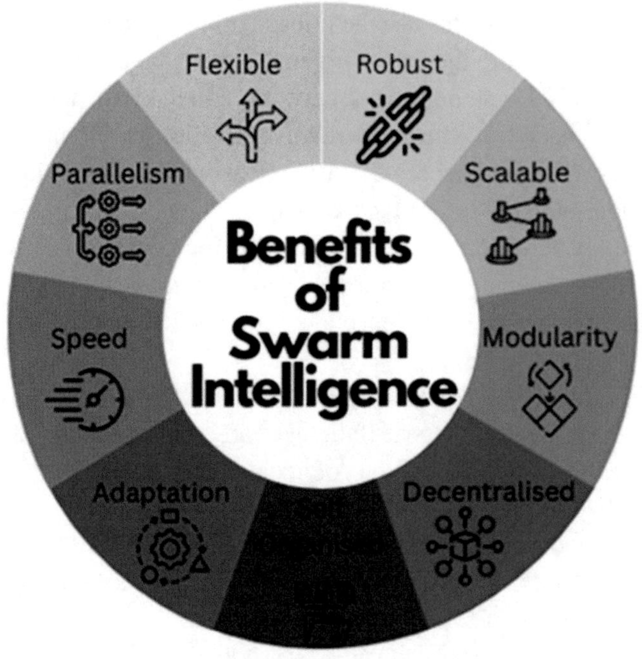

Ant Strategy

It is based on the phenomena known as stigmergy, which is the pheromone communication between a colony and a food source in an environment used by blind ants. In addition to pheromone intensity, another factor that affects the likelihood of an ant taking a certain path is its visibility, or how far it is from the target city. The strategy's goal is to use historical, pheromone-based, and heuristic data to build candidate solutions, each in a probabilistic step-by-step fashion, and incorporate the knowledge gained from doing so into the past. The likelihood of choosing a component is based on its heuristic contribution to the total cost of the solution, and the history and quality of the solution are updated proportionally to the quality of the best known solution.

Bees Algorithm

It takes its cues from honey bees' foraging habits. The colony sends out scout bees, who, after finding nectar (a sweet liquid secreted by flowers), return to the hive and, using a waggle dance, inform the other bees about the location, quality, distance, and direction of the food supply. The algorithm's goal is to find and investigate useful sites within a problematic search space. Numerous scout bees are dispatched, and each iteration is always looking for new, useful sites that can be used in local search applications (Kumar, Dixit, & Gayathri, 2020).

Scope of Swarm Intelligence

Systems made up of numerous individuals that cooperate by using decentralized control and self-organization are the focus of the field of swarm intelligence. It focuses particularly on the group behaviors that emerge from the local interactions of the individuals with one another and their surroundings. It is a rapidly expanding field that includes the work of academics from a variety of fields, including ethology, social science, operations research, and computer engineering. Due to its emphasis on group behavior, swarm intelligence can be applied across a wide range of industries.

Scope of SI in Healthcare Industry

Healthcare institutions have a wealth of data at their disposal. But there aren't enough sophisticated analytical techniques available to find hidden patterns and connections in data (Soni et al., 2011). Noisy data and issues with the sharing of medical data are a few of additional difficulties in health care data mining (Ahmad et al., 2015). A common method for making medical diagnoses is data mining. The possibility of missing values in medical data, which might reduce diagnostic accuracy, presents a significant difficulty in this sector (Nekouie & Moattar, 2018). Another difficulty is getting different healthcare institutions to share their data. Analysis of medical data is challenging due to its complexity. Data must consistently be accurate and of high quality if judgements are to be useful. Additionally, attributes in medical datasets may be duplicated or incorrect, which could slow down processing and reduce accuracy. Therefore, feature selection techniques are required to improve the efficiency and precision of classification models (Tomar & Agarwal, 2013). Swarm intelligence (SI) may show to be an effective strategy for this aim.

Healthcare datasets can include a wide variety of attributes and are often complex. High dimensional datasets are what these datasets are known as. There are several ways to gather healthcare data, such as pathology reports, surveys, and other methods that aid in disease diagnosis. However, it gets more challenging to interpret the data and make predictions as data size grows. The term "feature selection" refers to the first stage of classification, which aids in reducing the problem's dimensions, lowering noise levels, boosting processing speed, and removing redundant and irrelevant features (Aghdam et al., 2009). It is predicted that features made up of useful information and datasets must contain few features in order to construct coherent data mining models (Kaushik, 2016). Swarm intelligence (SI) can therefore be used to choose the most advantageous subset of traits. Additionally, the size of the data set between the training and testing sets as well as the features present in the dataset have a significant impact on the accuracy of data mining methods (Jothi & Husain, 2015). Therefore, it is a good idea to have the fewest possible features and to determine which features are essential for the dataset and can influence the result's correctness. Swarm based algorithms are developed based on the animal or insect behavioral traits. ACO (Ant colony optimization), PSO (Particle Swarm Optimization), firefly-based algorithm, fruit-fly, glowworm, Cuckoo search, Lion, Monkey, Bat, Wolf, etc. are some examples of Swarm Intelligence algorithms. Engineering, biology, research, and numerous industrial applications are just a few of the fields in which Swarm Intelligence (SI) techniques have recently been used.

Scope of SI in Social Media

Researchers from all over the world are becoming increasingly interested in real-time surveillance in the context of health informatics. Numerous public health informatics efforts have been introduced thanks to this field's evolution. For early detection of disease outbreaks and disease monitoring, surveillance systems in the field of health informatics have been developed using information from social media. Since a few years ago, real-time syndromic monitoring has been made possible by the availability of social media data, notably Twitter data. This allows people in charge of following up on and looking into potential outbreaks to receive fast analysis and feedback (Gupta & Katarya, 2020).

Through data obtained from a variety of sources before clinically validated data is available, syndromic monitoring has become a possible tool to forecast outbreaks for public health purposes. Reduced population dispersion and the implementation of preventative measures are the desired outcomes. Information from social media has been extensively used in recent years to calculate illness incidence and identify disease outbreaks. Public health experts could identify outbreaks earlier than using conventional approaches thanks to such data. The information is often presented as self-reported symptoms. According to studies, healthcare monitoring systems can be used to predict diseases that pose a threat to the public's health. Early warning and outbreak detection techniques have been applied to Twitter data in the prediction of diseases like syphilis (Young et al., 2018), swine flu (Kostkova et al., 2014), TB (Zhou & Ye, 2011), influenza (Chen et al., 2014), and Ebola (Yom-tov,). The Philippines recommended a different study that might look at typhoid and dengue fever occurrences in a region (Espina & Regina, 2017). In a similar vein, another study examined the use of social media data for illness detection via surveillance systems (Byrd et al., 2016).

The size of the issue can be estimated via surveillance systems. By predicting future disease levels, one may plan, allocate resources, provide treatments, and implement preventative measures. Assessments can be done in accordance with the analysis supplied by the surveillance systems to determine the severity of the disease over time.

Swarm Intelligence in Healthcare Industry

Today the healthcare sector is facing challenges such as detecting the cause of ailments, disease prevention, high operating costs, availability of skilled technicians and infrastructure bottlenecks. Intelligent healthcare management technologies are needed to manage these challenges. Healthcare organizations also need to continuously discover useful and actionable knowledge to gain insight from tons of data being generated for saving lives, reducing medical errors, enhancing efficiency, reducing costs and making the whole world a healthy place. Swarm Intelligence algorithms have been used for prognosis of major diseases like cancer, heart diseases, tumors, and cardiology (Smailhodzic et al., 2016). The Swarm Intelligence approaches have been applied in the areas of disease diagnosis and treatment.

One of the examples is SI based algorithms for Proteomic Pattern Detection of Ovarian Cancer (Meng, 2006). Multiple proteins can be resolved and analyzed simultaneously using modern protein profiling technology. To create distinctive proteome patterns that separate cancer from non-cancer, it will be necessary to evaluate a variety of proteins. To identify modifications in protein expressions and their connections to illness states, it is crucial to have sophisticated and intelligent analysis methods. To find the diagnostic proteomic patterns of biomarkers for early diagnosis of ovarian cancer, we employ a swarming-agent based intelligence system employing a blended or hybrid ant colony optimization/particle swarm optimization (ACO/PSO) algorithm.

A system that mimics the natural behavior of ants, including their systems for cooperation and adaptation, is known as an ACO algorithm. These concepts form the foundation of ACO algorithms. First, each route taken by an ant corresponds to a potential fix for a certain issue. Second, the caliber of the related decision variable for the target problem is proportional to the amount of pheromone deposit on the path that an ant chooses to follow. Third, the path(s) with a higher concentration of pheromones are more alluring to the ant when forced to choose among two or more options. The ants will finally congregate on a short path after a number of cycles, which is anticipated to be the ideal or almost ideal solution for the target problem

The population-based PSO algorithm develops a feasible solution (or group of feasible solutions) for a problem from a set of potential options. Determining the optimum solution of a real-valued function (fitness function) defined in a particular space is the goal of the optimization approach (search space). PSO can be viewed as a potent new search algorithm capable of optimizing a variety of N-dimensional problems rather than just as a social simulation. This algorithm's social metaphor can be summed up as follows: People who belong to a society have beliefs that are held by all potential people in a "belief space" (also known as the search space). This "opinion state" may be changed by people depending on three things: The first is environmental information (its fitness value), the second is a person's recall of their past experiences, and the third is their neighborhood's past experiences.

The "social network" of an individual can be configured in a variety of ways depending on how their neighborhood is defined. People in the population adjust their belief systems to those that are more effective inside their social network by adhering to particular standards of interaction. A culture forms through time in which people share closely linked viewpoints.

Each person is referred to as a "particle" in the PSO algorithm and is subject to moving in a multi - dimensional space that symbolizes the belief space. Due to the memory of particles, they can preserve some of their past states. Although there is no constraint on particles sharing the same position in belief space, their uniqueness is nevertheless protected. Individuality, the inclination to migrate back to one's best former stance, and sociality, the ability to move in the direction of one's neighborhood's best previous position, are the two randomly weighted effects that make up each particle's movement.

An agent is a free-standing processing unit that interacts with both the outside world and other agents in order to achieve a specific set of objectives. The ACO algorithm allows the individuals in the systems to coordinate their actions and exchange information through the shared dynamic environment of pheromone. These pheromone interactions can lead to the self-organizing and self-adapting system-level behaviors. Each agent's local sensors are limited to what they can see of the environment. In other terms, the agent can only detect the pheromone that is nearby and is unaware of the presence of other pheromones farther away. It's feasible that most agents could quickly lock into a local maximum in the absence of a central host. But on the other hand, PSO algorithm-using agents synchronize their actions through chance encounters with other agents. The agents in the population adapt their system of belief to those that are more effective inside their social network by adhering to a set of interactional rules. A global optimization can be attained throughout time. Consequently, a hybrid ACO/PSO algorithm is suggested in the paper for the swarming-agent based diagnosis system. This algorithm combines two collective and coordination processes, one based on the ACO algorithm, where the agents' local movements are guided by pheromones in the shared environment, and the other based on the PSO algorithm, where a global maximum of the attribute values can be obtained through random interaction between the agents.

Another illustration is the detection of brain cancers using image segmentation and particle swarm optimization (Mahalakshmi & Velmurugan, 2015). One of the most fundamental methods used in image processing is picture segmentation. The past few years have seen a significant increase in the use of image processing mechanisms in a variety of medical fields for the early stage detection, separation, and identity of diseases; in this context, the time consumption is a crucial factor to consider when determining the diseases for the patient. Here, we use Particle Swarm Optimization (PSO), a heuristic global optimization technique based on swarm intelligence, to identify and classify brain cancers using medical pictures obtained through Magnetic Resonance Imaging (MRI). Due to the algorithm's simplicity of usage, it has been developed quickly. The conversion, implementation, selection, and extraction phases of this work are divided into four steps.

In the past ten years, numerous techniques have been used to detect obstructions in the brain (tumor). The analysis of MRI brain data in this case is ideally suited for the PSO method. A brain tumor is an accumulation of aberrant cell development in the vicinity of the brain. There are numerous varieties of brain tumors. Early-stage benign brain tumors cannot spread to other parts of the body. However, the malignant cancer tumor expanded to other areas and body parts. Generally speaking, benign brain tumors do not spread cancer to other parts of the body, whereas malignant brain tumors do. This study examines the affected area of the brain tumor and the tumor itself.

PSO technique is used to handle a number of optimization issues in engineering due to its precision in optimization. PSO-based techniques are incredibly effective in picture segmentation applications right now. PSO is both an optimization algorithm based on swarm intelligence and a heuristic global optimization method. The social interaction and behavior of swarming particles served as the inspiration for the idea of PSO. The birds' natural tendency is to migrate in groups or to become dispersed when scavenging for food. The birds move from one location to another in search of food, and the birds closest to the food can smell it. The location of every one of the n swarm particles in PSO's fundamental algorithm represents a potential solution. In accordance with the three principles, the swarm particle adjusts its position. Keeping its momentum first, then updating the situation in light of its ideal position third, updating the situation in light of the swarm's ideal position.

Using a few picture segmentation techniques, the PSO algorithm is implemented. To acquire the affected brain tumor region, there are four steps. The primary goal is to remove the brain tumor on its own. This research determines if an MRI image is malignant or benign. There are four stages. The Digital Imaging and Communication in Medicine (DICOM) data file must first be converted into an image file format. The PSO method is implemented in a second stage using a variable's changed value as the default value. The best image is chosen from the segmentation results in the third step based on the amount of time that has passed. The algorithm for the fourth step, which separates the brain region impacted by the tumor, is as follows.

Based on swarm intelligence, the Particle Swarm Optimization (PSO) is a theoretical concept in engineering and scientific study. Without considering mutations or overlaps, the particle's speed is used to conduct the search. The best optimized particle can convey information to other particles at a very high speed and with great efficiency through to the new generations. The PSO accepts real number codes, uses a straightforward calculation, and shows the straightforward result with ease.

In conclusion, manually segmenting the brain is likely more accurate than totally automating it. However, the time commitment and subjectiveness of human segmentation are the main downsides of manual picture segmentation. To get over the limitations of manual segmentation, it is important to construct a trustworthy automated segmentation. There are numerous distinct ways as a result of the difficulties in automatically segmenting MRI brain pictures. Some of the criteria for automation are carried by the technique. The axial and coronal planes of the image have been identified; however, automation of the sagittal plane has not yet been completed in this study. It follows that the parameters of time elapsed and segmentation level are the foundation for the automating of MRI brain pictures to detect brain tumours. The coronal plane performs better than the axial plane when the PSO algorithm is used to segment the MRI brain image.

Figure 2. Scope of swarm intelligence in healthcare

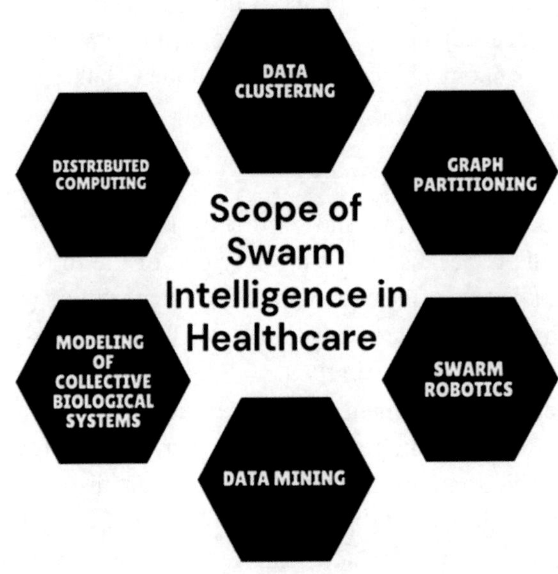
DATA CLUSTERING
DISTRIBUTED COMPUTING
GRAPH PARTITIONING
Scope of Swarm Intelligence in Healthcare
MODELING OF COLLECTIVE BIOLOGICAL SYSTEMS
SWARM ROBOTICS
DATA MINING

Overview of Swarm Intelligence in Healthcare Applications

For the prognosis of serious illnesses like cancer, heart disease, tumors, and cardiology, swarm intelligence techniques have been applied. Disease diagnosis and therapy have both benefited from the application of swarm intelligence techniques (Nayar, 2019). Health care is combined with various fields like social media, security, cloud, data mining and many more.

Breast Cancer

One of the worst illnesses that affect women is breast cancer, which necessitates early detection. Although the traditional diagnostic technique takes more time, using machine learning to detect illness can lead to a practical and simple approach. Technology advancements, however, produce a variety of high-dimensional data types, primarily cancer or medical information. It is more difficult for them to gain insight knowledge when the amount of data is staggering, and unrepresentative information might lead to skewed categorization results. Any of these problems can be resolved by using the attribute selection process to improve classification performance. This article suggests using Particle Swarm Optimization (PSO) to improve the effectiveness of the classification using the Decision Tree method on a dataset for Wisconsin Breast Cancer. The results show that the system performed with 92.26% accuracy when compared to current best practices. In conclusion, the system will aid health professionals in making decisions and will lessen the prevalence of breast cancer sickness by developing an early identification approach for diagnosis based on a machine learning technique (Chakraborty et al., 2022).

Heart Diseases

The biggest issue in identifying and predicting heart disease before it has any implications or kills is because it is currently one of the most prevalent diseases and many individuals are suffering from it. Since heart illness is spreading quickly throughout the cosmos, there are some strategies for predicting it. This method of prediction could even save lives. In the healthcare sector, especially in the area of cardiology, efficiency and time management are crucial factors in recognising cardiac disease. Using machine learning approaches, dynamic and precise algorithms for cardiac disease prediction have been developed. Heart disease can be recognised and predicted by two phases: 1) Selection of features 2) stage of categorisation. One way for choosing attributes and feature subsets is feature selection since it filters out irrelevant information and applies classification algorithms to a dataset that includes patient characteristics such age, gender, pulse rate, glucose levels, and blood sugar, among others. We can calculate the likelihood of developing heart disease by analyzing these characteristics. For the purpose of running supervised classification algorithms, optimization approaches like Grey Wolf Optimization, Particle Swarm Optimization, and Ant Colony Optimization are used. The hybrid proposed algorithm is implemented, the results are estimated, and the effectiveness and robustness are determined to determine the best solutions and good pathways (Shaik & Verma, 2022).

Drug Development

A swarm is a large group of uniform, straightforward agents cooperating locally with one another and their environment without any central supervision, allowing a fascinating pattern of behavior to emerge on a larger scale. Swarm-based algorithms are population-based algorithms with natural inspiration that are adept at coming up with the best answers to a variety of difficult combinatorial problems. The creation of products and other processes in the pharmaceutical sector can include a large number of independent variables and different limitations. It is particularly difficult to tackle challenges relating to the pharmaceutical sector using conventional methods since they call for precise solutions. A group of knowledge-based algorithms that can solve complicated issues and produce accurate or optimal solutions make up the swarm intelligence technique (Kittusamy, n.d.).

Real-time surveillance in the field of health informatics has emerged as a growing domain of interest among worldwide researchers. Evolution in this field has helped in the introduction of various initiatives related to public health informatics. Surveillance systems in the area of health informatics utilizing social media information have been developed for early prediction of disease outbreaks and to monitor diseases. In the past few years, the availability of social media data, particularly Twitter data, enabled real-time syndromic surveillance that provides immediate analysis and instant feedback to those who are charged with follow-ups and investigation of potential outbreaks (Gupta, 2020).

In the present scenario, the healthcare system procreates a huge amount of heterogeneous data. So, the AI healthcare system is an interactive or intelligent system that manages that data in a meaningful way. It gives various techniques to optimize the data. Basically, SI is a rising technique of AI that is based on the behavioral model of social insects. SI is a problem-resolving technique that comes from the information processing category. SI theory depends on multiplicity, dispensation, haphazardness, and untidiness. This technique solves problems, which relies on learning, creativity, and perception ability (Kumar, Dixit, & Gayathri, 2020).

The Healthcare industry has been quickly developing worldwide. A necessary quantity of mixed data has been produced through the healthcare industry. It has been critical for the healthcare industry to accomplish build-up and the data of mine in a productive way. Therefore, data mining could give huge latitude for the treatment of essential, diagnosis, and prediction. Data removal has played a crucial position in the medical field which has been an easier system towards examining the enormous data, so the outstanding practice has been functioning for the supplemental investigation as well as examining the patient's report. Swarm intelligent technology has been typically consisting of a population, which has simply interacted only with their environment. Data mining is concerned with the analysis of large-scale data (Narmatha, 2021).

Previous studies on social media use in healthcare identified different effects of social media use by patients for health related reasons within the healthcare system. Social media can serve as an aid to patients. For example, it fosters their autonomy by complementing the information provided by healthcare professionals (Rupert et al., 2014) and by providing psychosocial support (Ho et al., 2014). Social media use by patients can also be an aid to healthcare professionals by providing a tool to strengthen the organization's market position (McCaughey et al., 2014; Williams, 2011) and stimulating conversation for brand building and improved service delivery (Li & Bernoff, 2008; Williams, 2011). In fact, social media may have effects on both patients, and on the wider healthcare system (Hawn, 2009). In particular, it allows patients to receive support, and to complement offline information (Ho et al., 2014), which may lead to enhancing the empowerment of patients (Hawn, 2009). However, social media use by patients does not only provide beneficial effects. It may also constitute a challenge within the healthcare system to both patients and healthcare professionals. Since everybody with access to social media can post "advice" on how to deal with a certain health condition, it is important to create reliable online communication channels to prevent health problems from being exacerbated (Carter, 2014). For example, one misguided idea on Twitter urged Nigerians to drink excessive amounts of salt water to combat Ebola. However, this may have led to two deaths and more than 12 admissions to hospital (Carter, 2014). Thus, many healthcare professionals fear that social media use by patients for health-related purposes often spreads misinformation among patients (Rupert et al., 2014).

CONCLUSION

Several swarm-based algorithms (Kazadi, 2000) have been inspired by bees, ants, birds, bats, and other creatures, but the literature has yet to explain their distinctions and complicated behavior—a condition that may impede us from understanding and enhancing such algorithms. In the area, we frequently define the differences between approaches or versions by the performance obtained when tackling different issues. This black-box approach has allowed the sector to produce outstanding

Figure 3. Applications of swarm intelligence

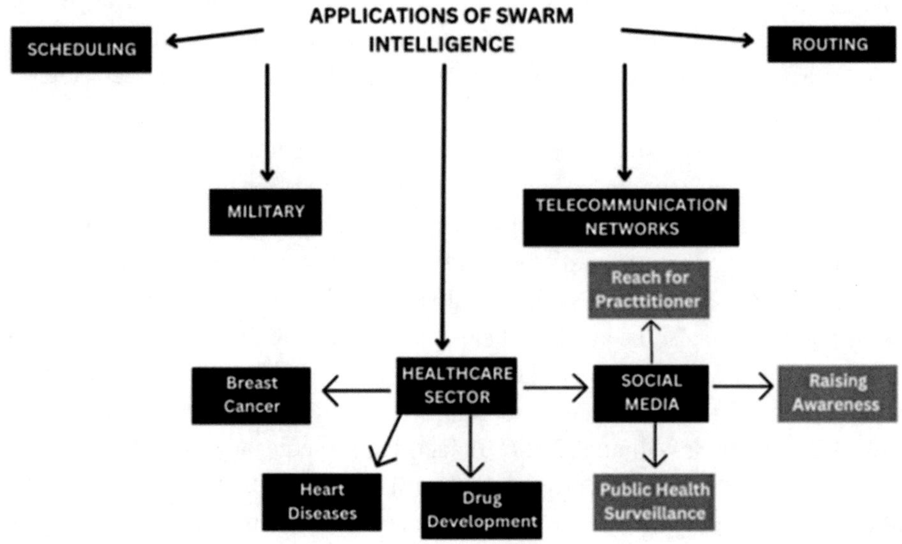

general-purpose tools throughout the years. This technique, on the other hand, lacks interpretability and explainability. The biggest challenge to comprehending swarm complex behavior is the gap between individual micro-level activities and swarm macro-level activity. In our study, we claim that the swarm interaction network operates at a meso level, which might aid in explaining and comprehending these systems. With this method (Kazadi, 2005), we may investigate a system through an intermediate structure that arises through social interaction inside the swarm. The patterns of these self-organized interactions may now be examined. The interaction network also provides an agnostic representation of swarm systems in the swarm interaction space, giving us a broader view of swarm-based algorithms.

REFERENCES

Afolayan, J. O., Adebiyi, M. O., Arowolo, M. O., Chakraborty, C., & Adebiyi, A. A. (2022). Breast Cancer Detection Using Particle Swarm Optimization and Decision Tree Machine Learning Technique. In C. Chakraborty & M. R. Khosravi (Eds.), *Intelligent Healthcare*. Springer. doi:10.1007/978-981-16-8150-9_4

Aghdam, M. H., Tanha, J., Naghsh-Nilchi, A. R., & Basiri, M. E. (2009). Combination of ant colony optimization and Bayesian classification for feature selection in a bioinformatics dataset. *Journal of Computer Science and Systems Biology*, *2*(3), 186–199. doi:10.4172/jcsb.1000031

Ahmad, P., Qamar, S., & Rizvi, S. Q. A. (2015). Techniques of data mining in healthcare: A review. *International Journal of Computer Applications*, *120*(15), 38–50. doi:10.5120/21307-4126

Byrd, K., Mansurov, A., & Baysal, O. (2016). O. Baysal Mining Twitter data for influenza detection and surveillance. *Proc. Int. Work. Softw. Eng. Healthc. Syst. - SEHS*, *16*, 43–49. doi:10.1145/2897683.2897693

Carter, M. (2014). Medicine and the media: How Twitter may have helped Nigeria contain Ebola. *BMJ (Clinical Research Ed.)*, 349.

Chen, Hossain, Butler, Ramakrishnan, & Prakash. (2014). *Flu Gone Viral: Syndromic Surveillance of Flu on Twitter using Temporal Topic Models.* . doi:10.1109/ICDM.2014.137

Datta, Barua, & Das. (2019). Application of artificial intelligence in modern healthcare system. *Alginates-Recent Uses of This Natural Polymer.*

Espina, K., & Regina, M. (2017). J.E. Estuar Infodemiology for Syndromic Surveillance of Dengue and Typhoid Fever in the Philippines Proc. *Procedia Computer Science*, *121*, 554–561. doi:10.1016/j.procs.2017.11.073

Garnier, S. (2007). *The Biological Principles of Swarm Intelligence - Swarm Intelligence*. SpringerLink. link.springer.com/article/10.1007/s11721-007-0004-y

Gupta. (2020, August). Social media based surveillance systems for healthcare using machine learning: A systematic review. *Journal of Biomedical Informatics, 108.*

Gupta, A., & Katarya, R. (2020, August). Social media based surveillance systems for healthcare using machine learning: A systematic review. *Journal of Biomedical Informatics*, *108*, 103500. doi:10.1016/j.jbi.2020.103500 PMID:32622833

Hawn, C. (2009). Take two aspirin and tweet me in the morning: How Twitter, Facebook, and other social media are reshaping health care. *Health Affairs (Project Hope)*, *28*(2), 361–368. doi:10.1377/hlthaff.28.2.361 PMID:19275991

Ho, Y. X., O'Connor, B. H., & Mulvaney, S. A. (2014). Features of online health communities for adolescents with type 1 diabetes. *Western Journal of Nursing Research*, *36*(9), 1183–1198. doi:10.1177/0193945913520414 PMID:24473058

Jothi, N., & Husain, W. (2015). Data mining in healthcare–a review. *Procedia Computer Science*, *72*, 306–313. doi:10.1016/j.procs.2015.12.145

Kaushik, S. (2016). *Introduction to feature selection methods with an example (or how to lead).* https://www.analyticsvidhya.com/blog/2016/12/introduction-tofeature-selection-methods-with-an-example-or-how-to-select-the-rightvariables

Kazadi, S. (2000). *Swarm Engineering* [Ph.D Thesis]. California Institute of Technology.

Kazadi, S. (2005). On the Development of a Swarm Engineering Methodology. *Systems, Man and Cybernetics, 2005 IEEE International Conference on, 2*, 1423-1428. 10.1109/ICSMC.2005.1571346

Kittusamy. (n.d.). Applications of Swarm Based Intelligence Algorithm in Pharmaceutical Industry: A Review. *International Research Journal of Pharmacy, 8*(11), 24-27.

Kostkova, P., Szomszor, M., & St Luis, C. (2014). #Swineflu: The Use of Twitter as an EarlyWarning and Risk Communication ACM Trans. *Manag. Inf. Syst.*, *5*, 1–25. doi:10.1145/2597892

Kumar, Dixit, & Gayathri. (2020). Healthcare data analytics using swarm intelligence. Swarm *Intelligence Optimization: Algorithms and Applications*, 101-121.

Li, C., & Bernoff, J. (2008). *Groundswell: Winning in a world transformed by social technologies*. Harvard Business School Press.

Mahalakshmi, & Velmurugan. (2015, September). Detection of Brain Tumor by Particle Swarm Optimization using Image Segmentation. *Indian Journal of Science and Technology*, *8*(22), IPL0246.

McCaughey, D., Baumgardner, C., Gaudes, A., LaRochelle, D., Jiaxin, K., Wu, K. J., & Raichura, T. (2014). Best practices in social media: Utilizing a value matrix to assess social media's impact on health care. *Social Science Computer Review*, *32*(5), 575–589. doi:10.1177/0894439314525332

Meng, Y. (2006). A Swarm Intelligence Based Algorithm for Proteomic Pattern Detection of Ovarian Cancer. *IEEE Symposium on Computational Intelligence and Bioinformatics and Computational Biology*. 10.1109/CIBCB.2006.331010

Narmatha. (2021). Data Mining and Swarm Intelligence in Healthcare Applications. *Journal of Computational and Theoretical Nanoscience, 18*(3), 1100-1106.

Nayar. (2019). Swarm intelligence and data mining: a review of literature and applications in healthcare. *Proceedings of the Third International Conference on Advanced Informatics for Computing Research*. 10.1145/3339311.3339323

Nayarw. (n.d.). *Swarm Intelligence and Data Mining: A Review of Literature and Applications in Healthcare*. Academic Press.

Nekouie, A., & Moattar, M. H. (2018). Missing value imputation for breast cancer diagnosis data using tensor factorization improved by enhanced reduced adaptive particle swarm optimization. *Journal of King Saud University Computer and Information Sciences*.

Phillips, A. (2021). *A History and Timeline of Big Data*. www.techtarget.com/whatis/feature/A-history-and-timeline-of-big-data

Rupert, D. J., Moultrie, R. R., Read, J. G., Amoozegar, J. B., Bornkessel, A. S., Donoghue, A. C., & Sullivan, H. W. (2014). Perceived healthcare provider reactions to patient and caregiver use of online health communities. *Patient Education and Counseling*, *96*(3), 320–326. doi:10.1016/j.pec.2014.05.015 PMID:24923652

Shaik, M. A., & Verma, D. (2022). Prediction of heart disease using swarm intelligence-based machine learning algorithms. *AIP Conference Proceedings*, *2418*(1), 020025. Advance online publication. doi:10.1063/5.0081719

Smailhodzic, E., Hooijsma, W., Boonstra, A., & Langley, D. J. (2016). Social media use in healthcare: A systematic review of effects on patients and on their relationship with healthcare professionals. *BMC Health Services Research*, *16*(1), 442. doi:10.118612913-016-1691-0 PMID:27562728

Soni, J., Ansari, U., Sharma, D., & Soni, S. (2011). Predictive data mining for medical diagnosis: An overview of heart disease prediction. *International Journal of Computer Applications*, *17*(8), 43–48. doi:10.5120/2237-2860

Tomar, D., & Agarwal, S. (2013). A survey on Data Mining approaches for Healthcare. *International Journal of Bio-Science and Bio-Technology*, *5*(5), 241–266. doi:10.14257/ijbsbt.2013.5.5.25

Williams, J. (2011). A new roadmap for healthcare business success. *J Healthc Financ Manage Assoc.*, *65*(5), 62–69. PMID:21634269

Yom-tov, E. (n.d.). *Ebola data from the Internet: An Opportunity for Syndromic Surveillance or a News Event?* Categories and Subject Descriptors. doi:10.1145/2750511.2750512

Young, S. D., Mercer, N., Weiss, R. E., Torrone, E. A., & Aral, S. O. (2018). Using social media as a tool to predict syphilis Prev. *Preventive Medicine*, *109*, 58–61. doi:10.1016/j.ypmed.2017.12.016 PMID:29278678

Zhou, X., & Ye, J. (2011). Y. Feng Tuberculosis surveillance by analyzing google trends. *IEEE Transactions on Biomedical Engineering*, *58*(8), 2247–2254. doi:10.1109/TBME.2011.2132132 PMID:21435969

Zhu & Tang. (2010). Overview of swarm intelligence. In *2010 International Conference on Computer Application and System Modeling (ICCASM 2010)* (vol. 9). IEEE.

Chapter 7
The AI-Based COVID-19 Personal Protective Equipment Is Smarty and Secure

Mohd Asif Shah
https://orcid.org/0000-0002-6166-8587
Chandigarh University, India

Ramesh Sekaran
Jain University (Deemed), India

ABSTRACT

Detecting SARs-COV'19 at early stages is essential for both providing suitable medical facility to the patients and also to safeguard the unaffected people. The dangerous part of COVID-19 infection occurs in patients with lower levels of immunity, say older people, patients with cardiovascular diseases, diabetes, chronic respiratory diseases, or cancer, in which case a serious illness develops and at last leads to the death of the patient. The chatper aims at monitoring the SpO_2*, heartbeat, and temperature of the COVID-19-infected patients in critical care units and takes immediate action by supplying oxygen or medicated aerosol to the needy patients. A supervised machine learning technique is used for effective prediction of the patient's condition based on the monitored parameters. Experimental results show that this model can predict the abnormal condition of the patient with an efficiency of 94% and revert back to normal conditions with an efficiency of 95%.*

1. INTRODUCTION

The SARs-CoV-2 a new strain of corona virus that shook the world belongs to the group of viruses that are responsible for mild to serious respiratory illness in human.

DOI: 10.4018/978-1-6684-6894-4.ch007

This SARs-CoV-2 virus was first identified in China's Wuhan city in the middle of December 2019. Since then, every country in the world reported positive COVID cases. Globally, as of June 2022, there are around 532,887,351 confirmed cases of COVID-19, which includes 6,307,021 deaths, reported to WHO. As of now, a total of 11,854,673,610 vaccines have already been administered. Though the fatality rate is very low compared to the Severe Acute Respiratory Syndrome (SARS) and Middle East Respiratory Syndrome (MERS), COVID-19 is very contagious and has spread to every part of the globe. The first weapon taken by the world to take hold of the situation is early detection of the infection and isolating the infected to nullify further spread. Considering the pandemic of COVID-19, it is important to detect COVID-19 early, which could facilitate the slowdown of viral transmission and thus disease containment. With COVID-19 the common symptoms include fever, dry cough, and tiredness accompanied by loss of taste or smell, sore throat, heart disease and respiratory problems. In spite of all the medical advancements in the twentieth century, COVID'19 has traumatized the whole world like never before so that it can be called a disaster. The debate is still on as to how to name this pandemic and some common descriptions include "Sanitary Crisis", "Health Emergency", "Natural Disaster", etc.

On the other hand, Science and Technological development leading the path towards Artificial Intelligence obviously playing a major role in every field in this 21st century. Though there are so many critics that it increases un-employment, when seen on the positive side, AI can be used effectively in scenarios that are harmful and dangerous for human interventions. A scenario aiding this argument is the COVID pandemic in which case complete isolation of the infected individual is highly recommended to avoid transmission of the virus. In such case where an individual is isolated, it is his right to get all medical aid for his well-being and that no one can stop. In spite of that, medical practitioners are highly vulnerable to the disease as they are always attending infected people. There are situations that we heard in televisions that Physicians attending COVID isolation ward are also quarantined to aid in containment of the disease. So, when it comes to a highly contagious disease like SARs-COV-19, there are two areas to be concentrated on, to handle the situation. They are i) Predicting the disease spread and contact tracing and ii) Effective healthcare monitoring and mitigation. Artificial Intelligence can be used for both the cases effectively and thus AI played a key role in handling the pandemic. This paper, proposes the most economical AI based patient monitoring system which can effectively monitor and mitigate the emergencies that arise with a COVID patient. With this small introduction let us have a look at the organization of the paper,

Section 1 is an Introduction to the current COVID scenario and the technologies that aid us in effective handling of the same. Section 2 briefs the different application of Artificial Intelligence in handling the COVID pandemic with limelight on i) Predicting, ii) Surveillance and iii) Minimizing human interventions to safeguard healthcare providers. It also elaborates the existing patient monitoring systems available for domestic personal care as well as a smart healthcare in a hospital setup throwing light on Internet of things and machine learning.

Section 3 explains the different blocks in the proposed system hardware along with their working.

Section 4 introduces the types of Machine Learning algorithms and their significances and depicts the ML algorithms used for the training and inference of a patient condition based on supervised learning algorithm whereas Section 5 discusses the effectiveness of the AI system in mitigating the risks based on the results obtained. The conclusion and future expansion of the work is discussed in Section 6 with the References cites being listed at the end.

2. HEALTHCARE INDUSTRY

Adding to the point that "Everyone Included" is portrayed in Woolhandler and Himmelstein (2020), where the "Annals of Internal Medicine" states that COVID pandemic has induced a surge of Joblessness and that in turn created loss of health insurance too. The article by Daniel Shu Wei Ting et al. (2000), elaborates on the benefits of using digital technologies such as IoT, Big data, AI and Blockchain for the effective deployment of healthcare and monitoring services to the general public during a health crisis like the COVID19. According to Daniel Shu Wei Ting et al, there are two major areas in healthcare services that benefit from this digital technology and they are 1) Surveillance of the infected crowd, early detection of infection and its prevention, Monitoring the patients and 2) Taking necessary action to lessen the Impact of the disease. In an article to "The Lancet", Joseph A Lewnard (2010) mentioned that Mathemetical modeling can be used in an effective way to determine the transmission of a novel infection like COVID'19. In addition, the authors quoted an example where mathematical modeling is effectively used by Koo and his colleagues in determining the consequences of social distancing intervention on the spread of COVID 19 in Singapore.

Penang Institute (2020) states that Artificial Intelligence can be effectively utilized in different ways during a pandemic situation like corona outbreak. In this article to Penang Institute Issues the author highlights the significance of AI based predictive analysis done by tools such as "BlueDot", "HealthMap" and "Metabiota" in predicting the outbreak of the COVID pandemic at the earliest. In addition to the predictive analysis, AI can be utilized in supporting the early detection and medication of disease and also to support in online education. Also Rafael (2020) depicts the importance of surveillance by digital contact tracing of patients with the help of AI during COVID'19 pandemic. A comprehensive survey of the different technologies that aid in the effective implementation of a medical rehabilitation system based on IoT is detailed in Yin et al. (2016). Such a rehabilitation system aids in sharing the available resources and thus enables flexible and convenient treatment to patients. Such a setup will maximize the utilization of the medical resources. Also, a limelight is shown on the future trends and directions of IoT field in healthcare division. Potential applications of IoT in healthcare system is detailed in Laplante and Laplante (2016) and Yin et al. (2016) and the three main challenges to effective implementation of IoT in healthcare is given in Laplante and Laplante (2016).

An IoT based remote elderly people monitoring platform, and (b) a smart ambulance system was discussed in Kotronis et al. (2017). Chang et al. (2016) explains an interactive system that provides real-time, two-way communication between diabetes patients and caregivers by utilizing Internet of Things. A GUI based Exercise or Workout recommendation system using IoT that can be used in gymnasiums, sports clubs to improve sportsman/women performance is detailed in Castillejo et al. (2013). In Chawathe (2018), location of person and devices in a locality are determined using a machine learning approach that classifies device locations based on strength of the Bluetooth signals. This idea of comparison can be used in other applications also. Having studied the importance of COVID care, IoT in Healthcare, and Machine learning in affective prediction in this paper we propose a Machine Learning and IoT based CoVID Care system that is capable of making decision based on acquired knowledge from training so as to supply Oxygen or Medicated aerosol or Continue Monitoring patient condition based on SpO2 and heart rate of patients.

3. EXISTING SYSTEM

Remote patient monitoring is an ideal application where Internet of Things can be utilized to the fullest. IoT systems have been efficiently applied to aid people with Parkinson's and Alzheimer's disease. In addition, such IoT systems can provide an early remote diagnosis to patients prior to hospitals as an effort towards providing initial preliminary treatment. Various health parameters of the patient, including temperature, respiratory rate and cough rate and blood oxygen saturation are monitored by an active IoT node and it then updates the smart phone application to display the health conditions. Raspberry Pi Zero (RPIZ) is used to develop the hardware nodes. Audio signal processing is another area - helpful for the diagnosis of many respiratory diseases.

Figure 1. IoT-based patient monitoring system

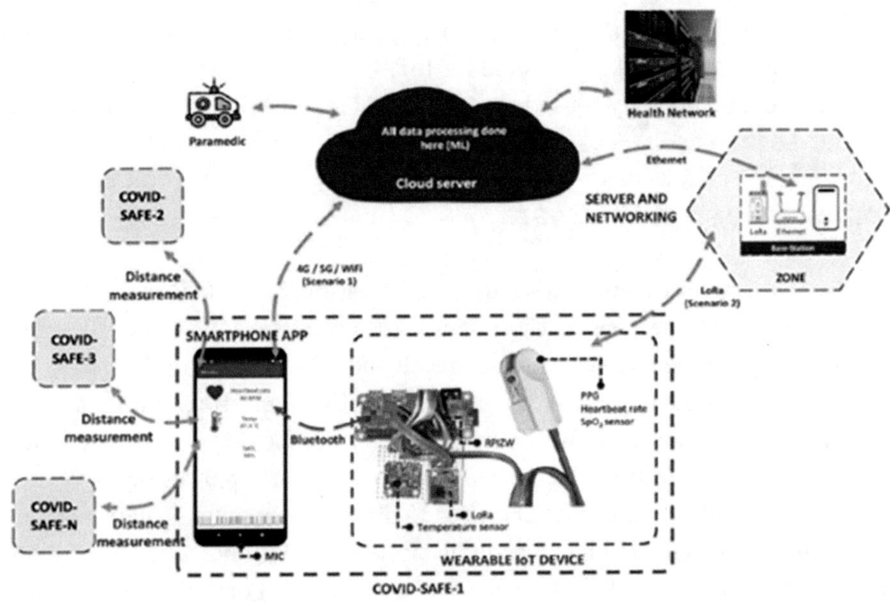

A software core consisting of two parts namely an Application Program Interface and a Fuzzy decision-making system is used for interacting with the users on a smart phone and the fog server respectively. There are three major constituents of the system which includes

i) wearable IoT device,
ii) smart phone app, and
iii) fog (or cloud) server.

The various health parameters of the patient are monitored by an IoT node and upgrades their decision-making rules such as i) doctor intervention needed, ii) maintain physical distance and iii) alerting high risk areas.

The distances between people are tracked using Bluetooth technology and individuals are warned in order to maintain a social distance between them. In such case, it is important to consider security and data management thoroughly to prevent misuse of personal information.

i) Bluetooth is available with every electronic device say from smart phones to smart watches. The primary issue with Bluetooth is the reflection of its signals, due to which it is difficult to acquire the exact distance prediction (Exposure Notifications, n.d.).

ii) The usage of GPS can be reduced by using orientation sensor and accelerometer for a low-power tracking method for IoT.

iii) Bluetooth technology is used by Apple and Google for contact tracing of iOS and Android users.

Proposed System Hardware

In the proposed system, there are various kinds of sensors like SpO2 Sensor, Heartbeat sensor and Temperature Sensor. These sensors can measure and identify the various body conditions of the patients who are unwell and it helps monitor them during the course of treatment and improve their health. ARDUINO is used to control and monitor the sensors. If a patient faces Respiratory problems or Low Oxygen content in the blood, they are preferred to use Nebulizer pump for Oxygen Supply using Driver Relay Circuit automatically and then LCD is used to display the required parameters in the entire system. The primary objective of this project is fully automatic observation of corona infected patients and handling the emergency need of oxygen in an economical way. 24X7 monitoring of a patient is guaranteed with mitigation measures.

Block Diagram

Figure 2. Proposed COVID-19 patient monitoring system

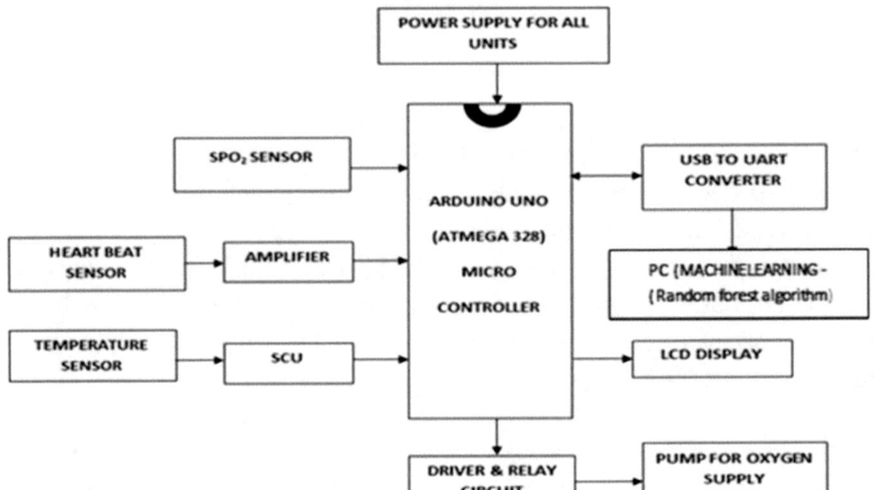

4. MACHINE LEARNING AND ALGORITHMS USED

Artificial Intelligence is imparted to a machine by training the machine with labelled (Supervised learning) or unlabelled (Unsupervised Learning) datasets. Learning algorithms are used in this training phase and once the machine learns then the machine will be able to predict the outputs for new datasets based on the knowledge gained by training. And as the machine predicts the results for new data it keeps on updating its knowledge base by some weight update algorithm. A broad classification of the machine learning algorithms and their types is given in Figure 3.

Learning Algorithms

Random Forest: A supervised machine learning algorithm uses labeled input data for training the model and then uses the acquired knowledge to infer the outputs for test data. Random Forest algorithm belongs to a type of supervised machine learning algorithm that can be used for both classification and regression problems. A significant feature of Random Forest algorithm is that it works on both continuous and discrete data sets. Random forest algorithm divides the entire dataset into a large number of individual decision trees and each tree learns individually using different classifier and then they are treated as a whole to solve a complex problem and improve the performance of the model. That is each decision tree works on a class prediction and the one with the most recommended optimal value becomes our model's prediction. Random forest model's efficiency is directly dependent on a large number of relatively uncorrelated or low correlated models operating together to give a result that will outperform individuals in the set. There are two main criteria for effective working of Random Forest algorithm, they are there should be some actual values in the feature variable of the dataset and also there should be low correlation between the trees considered for prediction.

Figure 3. Classification of machine learning algorithms

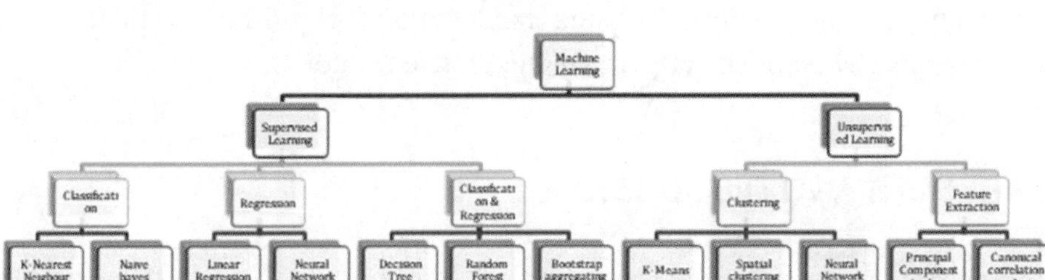

Breiman's Bagging and random selection of features are the two important ideas behind the Random Forest algorithm. A gradient boosting decision tree is one that uses XG Boost algorithm to update the gradient weights while inference and such a gradient boosting algorithm will be helpful in system optimization and enhancement. This algorithm uses the max depth feature/parameter and hence it prunes the tree in the backward direction. XGBOOST can be used in any of the three ways which may be Stochastic Gradient Boosting, Penalized Gradient Boosting, or Regularized Gradient Boosting

Algorithm used:

1. Import the required Python Libraries
2. Read the test dataset to a .csv file
3. Split the input features based on Labels and the corresponding outputs.
4. Split the data set into Test and Train datasets.
5. Build the model using XGB Classifier imported from xgboost. sklearn
6. Predict the XGB model function and plot it
7. Print the accuracy of the model.
8. Classify using Random Forest Classifier imported from sklearn
9. Predict the RF model function and plot it
10. Print the accuracy of the model.

System Optimization can be done by three ways namely, Tree Pruning, Parallelization and Hardware optimization. Whereas Algorithmic Enhancements can be done by utilizing Sparcity, Regularization, Cross-Validation.

Hardware Model

The Hardware contains Arduino UNO, Temperature sensor, Heartbeat sensor and SpO2 sensor, Power supply regulator circuit provide the continuous power supply to the circuit. The heartbeat sensor and SpO2 sensor are used to sense the heart rate and level of oxygen in blood hemoglobin. The temperature sensor is used to sense the body temperature and then sensor values given to Arduino UNO (ATmega328P microcontroller) and predicted by using Random Forest algorithm and then oxygen pump triggers ON automatically based on predicted conditions.

5. RESULTS AND DISCUSSION

The proposed smart monitoring system used Random Forest and XGBOOST algorithm for classifying the training data and for predicting the test data based on acquired

Figure 4. Image of the hardware model of the proposed system

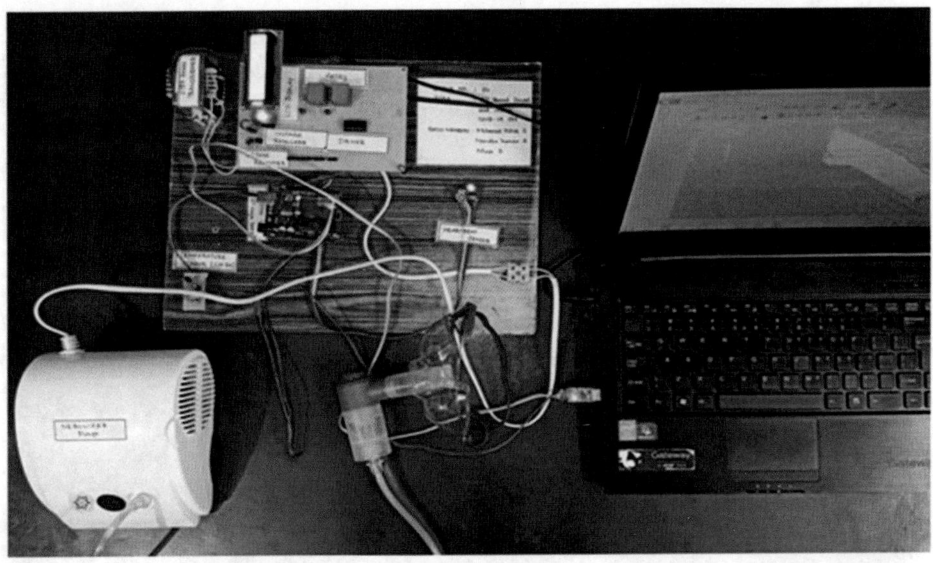

knowledge. It is found that the random forest classifier performs better compared to the XGBoost algorithm. The reason behind this the classification accuracy of the algorithm used is 99.3% and the prediction accuracy is 98.5% revealing a better model performance.

6. CONCLUSION

An exclusive study of the supervised and unsupervised machine learning techniques in the context of IoT based smart data analysis is done. The various algorithms were

Table 1. Sample dataset used for training phase in ML models

Normal Condition			Abnormal Condition		
Temperature Sensor (°C)	Heartbeat Sensor (BPM)	SPO_2 Sensor (%)	Temperature Sensor (°C)	Heartbeat Sensor (BPM)	SPO_2 Sensor (%)
33	39	94	42	112	103
34	49	95	46	116	107
36	69	97	50	120	111
38	89	99	54	124	115
40	109	101	58	128	119

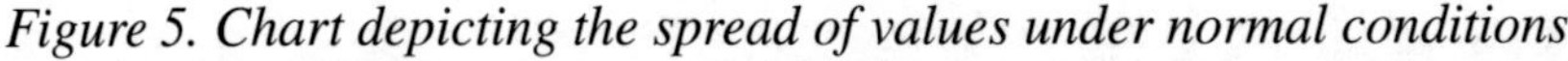

Figure 5. Chart depicting the spread of values under normal conditions

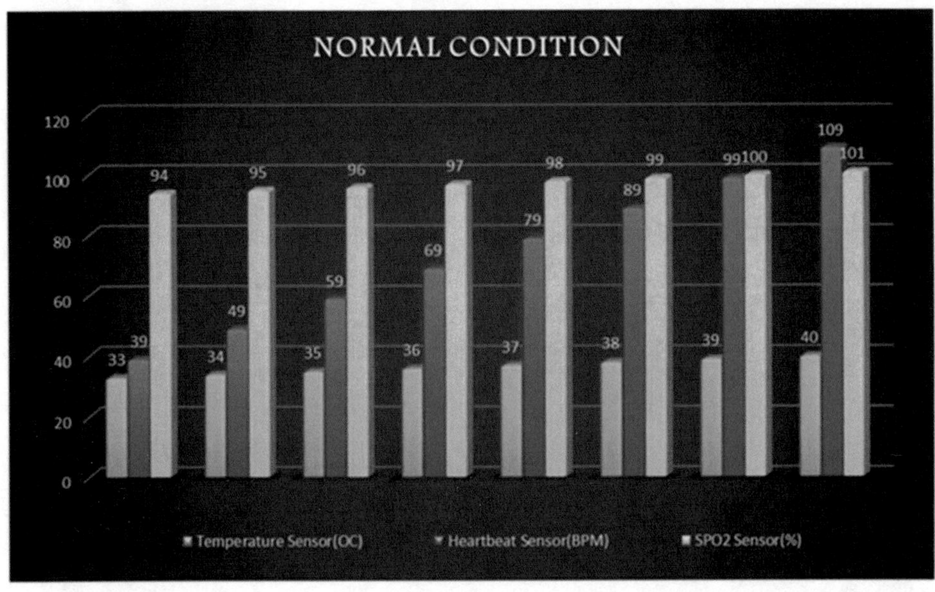

Figure 6. Chart depicting the spread of values under abnormal conditions

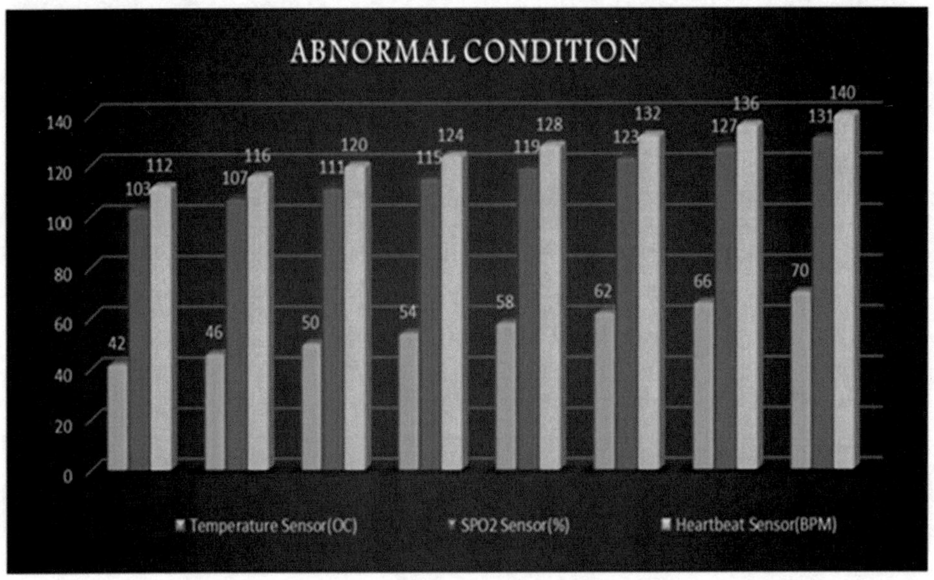

used in each of these techniques. These techniques are investigated based on their respective sub-domains, as well as advantages and limitations to achieving a precise,

Table 2. The range of various conditions

Sensors	Normal Condition	Abnormal Condition
Temperature Sensor (OC)	33 – 40	41 – 70
Heartbeat Sensor (BPM)	60 – 109	110 – 140
SpO_2Sensor (%)	96 – 100.9	101 – 131

Figure 7. Chart depicting the spread of test data

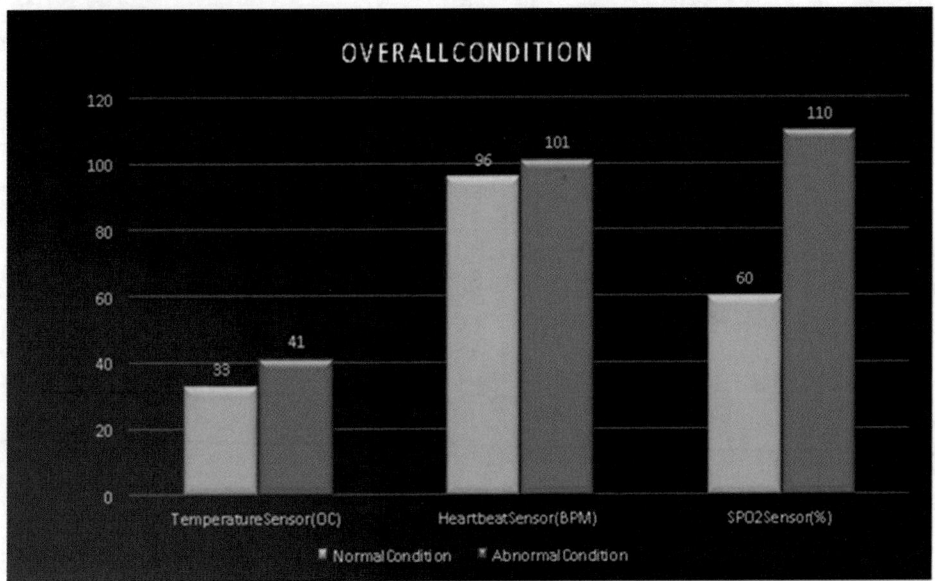

concrete, and concise conclusion. An AI powered IoT device has been utilized in many forms during the pandemic. To list a few includes 1) surveillance and image recognition for safety and security of the unaffected population, 2) Drug and food delivery using drones, 3) public alert systems based on contact tracing. The proposed device is cost effective at the same time performs better than the existing system in terms of efficiency in predicting a condition and responding quickly to need. This system can be expanded to monitor any physical condition of the patient and take emergency action in addition to alerting the hospital staff.

REFERENCES

Castillejo, Martinez, Rodriguez-Molina, & Cuerva. (2013). Integration of wearable devices in a wireless sensor network for an E-health application. *IEEE Wireless Communications, 20*(4), 38–49. doi:10.1109/MWC.2013.6590049

Chang, Chiang, Wu, & Chang. (2016). A Context-Aware, Interactive M-health system for Diabetics. *IT Professional, 18*(3), 14–22. doi:10.1109/MITP.2016.48

Chawathe, S. S. (2018). Indoor Localization Using Bluetooth-LE Beacons. *Proc. 9th IEEE Annu. Ubiquitous Computing, Electronics and Mobile Communication Conference (UEMCON),* 262–268. 10.1109/UEMCON.2018.8796600

Exposure Notifications. (n.d.). *Helping fight COVID-19.* https://www.google.com/covid19/exposurenotifications/

Kotronis, C., Minou, G., Dimitrakopoulos, G., Nikolaidou, M., Anagnos, D., Amira, A., Bensaali, F., Baali, H., & Djelouat, H. (2017). Managing Criticalities of e-Health IoT systems. *IEEE 17th International Conference on Ubiquitous Wireless Broadband (ICUWB),* 1–5. 10.1109/ICUWB.2017.8251004

Laplante, P. A., & Laplante, N. (2016, May-June). The Internet of Things in healthcare: Potential applications and challenges. *IT Professional, 2–4*(3), 2–4. Advance online publication. doi:10.1109/MITP.2016.42

Lewnard, Nathan, & Lo. (2020). Scientific and ethical basis for social distancing interventions against COVID-19. *Lancet Infect Disease, 20,* 631–633. doi:10.1016/S1473-3099(20)30190-0

Penang Institute. (2020). *Smart City Technologies Take on COVID-19.* https://penanginstitute.org/publications/issues/smart-city-technologies-take-on-covid-19/

Rafael, A. (2020, April 6). Health Surveillance during covid-19pandemic. *BMJ (Clinical Research Ed.), 369,* m1373. doi:10.1136/bmj.m1373

Ting, D. S. W., Carin, L., Dzau, V., & Wong, T. Y. (2020, April). Digital Technology and COVID19. *Nature Medicine, 459–461*(4), 459–461. Advance online publication. doi:10.103841591-020-0824-5 PMID:32284618

Woolhandler, S., & Himmelstein, D. U. (2020, July). Intersecting U.S. epidemics: COVID-19 and lack of health insurance. *Annals of Internal Medicine, 63–64*(1), 63–64. Advance online publication. doi:10.7326/M20-1491 PMID:32259195

Yin, Zeng, Chen, & Fan. (2016). The Internet of Things in healthcare: An overview. *Journal of Industrial Information Integration, 1,* 3–13. doi:10.1016/j.jii.2016.03.004

Chapter 8
Internet of Things-Integrated Remote Patient Monitoring System:
Healthcare Application

Sampath Boopathi
Muthayammal Engineering College, India

ABSTRACT

Remote monitoring technologies are required to remotely monitor patients. The internet of things allows for remote monitoring of smart devices and apps, but sensors are used to track ECG, pressure, weight, and cardiac rate. IoT infrastructure enables intelligent devices to remotely monitor health and advise on medical concerns in an emergency. Heart disease is the leading cause of mortality, and in order to enhance medical services and lower the death rate, social insurance must be made mandatory. This chapter presents a low-cost, portable remote system for patient monitoring based on the ESP32 MCU and WiFi.

INTRODUCTION

The Internet of Things (IoT) is a network of intelligent machines that interact and communicate with one another, as well as with other devices, objects, surroundings, and infrastructures. The internet is the most widely used form of communication, connecting individuals all over the world. The world is being electrified, with practically every produced object including an embedded processor and user interfaces that enable programmability and deterministic "command and control" capabilities.

DOI: 10.4018/978-1-6684-6894-4.ch008

These skills may be leveraged to develop new services that improve the lives of users. In the last decade, the phrase "Internet of Things" has become increasingly comprehensive, including a wide range of applications (Abawajy & Hassan, 2017).

Technology has progressed to the point that a network of networked things gathers information from the environment and interacts with the actual world, utilizing current Internet protocols to provide services for information transmission, analytics, applications, and communications. IoT has progressed from its infancy to the point where it is on the verge of changing the existing static Internet into a fully integrated Future Internet. The Internet revolution enabled people to connect, and the next revolution will enable objects to connect to create a smart environment (Nduka et al., 2019).

With Cloud computing as the unifying framework, the Internet of Things is a unified framework for sharing information across platforms, enabling innovative applications through seamless sensing, data analytics, and representation. Home security, robot control, DC motor control, stepper motor control, and voting machine control are just a few of the novel uses for GSM MODEM. The goal of this project is to create a GSM-based electronic notice display system that can automatically convey information to students or retail centers such as results, circulars, timetables, and time tables. It may show critical information via a web server and deliver it to registered mobile phone numbers (Raviteja & Supriya, 2020).

TECHNOLOGICAL BACKGROUND

The most crucial elements are that a system with numerous wireless sensors is being developed to monitor and transmit health-related data such as body temperature, blood pressure, saline level, and heart rate via the internet for other users to access. This will allow for the creation and documentation of a patient's health database, which will be important for doctor analysis. Based on past database readings, this study proposes a health-monitoring system that analyses parameters and diagnoses health concerns. When certain threshold values are exceeded in an emergency, alerts are generated to assist doctors in taking the essential steps (Imtyaz Ahmed & Kannan, 2022).

Sensors in next-generation smart phones and intelligent devices measure ECG, systolic pressure, diastolic pressure, and pulse rate. This study examines current works on health assessment systems and IOT, which entail connecting devices to automatically gather and analyse data in order to produce intelligent data. The Internet of Things (IoT) is a concept that entails linking objects in order for data to be automatically retrieved and processed. Advances in medical science technology will assist doctors in taking proper steps to avoid deterioration and keep patients from acquiring health issues. Because of poor socioeconomic position, a lack of knowledge about health practices, and limited access to medical services, rural regions have a higher mortality rate (Philip et al., 2021). Rural public health centers lack medical practitioners and facilities, resulting in frequent diseases and serious health concerns. This has occurred in rural regions. IoT has enhanced the use of technology in healthcare, with low-cost wearable sensors and healthcare systems now readily available for personalized application. This is the outcome of extensive research and significant financial investment (Habib et al., 2015).

Sensor data is stored in the cloud and may be accessed using online tools to get insights. They are beneficial for enhancing health and delivering practical healthcare applications in remote places, such as remote patient health monitoring, which assists health staff in better monitoring their patients and preventing medical diseases from increasing. Remote monitoring enables doctors to access current or historical health data at any time, allowing for more accurate diagnosis and treatment. However, adoption of such platforms in rural areas is lower than in urban areas, resulting in little impact on the medical and clinical sectors in rural India (Mohammed et al., 2014). To satisfy healthcare needs and educate and inform individuals about illnesses, treatments, and personal hygiene, an easy-to-use system for personal health monitoring is being created.

IOT can gather data from sensors in the healthcare environment that detect crucial health-related elements, which can then be utilized to deliver useful insights to physicians and medical experts hundreds of kilometers away. Amrita Jeevanam provides remote health monitoring and medical intervention using the Internet of Things (IoT). A Medical Interface Unit collects important data using low-cost health sensors, which is subsequently analyzed. This information is utilized to predict the presence of any illness problems in the patient's body, resulting in personalized medical recommendations as well as greater awareness and avoidance of future concerns (Stone et al., 2022).

IoT solutions are available for a variety of applications, including traffic control, industry management, emergency services, and health care. IoT-based healthcare apps are gaining popularity as a tool to monitor remote patient health, and medical sensors are becoming more widely available, allowing them to be utilized in a wide range of medical applications. The Internet of Things and cloud computing combine to produce a powerful platform for remotely monitoring patients and sending continuous health information to doctors and caregivers, enabling for more precise illness detection.

REQUIREMENTS FOR MEASURING BODY TEMPERATURE

Body temperature measurement is significant in medicine because it allows clinicians to assess the efficacy of therapies based on body temperature. Fever is the most prevalent type of disease-related rise in body temperature, and it occurs as a result of a response to disease-specific stimuli. There is no such thing as a universal normal body temperature since it varies depending on the portion of the body being monitored. Body temperature fluctuates throughout the day, peaking in the evening due to physiological factors and physical exercise. Surface temperature is measured on the skin's surface, whereas core temperature is obtained by inserting a thermometer into a body opening (Kang et al., 2018).

Pulse oximetry measures the amount of oxygen in the blood and is useful for persons with respiratory or cardiovascular disorders, very young newborns, and certain illnesses. Because it can cause cell death and organ failure, oxygen is critical for the body's survival. It travels through the lungs and into the bloodstream via hemoglobin proteins in red blood cells. The proportion of oxygen in hemoglobin proteins measured by pulse oximetry is known as oxygen saturation. Normal values range from 95 to 100 percent, but anything less than 90 percent is regarded unusually low and might result in a clinical emergency. Pulse oximeters are portable oxygen saturation meters. Suffocation, choking, drowning, illnesses, dangerous substances, heart failure, allergic responses, general anesthesia, sleep apnea, and pulse oximeters can all produce a decline in oxygen saturation. By beaming light onto a detector on the other side of the skin, pulse oximeters assess oxygen saturation. The quantity of light absorbed by the blood reveals the saturation level of oxygen. Pulse oximeters, which are powered by Rubicon Project, are beneficial for those who have conditions that alter oxygen saturation.

Pulse oximetry is used to monitor oxygen saturation levels, evaluate the safety of physical exercise, and determine the efficacy of breathing therapies. It can also be used to determine the safety of physical activity in persons with cardiovascular or pulmonary disorders, as part of a stress test, and in patients who are particularly susceptible, such as new-borns in neonatal intensive care units. Pulse oximetry gives persons with respiratory or cardiovascular disorders peace of mind by determining the requirement for supplementary oxygen, monitoring oxygen saturation levels in people under anaesthesia, and warning of potentially serious side effects in those using medicines that impact breathing. Although pulse oximeters are widely available for purchase online, no research has been conducted to support their claim of preventing SIDS or accidents. Companies promote them to the parents of

Although pulse oximeters are noninvasive and pose no serious risks, they can cut off oxygen from surrounding vessels if used too tightly and for an extended period of time. Pulse oximetry is susceptible to misleading results owing to simple changes in posture, such as sleeping turning over. Because of changes in sleeping posture or breath-holding, oxygen saturation may drop for brief intervals. Even if the dip is momentary and innocuous, a pulse oximeter will notify you. Pulse oximeters might induce undue stress and false security in persons who are anxious about their health. People should see a doctor about the hazards and keep a record of their readings over time. Changes in readings, especially in reaction to environmental changes, might indicate a health issue. Before purchasing a consumer-grade pulse oximeter, people should consult with a doctor about their goals.

Need for ECG (Electrocardiogram)

An ECG (electrocardiogram) is a test that records the electrical activity of the heart while it is completely still. It can reveal if the heart has been augmented owing to hypertension or if there has been a previous respiratory failure. It is not the same as a blood pressure, exercise, or cardiovascular imaging test. It may be necessary if you have risk factors for or signs of coronary artery disease, or if you already have coronary artery disease.

An ECG is not required if there are no risk factors or symptoms of coronary artery disease. The ECG is not beneficial for persons who do not have risk factors for coronary artery disease, although it might occasionally indicate minor anomalies that are not related to fundamental coronary artery disease, leading to stress and follow-up tests and medications. ECGs are not the best way to avoid coronary artery disease(AlGhatrif & Lindsay, 2012).

Fundamental of ECG

The electrocardiogram (ECG) is a non-invasive diagnostic procedure that assesses cardiac illness by evaluating the electrical system of the heart. It detects electrical charges created by the heart as it beats using flat metal electrodes inserted on the chest, which are then graphed(Becker, 2006).

Usages: An ECG is a machine that monitors the electrical rhythm of the heart and generates a wave tracing. If the waves are inconsistent or do not develop as expected, this is an indication of cardiac problems. Many doctors will order an ECG as part of a yearly physical to screen for heart disease. If you have indications or symptoms of heart illness, such as chest discomfort, shortness of breath, light-headedness, dizziness, or fainting episodes, an ECG may be indicated. In addition, if you experience symptoms of a TIA or stroke, such as visual abnormalities, numbness, weakness, or speech difficulties, you will most certainly require an ECG. ECG testing is required to diagnose cardiac problems and monitor therapy outcomes. It is also necessary before any form of heart surgery, including pacemaker insertion and pre-operative screening. Prior to general anaesthesia, an ECG is necessary. This assists anaesthesiologists in the planning of aesthetic medicines and operative monitoring (Ru et al., 2021).

Conditions: Tachycardia, bradycardia, and arrhythmia can all be detected using EKG wave patterns. These variations in wave shape reveal information regarding the type of cardiac illness and the afflicted location.

Limitations: The ECG is a common medical test because of its capacity to screen for a number of heart problems, as well as its ease, safety, and cost. An ECG has limitations, such as exposing the heart rate and rhythm for just a few seconds while the tracing is being recorded. It is frequently normal or virtually normal in many forms of cardiac illness, and sometimes ECG abnormalities have little medical importance.

Requirements: If you have risk factors for an enlarged heart, such as hypertension or symptoms of coronary sickness, an ECG test is recommended. It can also be utilized for screening or word-related needs, or if you have a personal or family history of cardiovascular disease, diabetes, or other risks. These tests can help protect your heart, whether you have coronary disease or want to avoid it. Understand your risk of coronary artery disease and utilize the risk appraisal exam to determine your risk.

The most important details to reduce your risk of coronary illness are to be aware of your risk factors, quit smoking, be active, control your circulatory strain, eat a healthy diet, achieve and maintain a healthy weight, manage diabetes, limit alcohol use, reduce stress, visit your medical care provider on a regular basis, and control your blood cholesterol.

ECG Interpretation

To assess your risk of coronary sickness, check your pulse, blood cholesterol, and glucose levels (Palanisamy et al., 2019).

Circulatory Strain: The pulse should be tested once a year, but if you have hypertension, you should have it checked more regularly. Inquire with your medical care provider about how frequently it should be examined.

Cholesterol: If you are male and over 40, female and over 50, or postmenopausal, have coronary illness, stroke, diabetes, or hypertension, have circumferences more than 102 cm or 88 cm, and have a family history of coronary illness or stroke, you should undergo a cholesterol blood test.

Glucose: A glucose test once a year is recommended for older persons with diabetes risk factors or who are pregnant, and should be reviewed with a medical care provider. Work with your medical physician to lower your cholesterol, pulse, and glucose levels to lessen your risk of cardiovascular failure and stroke.

Risks and Contraindications of ECG

ECG is a safe test that has no negative health consequences (Kang et al., 2018; Stone et al., 2022).

Before the Test: ECGs can be performed at the doctor's office provided time, room, and equipment are available. Some medications, however, may need to be stopped for a day or two before the test.

Timing: Expect an ECG test to take an additional 10-15 minutes if it is part of a doctor's appointment, and longer if it is a special visit.

Location: ECGs are frequently performed at the doctor's office, although they may also be performed in a different location.

What to Wear: You must change into a hospital gown and remove any heavy necklaces/chains that are in the way, but no metal jewelry.

Food and Drink: You can eat or drink whatever you want before the test, however caffeine should be avoided for 6-10 hours.

SCOPE OF REMOTE MONITORING SYSTEM

The COVID-19 pandemic in India is critical for the worldwide COVID-19 pandemic produced by SARS-CoV-2. India has the most confirmed cases in Asia and the second most confirmed cases on the world, with over millions of illnesses and deaths.

By mid-2020, India had the largest number of daily tests on the world, resulting in a high number of positive instances. COVID-19 is a lethal virus that has reached the twenty-first century, and the World Health Organization suggests using oxidation level and body temperature to detect it. Humans employ SPO2, Body Temperature, and ECG equipment, however they cannot provide data to medical experts who can readily grasp the data values.

RESEARCH OBJECTIVES

This book chapter highlights the importance of smart technology research. It is vital to highlight that there is a shortage of real-time monitoring devices in medical equipment, such as ambulances, which cannot give doctors with real-time health status. This thesis offers a system that may give real-time data at a cheap cost and with great efficiency.

The work goals are to minimize device costs, hardware complexity, form factor complexity, obtain better parameter values, high-speed data transmission, web-based platform, no connectivity difficulties, emergency alert message, Wi-Fi connectivity, and SPO2 parameters used to monitor blood pressure. These goals will be addressed by utilizing real-world parameters, high-speed data transfer, a web-based platform, Wi-Fi connectivity, and SPO2 parameters. India is the world's second most populous country, yet monetary and geographical inequalities result in limited access to healthcare. Low financial status, a lack of understanding of wellness measures, and a lack of access to healthcare offices all contribute to a rise in provincial death rates.

METHODOLOGY

The Remote Monitoring Emergency Medical System is explained, algorithms are employed, and research is undertaken to compare and implement approaches(Figure 1).

Basic Remote Monitoring System

This study presents a method for remote monitoring of medical parameters utilizing Zigbee and GSM technologies, divided into two sections: receiver & transmission,

Figure 1. Remote patient monitoring system using IoT

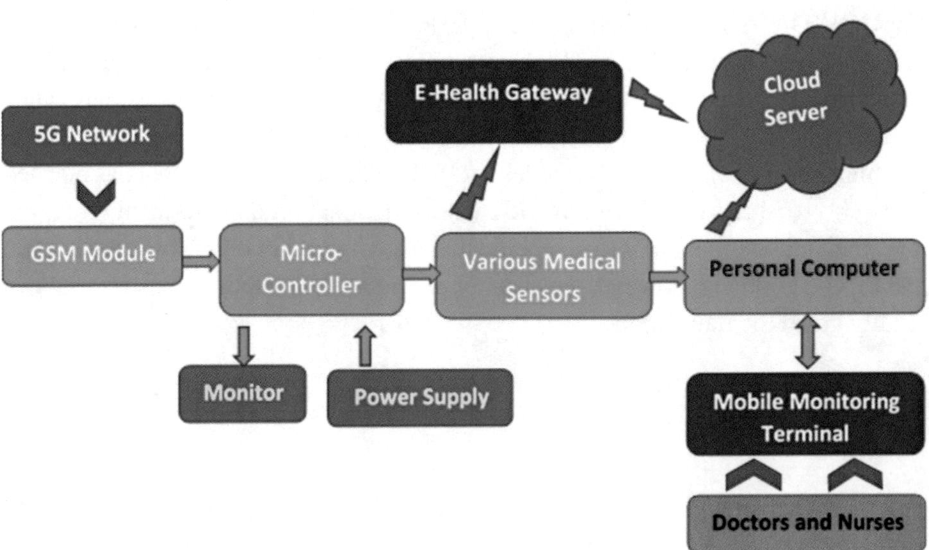

data reception, and data transfer to a web server. This research presented an Internet of Things-based cardiac sickness monitoring architecture that screens physical symptoms and offers four distinct information transmission mechanisms to balance medical services demand and interest. The framework was reviewed using a model. An MCU, Light Emitting Diode, LED Light Emitting Diode, Infrared Light Emitting Diode, BLE, 0.96 inch OLED display, and buttons for user input and power supply comprise the SPO2 System (Mohammed et al., 2014; Xu, 2020).

Remote SPO2: The system built employs an ESP32 MCU and Wi-Fi module, a MAX30100 SPO2 sensor, a 180mah battery for long life, and Think Speak, a free cloud server platform powered by MathWorks. It can obtain SPO2 and Heart Rate data in less time and with greater precision. The development cost is minimal, and the battery backup capacity is 180mah.

Remote Body Temperature Monitor: The built system makes use of an ESP32 MCU and Wi-Fi module, a DS18B20 sensor, a 180mah battery, and Think Speak, a free cloud server platform powered by MathWorks. It can obtain body temperature data rapidly and precisely, and it has a cheap development cost and a long battery life.

Remote ECG Monitor: The built system makes use of an ESP32 MCU and Wi-Fi module, an AD8232 sensor, a 180mah battery, and Think Speak, a free cloud server platform powered by Mathwork. It can get ECG data rapidly and correctly, with a low development cost and a long battery backup life.

Hardware Details

ESP-8266 Family (ESP32): The Espressif Systems ESP-8266 is a low-effort Wi-Fi central processor designed in Shanghai, China. It enables microcontrollers to connect to a Wi-Fi network and simplify TCP/IP communications by using Hayes-style instructions. The cheap cost and absence of exterior segments on the module, implying a limited volume, encouraged programmers to explore the module, chip, and product. They also had to translate Chinese documents. The ESP8285 is an ESP8266 with 1 MiB of internal flash memory that allows single-chip devices to connect to Wi-Fi. It has a 32-bit RISC processing core and memory running at 80 MHz. The device supports up to 16 MiB of external QSPI flash, IEEE 802.11 b/g/n Wi-Fi, and integrated TR switches, LNAs, power-amplifiers, baluns, and matching networks, which is the most essential concept(Deshpande & Kulkarni, 2017; Krishnan et al., 2018; Vijay Kumar et al., 2018).

Pinout of ESP-0: GND, GPIO 2, GPIO 0, RX, VCC, RST, CH PD, TX are the pinouts for the ESP-01 module.

ESP32: The ESP32 is a 2.4 GHz Wi-Fi plus Bluetooth chip manufactured in TSMC's 40 nm process. It provides the most power in a variety of applications and power situations, proving longevity, adaptability, and dependability. The ESP32 chip family is built on the ECO V3 wafer. With 20 external components such as an antenna knob, power amplifier, noise reception amplifier, and so on, the ESP32 is a highly integrated solution for Wi-Fi and Bluetooth IoT applications. It is equipped with cutting-edge low-power semiconductor capabilities.

BT Key Features: NZIF receiver with -94 dBm BLE sensitivity and class-1, class-2, and class-3 transmitters with Enhanced Power Control. Bluetooth 4.2, SCO/eSCO, CVSD and SBC, Bluetooth Piconet and Scatternet, multi-connections in Classic BT and BLE, simultaneous advertising and scanning are all supported.

MCU and Advanced Features

CPU and Memory: QSPI supports various flash/SRAM chips, Xtensa® LX6 CPU, 448 KB ROM, 520 KB SRAM, 16 KB RTC, Espressif Systems 9 Please provide feedback on the documentation.

Clocks and Timers: External 2 MHz-60 MHz crystal oscillator, external 32 kHz crystal oscillator, two timer groups, one RTC timer, one RTC watchdog.

Advanced Peripheral Interfaces: 34 programmable GPIOs, 12 bit SAR ADC, 8 bit DAC, 10 touch sensors, 4 SPI, 2 I2S, 2 I2C, 3 UART, 1 host, 1 slave, Ethernet MAC interface, Two-Wire Automotive Interface, IR, Motor PWM, LED PWM, Hall sensor, and so on.

Security: Secure boot, flash encryption, 1024-bit OTP, and cryptographic hardware acceleration, including AES, SHA-2, RSA, ECC, and RNG, are all available in Systems 10.

Applications: It is possible to buy generic low-power IoT Sensor Hubs, Data Loggers, Cameras, OTT Devices, Speech Recognition, Image Recognition, and Mesh Networks.

Home Automation, Industrial Automation, Smart Agriculture, Audio Applications, Health Care Applications, Wi-Fi-enabled Toys, Wearable Electronics, Retail & Catering Applications, POS Machines, and Service Robots are some of the applications being developed. These include home automation, light control, smart plugs, smart door locks, industrial automation, smart agriculture, audio applications, health care applications, Wi-Fi-enabled toys, remote control toys, proximity sensing toys, educational toys, wearable electronics, retail & catering applications, POS machines, and service robots (Nookhao et al., 2020; Xu, 2020; Yang et al., 2016).

SPO2 Sensor

The MAX30100 sensor uses LEDs, better optics, a photodetector, and low-noise analogue signal processing to combine pulse oximetry with a heart rate monitor. It may be turned off by software using a negligible standby current. Wearable Devices, Fitness Assistant Devices, and Medical Monitoring Devices with Integrated LEDS, Photo Sensor, and High-Performance Analog Front-End System-in-Package. With configurable sampling rate and LED current, Ultra-Low-Power Operation extends battery life for wearable devices. High SNR and Advanced Functionality Improve Measurement Performance Robust motion artifact resilience, ambient light cancellation, high sample rate, and fast data output are all provided.

ECG Sensor

The AD8232 ECG Module is a single-chip intended to extract, amplify, and filter biopotential signals for biopotential measuring applications, as well as operate as an Op-amp to collect a clear signal from PR and QT Intervals.

Features of the AD8232 ECG Module: A single-lead ECG front end with two or three electrode configurations, an 80 dB common-mode rejection ratio, single-supply operation, quick restoration, and footprint. The AD8232 ECG Module is a low-cost board that monitors and displays the electrical activity of the heart. It has pins for connecting custom sensors, an LED indication, and functions such as rapid restoration to shorten the duration of lengthy HPFs.

Interfacing Diagram: For output and control activities, the AD8232 ECG module requires one analogy and three digital pins. Interconnected are heart rate monitors, ECGs, bio-potential signal gathering, remote health monitoring, and gaming accessories. Analog Devices' AD8232 ECG Module and IC are intended to collect, amplify, and filter biopotential signals for biopotential measuring applications. The iAD8232 Single Lead Heart Rate Monitor acts as an operational amplifier to generate a clear signal from PR and QT intervals.

Temperature Sensor

The DS18B20 is an aphorism integrated one-wire programmable temperature sensor that can measure temperatures ranging from -55°C to +125°C with a 5°C precision. It offers temperature measurements ranging from 9 to 12 bits, indicating the temperature of a specific device. To connect with an internal CPU, a one-wire bus protocol is employed.

The customizable Digital Temperature Sensor communicates via 1-Wire. When the bus is not in use, the sensor maintains the line high with a pull-up resistor. The temperature is stored in a 2-byte register and may be read using just one wire. Two types of commands must be provided to read the values: ROM and function. The datasheet specifies the address value of each ROM memory and sequence. Arduino may be used to interact with a library to measure temperature in harsh conditions, liquid temperatures, and many sites (Babu et al., 2023; Boopathi, Arigela, et al., 2023; Jeevanantham et al., 2023).

Software Details

The following tools are required to construct the proposed system: Eagle, Ardunio IDE, Thing Speak, and Bulk SMS Service.

EAGLE

EAGLE is setup using two sets of rules: Design Rule Check (DRC) rules that specify minimum item sizes and separations, and Auto Router Setup rules that optimize routing. Menus or.CTL files can be used to modify rules. A.DRU file and a.CTL file together generate a board layout for a certain PCB process, which may be saved to a new file if necessary. This article focuses on how to utilize EAGLE with low-quality processes that lack PTH and favour one side. Copper pouring must be used with caution for routing and electrical screening, and there are several interdependent choices available.

The EAGLE DRC rules may be adjusted to vary the size of the track and pads. Many PCB manufacturers have their own DRC rules, which can be downloaded from the internet or manually entered. Custom DRC rules may be required owing to poor PCB etching or a lack of a solder mask. The exact measurements can be modified on an individual basis. The main concept is to have a single minimum dimension for all dimensions.

Clearance Tab: Setting all settings equal to determine clearance between objects.
Sizes Tab: Minimum track width is usually set equal to clearance.
Restring Tab (pronounced rest ring: The DRC files ee rules 20mil.dru and ee rules 15mil.dru demonstrate this with 20mil and 15mil dimensions, respectively. Small changes in these values can have a big impact on layout, such as whether tracks on an IC can go between pads. This is also dependent on the IC pin hole drill size.

Arduino IDE

Arduino was dubbed by Massimo Banzi, David Mellis, and David Cuartielles following the Wiring stage, which comprised a PCB with an ATmega168 microprocessor, an IDE, and library capabilities. They also provided support for the lower-cost ATmega8 microprocessor. Musto held a PhD from Massachusetts Institute of Technology and an MBA from New York University, but neither had any record of his involvement. Massimo Banzi stated that the Arduino Foundation will be a new beginning for Arduino. Musto then confessed that he never received such degrees(Jeevanantham et al., 2023; Reddy et al., 2023; S. et al., 2022; Sahal et al., 2022; Sampath et al., 2022).

Due to Musto's reported removal of Open source licenses, schematics, and code from the site, Arduino has not established a Foundation in over a year. In October 2017, Arduino announced its partnership with ARM Holdings, stating that ARM saw autonomy as a key belief of Arduino. Arduino is devoted to collaborating with all innovators and designs. The Arduino IDE includes a Wiring project software library that enables standard input and output operations. The GNU toolchain compiles and links user-written code into an executable application. The Arduino IDE employs avrdude to transform executable code into a text file that a loader software loads into the Arduino board(Harikaran et al., 2023; Janardhana, Singh, et al., 2023; Selvakumar et al., 2023)(Domakonda et al., 2023; Kumara et al., 2023; Mohanty et al., 2023; Samikannu et al., 2023).

Thing Speak: Web API

Thing Speak is an open-source Internet of Devices API that allows the development of sensor recording applications, area tracking apps, and an informal community of things providing status updates. Thing Speak was introduced in 2010 by io Bridge and has a tight partnership with Math Works, Inc., where the majority of the documentation is integrated into their Matlab documentation portal. The Internet of Things (IoT) is a network of many linked devices that can communicate data via the internet. It is conceivable to make everything, from a pill to a jet, into an IoT device capable of transmitting continuous data without the involvement of a human. It is altering our everyday environments, making them smarter and more sensitive, and linking the real and virtual worlds.

The Internet of Things and Healthcare

IoT is a new technology with several applications in industries such as healthcare. Due to a lack of surveillance, 30% of medical patients are readmitted to the hospital following surgery. With the participation of IoT, remote patient monitoring may be conceivable, with wearable devices with integrated sensors monitoring patient state and alerting the doctor. IoT solutions can assist poor rural residents gain access to physicians while also lowering travel and hospitalization costs. This application's potential is enhanced by timely access to data by medical workers, and it sends reminders to doctors if a patient does not take medicine on a regular basis.

The Internet of Things (IoT) is gaining popularity, and RFID labels are being utilized to aid navigation. Sensors and internet connections are getting more affordable, allowing practically everything to be linked to the internet.

The Internet of Things (IoT) raises serious privacy and security concerns. A smart home, for example, may detect when you wake up, how well you clean your teeth, which radio station you listen to, what sorts of foods you eat, your children's thoughts, and when someone arrives to your house and passes by. Not all smart home firms rely their business strategies on gathering and selling your data. IoT data may be combined with information from other sources to create a reasonably complete image of you, such as what you ate for dinner. IoT devices are a security ticking time bomb for enterprises. The Internet of Things (IoT) is a workplace technology that is becoming increasingly significant(Boopathi, Siva Kumar, et al., 2023; Vanitha et al., 2023; Vennila et al., 2023). Consumers must be informed of their transaction and whether or not they are happy with it. IoT devices that are not properly configured might easily expose business networks to cyber-attacks or leak data. Because unused IoT devices will leave a catastrophic and hazardous legacy, the smart office is the future security nightmare. Businesses must be aware of the hazards involved with IoT in order to protect themselves.

The IoT and Cyber Warfare

IoT devices are susceptible to cyber assaults, which governments are taking into account while developing cyber warfare tactics. According to US intelligence briefings, the country's adversaries may be inflicting damage to its infrastructure, such as the Internet of Things, by hacking thermostats, cameras, and stoves that are connected to the internet. If they are hacked, this might result in eavesdropping or pandemonium, thus security should be as rigorous as feasible. Cyberwarfare is becoming a more serious concern, with the internet serving as a battleground and your smart toaster eavesdropping on you.

The Internet of Things and Data

Sensors in IoT devices will capture data such as temperature, pressure, sound, video, and humidity. This data will need to be transmitted somewhere, so IoT devices will use 5G, 4G, Wi-Fi, and other technologies to do so. In the next five years, IoT devices will create 79.4 zettabytes of data, some of which will be "small and rusty," such as temperature measurements from sensors or smart meters. In the future, IoT devices will create more data, mostly from video surveillance and other industrial and medical applications. Drones and self-driving vehicles will create massive volumes of data in the future, including audio, video, and automobile sensor data.

Big Data Analytics

The Internet of Things (IoT) is a significant contributor to big data by allowing organizations to collect and analyze enormous data sets. It can assist planners in improving traffic flow by gathering data from sensors in metropolitan areas. IoT metadata is a rising source of data that may be utilized to structure unstructured material or to add new degrees of comprehension, intelligence, and order to random environments. It may be fed into NoSQL databases or cognitive systems to improve understanding, intelligence, and organization.

The Internet of Things, in particular, will deliver massive volumes of real-time data. Machine-to-machine links that facilitate IoT applications, according to Cisco. An implanted framework is a chip-based PC equipment framework with code that is meant to perform a certain function. It can vary from a single microcontroller to a cluster of processors with accompanying peripherals and organizations, with implanted frameworks accounting for 98 percent of all chips made.

Embedded System

Microcontrollers, ASICs, FPGAs, GPUs, and door exhibitions manage installed frameworks. Programming instructions are kept in read-only memory or blaze memory chips, and they communicate with the outside world via peripherals, which link information and generate devices(Boopathi, Khare, et al., 2023; Imtyaz Ahmed & Kannan, 2022; Raviteja & Supriya, 2020; Ru et al., 2021).

Structure of Embedded System

Sensor: The sensor measures and transforms the real quantity to an electrical indication that can be read by an electronic device (Figure 2).

A-D Converter: A sensor signal is converted into an advanced signal by a basic to computerized converter.
Processor and ASICs: Processors measure yield and store it in memory using data.
D-A Converter: An advanced to basic converter translates computerized data to simpler data.

Figure 2. Structure of embedded system

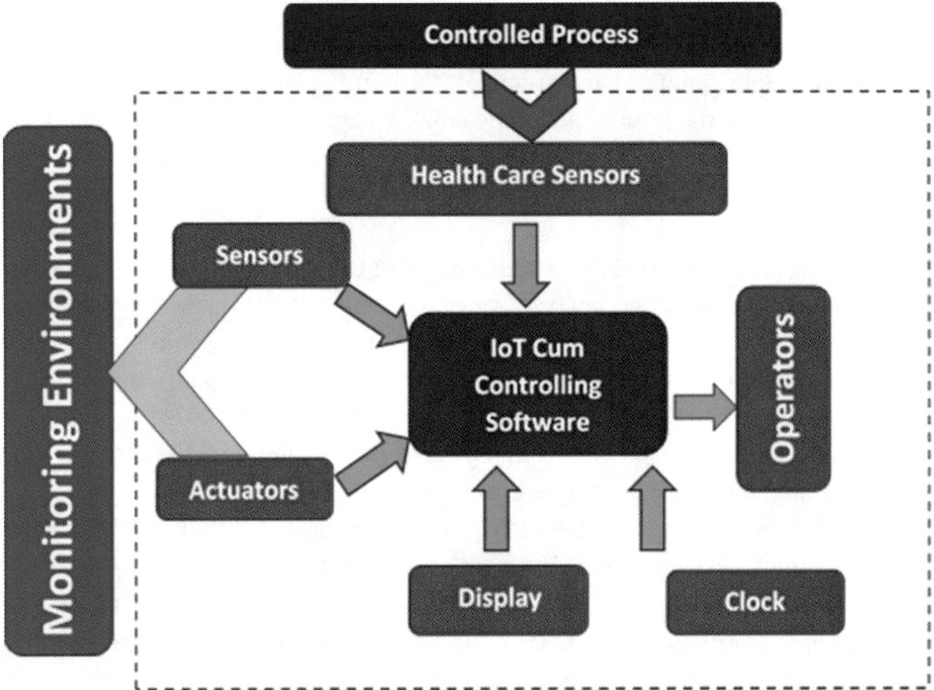

Actuator: Analyzing D-A Converter yield in order to save confirmed yield.

Because of AI, VR, AR, AI, deep learning, and IoT, the market for embedded frameworks is quickly expanding. These frameworks will be critical for trends such as reduced energy consumption, greater security, cloud availability, deep learning applications, and perception devices with continuous information.

IoT and Embedded System

Embedded systems are pieces of hardware and software that are designed to execute specialized tasks within a larger system. The Internet of Things (IoT) represents a massive growth opportunity for the installation enterprise. It is utilized in a variety of applications ranging from plant robotization to on-demand entertaining. However, IoT programming arrangements must be tailored to specific needs, which raises costs and discourages competitors from entering the market. Benison Technologies is creating innovative arrangements to decrease the expenses involved with constructing the fundamental foundation of IoT solutions, allowing them to focus on simplifying the center usefulness and selling answers faster and at a lower cost(Deshpande & Kulkarni, 2017; Xu, 2020).

Inserted Systems and Real-time Operating Systems (RTOS)

Installed frameworks are electrical components that include a microprocessor, peripherals, a memory card, and a programming software that executes instructions, a functioning framework, and apparatuses. Because of their distinct quality and features such as continuous processing, low force usage, minimal support, and high accessibility, they are becoming increasingly significant in the Internet of Things (IoT).

Installed frameworks are electrical components that include a microchip, peripherals, a memory card, and a programming software that runs instructions, a functioning framework, and apparatuses. They are becoming increasingly significant in the Internet of Things (IoT) because to their distinct quality and features such as continuous processing, low force usage, minimal support, and high accessibility.

RTOS is an operating system that continuously maintains equipment assets, applications, and information cycles, enabling for longer period dependability of both equipment and programs for low-powered and memory-constrained gadgets and organizations. In terms of planning between application acceptance and execution, RTOS has a high level of quality and consistency. Prior to the Internet of Things, patients' interactions with experts were restricted to visits and phone and text correspondences.

Web of Things (WoT)

The Internet of Things (IoT) is transforming the medical care industry by enabling remote monitoring, increasing patient commitment and satisfaction, and cutting medical service costs. Remote monitoring shortens emergency clinic visits and eliminates re-affirmations. The Internet of Things (IoT) provides medical applications that assist patients, families, physicians, emergency clinics, and insurance companies.

IoT for Patients: Wearables and remotely linked gadgets provide patients with tailored care by reminding them of carbohydrate levels, practice checks, arrangements, and pulse patterns. The Internet of Things has transformed people's lives by offering frequent illness monitoring, allowing families and health practitioners to spot any changes in an individual's behaviors (Jeevanantham et al., 2023; Reddy et al., 2023; S. et al., 2022; Samikannu et al., 2023).

IoT for Physicians: IoT allows medical practitioners to be more attentive and proactive in their contacts with patients, allowing them to choose the best treatment choice and achieve the desired results. Wearables and other IoT-enabled home monitoring technology can assist doctors in monitoring the health of their patients.

IoT for Hospitals: IoT devices in medical clinics may help with tracking the whereabouts of clinical equipment, dispatching healthcare professionals, monitoring cleanliness, resource management, natural observation, and mugginess and temperature adjustment, among other things. Sensor-enabled Internet of Things devices are utilized to track healthcare equipment's position, evaluate real-time dispatches, and keep patients safe.

IoT for Health Insurance Companies: IoT-connected smart devices let health insurance carriers to use data provided by health-monitoring devices to identify deceptive claims and identify opportunities for improving. In light of IoT-caught information driven selections, clients will have adequate deception into the basic principle behind each decision chosen and cycle consequences. Backup plans can reward consumers who use IoT devices to document their everyday activities and adherence to treatment regimens, reducing cases and allowing insurance companies to grant claims.

Reclassifying Healthcare: IoT devices have the potential to transform medical treatment by recording or processing data at one level and then passing it on to the next. The Internet of Things (IoT) features a four-stage engineering cycle that evokes intuition and conveys dynamic business potential.

- Create a data collection network of networked devices.
- For further processing, data obtained from sensors and devices must be translated to a more complex format.
- Data is pre-processed, normalized, and sent to a server farm or the cloud.
- By monitoring and analyzing data at the proper level, advanced analytics may deliver significant business insights.
- The Internet of Things is transforming medical treatment by giving better consideration, greater therapeutic outcomes, and cheaper patient expenses.

Some of the primary benefits of IoT in medical care are as follows:

Cost-Cutting: IoT allows for continuous patient monitoring, minimizing the need for needless travels.

Faster Disease Diagnosis: Early indications of infection can be detected by patient monitoring and information.

Medications and Equipment Management: Linked devices provide for more efficient medication and clinical equipment management, resulting in decreased costs. Linked devices provide for more efficient medication and clinical equipment management, resulting in decreased costs.

Blunder Reduction: Data supplied by IoT devices aids in the development of strong dynamic as well as the smooth operation of medical care tasks with fewer mistakes, waste, and system expenditures.
Improved Treatment: Clinicians can base their judgments on evidence.

Because it collects massive amounts of data and raises concerns about data security, the Internet of Things poses a significant challenge for medical service providers. This data, on the other hand, may be utilized to improve patient well-being and relationships while also raising income and enhancing medical care operations. Being set up to outfit this digital army would be in a connected universe.

CONCLUSION

Despite advances in medical knowledge, there is still a paucity of remote monitoring technologies for patients to use. Sensors are used for ECG monitoring, pressure, weight, and heartbeat rate estimation; however, no remote monitoring is available. Devices and apps have advanced thanks to the Internet of Things. The Internet of Things infrastructure provides a platform for availability and innovation, allowing intelligent gadgets to remotely check on people's well-being and advise on medical problems in an emergency. Although heart disease is the leading cause of death, the consequences are permanent. This work describes a low-power remote system for monitoring ECG, Heart Rate, SPO2, and Body Temperature, with effective results.

FUTURE SCOPE

By combining advanced facilities, mobile apps, and the Internet of Things, the Internet of Things is revolutionizing healthcare (IoT). IoT has been utilized in many areas, including corporate, retail, government, and industrial, and it is now being used in healthcare. The Internet of Things is a booming force for physicians, researchers, patients, and insurers, and it is transforming how hospitals operate. Healthcare is one of the most fascinating and difficult businesses to update using IoT. The creation of IoT apps is also gaining pace in the healthcare business. This work have been extended that the performances and various parameters of IoT monitoring Patient system have been monitored and optimized using Multi-criteria optimization techniques(Boopathi, 2019, 2021; Boopathi, Balasubramani, et al., 2023; Boopathi, 2022e, 2022d, 2022a, 2022f, 2022b, 2022c; Boopathi et al., 2021, 2022; Gunasekaran et al., 2022; Janardhana, Anushkannan, et al., 2023; Trojovský et al., 2023; Yupapin et al., 2023). To understand how technology is transforming healthcare, it is critical to examine IoT market trends and expand the system to include diverse categories such as home care patients, elderly patients, ICU patients, and others. To decrease problems and increase security, remote monitoring health care systems should be built with robust security and privacy safeguards.

REFERENCES

Abawajy, J. H., & Hassan, M. M. (2017). Federated Internet of Things and Cloud Computing Pervasive Patient Health Monitoring System. *IEEE Communications Magazine*, *55*(1), 48–53. doi:10.1109/MCOM.2017.1600374CM

Abolfaz Mehbodiya, Kumar, Rane, Bhatia, & Singh. (2021). Smartphone-Based mHealth and Internet of Things for Diabetes Control and Self-Management. *Journal of Healthcare Engineering*. doi:10.1155/2021/2116647

AlGhatrif, M., & Lindsay, J. (2012). A brief review: History to understand fundamentals of electrocardiography. *Journal of Community Hospital Internal Medicine Perspectives*, *2*(1), 14383. doi:10.3402/jchimp.v2i1.14383 PMID:23882360

Babu, B. S., Kamalakannan, J., Meenatchi, N., M, S. K. S., S, K., & Boopathi, S. (2023). Economic impacts and reliability evaluation of battery by adopting Electric Vehicle. *IEEE Explore*, 1–6. doi:10.1109/ICPECTS56089.2022.10046786

Becker, D. E. (2006). Fundamentals of electrocardiography interpretation. *Anesthesia Progress*, *53*(2), 53–64. doi:10.2344/0003-3006(2006)53[53:FOEI]2.0.CO;2 PMID:16863387

Boopathi, S. (2019). Experimental investigation and parameter analysis of LPG refrigeration system using Taguchi method. *SN Applied Sciences*, *1*(8), 892. doi:10.100742452-019-0925-2

Boopathi, S. (2021). Improving of Green Sand-Mould Quality using Taguchi Technique. *Journal of Engineering Research*. doi:10.36909/jer.14079

Boopathi, S. (2022a). An experimental investigation of Quench Polish Quench (QPQ) coating on AISI 4150 steel. *Engineering Research Express*, *4*(4), 45009. doi:10.1088/2631-8695/ac9ddd

Boopathi, S. (2022b). An Extensive Review on Sustainable Developments of Dry and Near-Dry Electrical Discharge Machining Processes. *Journal of Manufacturing Science and Engineering*, *144*(5), 50801. doi:10.1115/1.4052527

Boopathi, S. (2022c). An investigation on gas emission concentration and relative emission rate of the near-dry wire-cut electrical discharge machining process. *Environmental Science and Pollution Research International*, *29*(57), 86237–86246. doi:10.100711356-021-17658-1 PMID:34837614

Boopathi, S. (2022d). Cryogenically treated and untreated stainless steel grade 317 in sustainable wire electrical discharge machining process: A comparative study. *Environmental Science and Pollution Research International*, 1–10. doi:10.100711356-022-22843-x PMID:36057706

Boopathi, S. (2022e). Experimental investigation and multi-objective optimization of cryogenic Friction-stir-welding of AA2014 and AZ31B alloys using MOORA technique. *Materials Today. Communications*, *33*, 104937. doi:10.1016/j.mtcomm.2022.104937

Boopathi, S. (2022f). Performance Improvement of Eco-Friendly Near-Dry Wire-Cut Electrical Discharge Machining Process Using Coconut Oil-Mist Dielectric Fluid. *Journal of Advanced Manufacturing Systems*, 1–20. Advance online publication. doi:10.1142/S0219686723500178

Boopathi, S., Arigela, S. H., Raman, R., Indhumathi, C., Kavitha, V., & Bhatt, B. C. (2023). Prominent Rule Control-based Internet of Things: Poultry Farm Management System. *IEEE Explore*, 1–6. doi:10.1109/ICPECTS56089.2022.10047039

Boopathi, S., Balasubramani, V., Kumar, R. S., & Singh, G. R. (2021). The influence of human hair on kenaf and Grewia fiber-based hybrid natural composite material: An experimental study. *Functional Composites and Structures*, *3*(4), 45011. doi:10.1088/2631-6331/ac3afc

Boopathi, S., Balasubramani, V., & Sanjeev Kumar, R. (2023). Influences of various natural fibers on the mechanical and drilling characteristics of coir-fiber-based hybrid epoxy composites. *Engineering Research Express*, *5*(1), 15002. doi:10.1088/2631-8695/acb132

Boopathi, S., Haribalaji, V., Mageswari, M., & Asif, M. M. (2022). Influences of Boron Carbide Particles on the Wear Rate and Tensile Strength of Aa2014 Surface Composite Fabricated By Friction-Stir Processing. *Materiali in Tehnologije*, *56*(3), 263–270. doi:10.17222/mit.2022.409

Boopathi, S., Khare, R., Jaya Christiyan, K. G., Muni, T. V., & Khare, S. (2023). Additive manufacturing developments in the medical engineering field. In Development, Properties, and Industrial Applications of 3D Printed Polymer Composites (pp. 86–106). IGI Global. doi:10.4018/978-1-6684-6009-2.ch006

Boopathi, S., Siva Kumar, P. K., & Meena, R. S. J., S. I., P., S. K., & Sudhakar, M. (2023). Sustainable Developments of Modern Soil-Less Agro-Cultivation Systems. In Human Agro-Energy Optimization for Business and Industry (pp. 69–87). IGI Global. doi:10.4018/978-1-6684-4118-3.ch004

Deshpande, U. U., & Kulkarni, M. A. (2017). IoT based Real Time ECG Monitoring System using Cypress WICED. *International Journal of Advanced Research in Electrical*, *6*(2), 710–720.

Domakonda, V. K., Farooq, S., Chinthamreddy, S., Puviarasi, R., Sudhakar, M., & Boopathi, S. (2023). Sustainable Developments of Hybrid Floating Solar Power Plants. In *Human Agro-Energy Optimization for Business and Industry* (pp. 148–167). IGI Global. doi:10.4018/978-1-6684-4118-3.ch008

Gunasekaran, K., Boopathi, S., & Sureshkumar, M. (2022). Analysis of a Cryogenically Cooled Near-Dry Wedm Process Using Different Dielectrics. *Materiali in Tehnologije*, *56*(2), 179–186. doi:10.17222/mit.2022.397

Habib, K., Torjusen, A., & Leister, W. (2015). Security Analysis of a Patient Monitoring System for the Internet of Things in eHealth. *Researchgate.Net, 335*(c), 73–78. https://www.researchgate.net/profile/Wolfgang_Leister/publication/320596844_Security_Analysis_of_a_Patient_Monitoring_System_for_the_Internet_of_Things_in_eHealth/links/59efaa13458515c3cc4369d0/Security-Analysis-of-a-Patient-Monitoring-System-for-the-Inte

Harikaran, M., Boopathi, S., Gokulakannan, S., & Poonguzhali, M. (2023). Study on the Source of E-Waste Management and Disposal Methods. In *Sustainable Approaches and Strategies for E-Waste Management and Utilization* (pp. 39–60). IGI Global. doi:10.4018/978-1-6684-7573-7.ch003

Imtyaz Ahmed, M., & Kannan, G. (2022). Secure and lightweight privacy preserving Internet of things integration for remote patient monitoring. *Journal of King Saud University - Computer and Information Sciences, 34*(9), 6895–6908. doi:10.1016/j.jksuci.2021.07.016

Janardhana, K., Anushkannan, N. K., Dinakaran, K. P., Puse, R. K., & Boopathi, S. (2023). *Experimental Investigation on Microhardness, Surface Roughness, and White Layer Thickness of Dry EDM*. Engineering Research Express. doi:10.1088/2631-8695/acce8f

Janardhana, K., Singh, V., Singh, S. N., Babu, T. S. R., Bano, S., & Boopathi, S. (2023). Utilization Process for Electronic Waste in Eco-Friendly Concrete: Experimental Study. In Sustainable Approaches and Strategies for E-Waste Management and Utilization (pp. 204–223). IGI Global.

Jeevanantham, Y. A., A, S., V, V., J, S. I., Boopathi, S., & Kumar, D. P. (2023). Implementation of Internet-of Things (IoT) in Soil Irrigation System. *IEEE Explore*, 1–5. doi:10.1109/ICPECTS56089.2022.10047185

Kang, M., Park, E., Cho, B. H., & Lee, K. S. (2018). Recent patient health monitoring platforms incorporating Internet of Things-enabled smart devices. *International Neurourology Journal*, *22*(Suppl 2), S76–S82. doi:10.5213/inj.1836144.072 PMID:30068069

Krishnan, D. S. R., Gupta, S. C., & Choudhury, T. (2018). An IoT based Patient Health Monitoring System. *Proceedings on 2018 International Conference on Advances in Computing and Communication Engineering, ICACCE 2018*, 1–7. 10.1109/ICACCE.2018.8441708

Kumara, V., Mohanaprakash, T. A., Fairooz, S., Jamal, K., Babu, T., & B., S. (2023). Experimental Study on a Reliable Smart Hydroponics System. In *Human Agro-Energy Optimization for Business and Industry* (pp. 27–45). IGI Global. doi:10.4018/978-1-6684-4118-3.ch002

Mohammed, J., Lung, C. H., Ocneanu, A., Thakral, A., Jones, C., & Adler, A. (2014). Internet of things: Remote patient monitoring using web services and cloud computing. *Proceedings - 2014 IEEE International Conference on Internet of Things, IThings 2014, 2014 IEEE International Conference on Green Computing and Communications, GreenCom 2014 and 2014 IEEE International Conference on Cyber-Physical-Social Computing, CPS 20*, 256–263. 10.1109/iThings.2014.45

Mohanty, A., Venkateswaran, N., Ranjit, P. S., Tripathi, M. A., & Boopathi, S. (2023). Innovative Strategy for Profitable Automobile Industries: Working Capital Management. In Handbook of Research on Designing Sustainable Supply Chains to Achieve a Circular Economy (pp. 412–428). IGI Global.

Nduka, A., Samual, J., Elango, S., Divakaran, S., Umar, U., & Senthilprabha, R. (2019). Internet of Things Based Remote Health Monitoring System Using Arduino. *Proceedings of the 3rd International Conference on I-SMAC IoT in Social, Mobile, Analytics and Cloud, I-SMAC 2019*, 572–576. 10.1109/I-SMAC47947.2019.9032438

Nookhao, S., Thananant, V., & Khunkhao, T. (2020). Development of IoT Heartbeat and Body Temperature Monitoring System for Community Health Volunteer. *2020 Joint International Conference on Digital Arts, Media and Technology with ECTI Northern Section Conference on Electrical, Electronics, Computer and Telecommunications Engineering, ECTI DAMT and NCON 2020*, 106–109. 10.1109/ECTIDAMTNCON48261.2020.9090692

Palanisamy, R., Hiteshkumar, M. K., Sahasrabuddhe, R., Puranik, J. A., & Vaidya, A. (2019). IoT based patient monitoring system. *International Journal of Recent Technology and Engineering, 8*(2), 2559–2564. doi:10.35940/ijrte.B1304.0982S1119

Philip, N. Y., Rodrigues, J. J. P. C., Wang, H., Fong, S. J., & Chen, J. (2021). Internet of Things for In-Home Health Monitoring Systems: Current Advances, Challenges and Future Directions. *IEEE Journal on Selected Areas in Communications, 39*(2), 300–310. doi:10.1109/JSAC.2020.3042421

Raviteja, K., & Supriya, M. (2020). Greenhouse Monitoring System Based on Internet of Things. *Lecture Notes in Electrical Engineering, 637*, 581–591. doi:10.1007/978-981-15-2612-1_56

Reddy, M. A., Reddy, B. M., Mukund, C. S., Venneti, K., Preethi, D. M. D., & Boopathi, S. (2023). Social Health Protection During the COVID-Pandemic Using IoT. In *The COVID-19 Pandemic and the Digitalization of Diplomacy* (pp. 204–235). IGI Global. doi:10.4018/978-1-7998-8394-4.ch009

Ru, L., Zhang, B., Duan, J., Ru, G., Sharma, A., Dhiman, G., Gaba, G. S., Jaha, E. S., & Masud, M. (2021). A Detailed Research on Human Health Monitoring System Based on Internet of Things. *Wireless Communications and Mobile Computing, 2021*, 1–9. doi:10.1155/2021/5592454

S., P. K., Sampath, B., R., S. K., Babu, B. H., & N., A. (2022). Hydroponics, Aeroponics, and Aquaponics Technologies in Modern Agricultural Cultivation. In *Trends, Paradigms, and Advances in Mechatronics Engineering* (pp. 223–241). IGI Global. doi:10.4018/978-1-6684-5887-7.ch012

Saha, B. C., R, D., A, A., Thrinath, B. V. S., Boopathi, S., J. R., & Sudhakar, M. (2022). *IoT based smart energy meter for smart grid.* Academic Press.

Samikannu, R., Koshariya, A. K., Poornima, E., Ramesh, S., Kumar, A., & Boopathi, S. (2023). Sustainable Development in Modern Aquaponics Cultivation Systems Using IoT Technologies. In *Human Agro-Energy Optimization for Business and Industry* (pp. 105–127). IGI Global. doi:10.4018/978-1-6684-4118-3.ch006

Sampath, B. C. S., & Myilsamy, S. (2022). Application of TOPSIS Optimization Technique in the Micro-Machining Process. In Trends, Paradigms, and Advances in Mechatronics Engineering (pp. 162–187). IGI Global. doi:10.4018/978-1-6684-5887-7.ch009

Selvakumar, S., Adithe, S., Isaac, J. S., Pradhan, R., Venkatesh, V., & Sampath, B. (2023). A Study of the Printed Circuit Board (PCB) E-Waste Recycling Process. In Sustainable Approaches and Strategies for E-Waste Management and Utilization (pp. 159–184). IGI Global.

Stone, D., Michalkova, L., & Machova, V. (2022). Machine and Deep Learning Techniques, Body Sensor Networks, and Internet of Things-based Smart Healthcare Systems in COVID-19 Remote Patient Monitoring. *American Journal of Medical Research (New York, N.Y.)*, *9*(1), 97. doi:10.22381/ajmr9120227

Suresh Kumar, Kumar, Gupta, Shrivastava, Kumar, & Jain. (2022). IoT Communication for Grid-Tie Matrix Converter with Power Factor Control Using the Adaptive Fuzzy Sliding (AFS) Method. *Scientific Programming*, 3.

Trojovský, P., Dhasarathan, V., & Boopathi, S. (2023). Experimental investigations on cryogenic friction-stir welding of similar ZE42 magnesium alloys. *Alexandria Engineering Journal*, *66*(1), 1–14. doi:10.1016/j.aej.2022.12.007

Vanitha, S. K. R., & Boopathi, S. (2023). Artificial Intelligence Techniques in Water Purification and Utilization. In *Human Agro-Energy Optimization for Business and Industry* (pp. 202–218). IGI Global. doi:10.4018/978-1-6684-4118-3.ch010

Vennila, T., Karuna, M. S., Srivastava, B. K., Venugopal, J., Surakasi, R., & B., S. (2023). New Strategies in Treatment and Enzymatic Processes. In *Human Agro-Energy Optimization for Business and Industry* (pp. 219–240). IGI Global. doi:10.4018/978-1-6684-4118-3.ch011

Vijay Kumar, G., Bharadwaja, A., & Nikhil Sai, N. (2018). Temperature and heart beat monitoring system using IOT. *Proceedings - International Conference on Trends in Electronics and Informatics, ICEI 2017*, 692–695. 10.1109/ICOEI.2017.8300791

Xu, G. (2020). IoT-Assisted ECG Monitoring Framework with Secure Data Transmission for Health Care Applications. *IEEE Access : Practical Innovations, Open Solutions*, *8*, 74586–74594. doi:10.1109/ACCESS.2020.2988059

Yang, Z., Zhou, Q., Lei, L., Zheng, K., & Xiang, W. (2016). An IoT-cloud Based Wearable ECG Monitoring System for Smart Healthcare. *Journal of Medical Systems*, *40*(12), 1–11. doi:10.100710916-016-0644-9 PMID:27796840

Yupapin, P., Trabelsi, Y., Nattappan, A., & Boopathi, S. (2023). Performance Improvement of Wire-Cut Electrical Discharge Machining Process Using Cryogenically Treated Super-Conductive State of Monel-K500 Alloy. *Iranian Journal of Science and Technology. Transaction of Mechanical Engineering*, *47*(1), 267–283. doi:10.100740997-022-00513-0

Chapter 9
An IoMT and Machine Learning Model Aimed at the Development of a Personalized Lifestyle Recommendation System Facilitating Improved Health

Guru Prasad
https://orcid.org/0000-0002-1811-9507
Graphic Era University (Deemed), India

A. Suresh Kumar
https://orcid.org/0000-0001-7145-6337
Jain University (Deemed), India

Sakshi Srivastava
Graphic Era University (Deemed), India

Ananya Srivastava
Graphic Era University (Deemed), India

Aditi Srivastava
Graphic Era University (Deemed), India

ABSTRACT

The machine learning-based internet of medical things (IoMT) has recently gained traction in the healthcare industry because of its ability to reduce costs while simultaneously improving care quality through real-time and continuous monitoring.

DOI: 10.4018/978-1-6684-6894-4.ch009

The advent of cutting-edge technologies has sparked a surge in interest in and demand for a more sophisticated healthcare delivery system. The chapter also shows software integration designs that are extremely important for the creation of smart healthcare systems. The developed systems are discussed in terms of their contributions, working procedures, results, and comparative merits and limits, all of which are included in the explanations. Existing system flaws and new framework introduction strategies are discussed, as well as current research difficulties and potential future paths. The goal is to give readers a thorough understanding of the most current advancements in the field of smart healthcare systems.

INTRODUCTION

People are finding it increasingly challenging to access information of high quality and significant value as a result of the enormous expansion of information available online Nasr et al. (2021). As an effective information filtering tool that can assist consumers in coping with information overload, recommendation systems have seen widespread use in a variety of areas, including e-commerce, film, music, and news, amongst others Calvaresi et al. (2017). Using recommendation techniques to understand user requirements from huge amounts of user activity data, a recommendation system has the potential to successfully deliver individualized recommendations to users. At the moment, there are three main ways to make recommendations: collaborative filtering, content-based filtering, and hybrid filtering Charulatha A. et al (2020).

As a result of the rapid growth of modern civilization and the significant improvement in people's living conditions, the topic of health has attracted an increasing amount of attention from people all over the world. More and more people today are interested in leading a healthy lifestyle and keeping their bodies in a healthy state. According to the contemporary conception of health, being disease-free is no longer the only criterion for being healthy. The World Health Organization (WHO) describes "health" as a state that encompasses total mental, physical, and social well-being Patton M. et al. (2015). People who take care of their health can expect to live longer, and this has a direct bearing not just on the quality of life they enjoy but also on the amount of professional success they find themselves capable of achieving. At this time, non-communicable diseases are the primary causes of death that put a strain on human health. Non-communicable diseases account for more than 63 percent of all deaths worldwide, with heart disease, cancer, chronic lung diseases, diabetes, and others being the most common. Occupational, environmental, nutritional, and lifestyle variables are the primary contributors to the development of these disorders. In general, it is possible to avoid the majority of the problems caused. Alterations in one's pattern of behavior can also be an effective means of bettering one's health Baker et al. (2017).

When it comes to eating, more and more individuals are opting for organic and healthier options. Additionally, there has been an increase in the frequency of various health checkups as well as physical activities Rghioui et al. (2018). People are unable to live healthy lives and frequently make decisions that negatively impact both their physical and mental health because of factors such as their hectic work schedules, unhealthy habits, inadequate health awareness, unclear health-related knowledge, and a variety of other factors. Although different people have different ideas about what constitutes a balanced life, it is a widely held belief that the most important aspects of maintaining one's health are maintaining an optimistic mood, eating good food, and exercising on a regular basis. This is despite the fact that different people have different ideas about what constitutes a healthy lifestyle. Clearly, needs and standards pertaining to one's health change, depending on one's age as well as gender. The ideal state of health that each person strives for is likewise unique to them as an individual. So, one of the biggest challenges is figuring out how to give people advice that is both scientific and personalized, so that it fits their needs and helps them promote, maintain, and improve their current state of health Zhu et al. (2019).

As a result of the proliferation of digital health, both patients and medical professionals are now confronted with an overwhelming quantity of health data, which results in a large rise in the amount of time required to make decisions. In recent years, the field of recommended systems has noticed a rise in the amount of interest in the subject of recommended systems for health. They believe that a recommended system can help patients and doctors cope with information overload by providing useful and accurate advice on, for example, disease severity estimation, disease diagnosis, treatment, health management, and behavioral change due to the recommended system's unique advantages that have emerged rapidly over the years Dash et al. (2019). This is owing to the unique benefits and rapid development of the recommended system over the decades. The community developing the recommended system faces unprecedented difficulties as it attempts to apply the recommended system to the field of healthcare. Accuracy in estimating, diagnostic reliability, patient satisfaction, and a wide range of suggestions are just a few of the issues that need to be addressed Bahri et al. (2018).

Because the health recommendation system is continually being developed and its applications are continually being broadened, new application scenarios and issues continue to emerge one after the other. This brings not only new opportunities, but also new challenges for the community that has been advocating for the health recommendation system. This article's goal is to provide readers with an overview of various recommendation tactics and explain how such techniques may be applied to a range of different healthcare contexts. Additionally, the paper will demonstrate how such techniques can be used. In order to be more particular, the first thing that happens is that three well-known suggestion tactics are offered, and then each one is followed by a detailed description of itself Ali et al. (2018). We will go over a few different variations in order to provide an overall view of the development of these algorithms. Then, when I was thinking about the past studies, I recalled that many of the findings were published under the heading "suggested solutions for healthcare." According to the findings, researchers focus the majority of their attention on the following areas: making recommendations concerning diet and lifestyle; making recommendations concerning training; making recommendations concerning decision-making for patients and physicians; and making recommendations concerning disease-related prediction. There have been some tough problems with the recommended health system, and these problems need to be solved quickly so that the recommended health system can be better in the future.

2. INTERNET OF MEDICAL THINGS

IoMT Wood et al. (2020) is a key component of today's healthcare infrastructure. More and more healthcare services, including disease diagnosis, can be provided by the Internet of Medical Things (IoMT). Remote monitoring and full chronic disease diagnosis can be improved by utilizing new technologies. Researchers are taking advantage of various wearable sensors. Remote monitoring will be improved, as will the ability to diagnose chronic conditions more quickly and thoroughly. Pulse rate, body temperature, and respiratory values are all recorded by these sensors. Several subcategories of remote health monitoring are shown in Figure 1.

Figure 1. IoMT environment

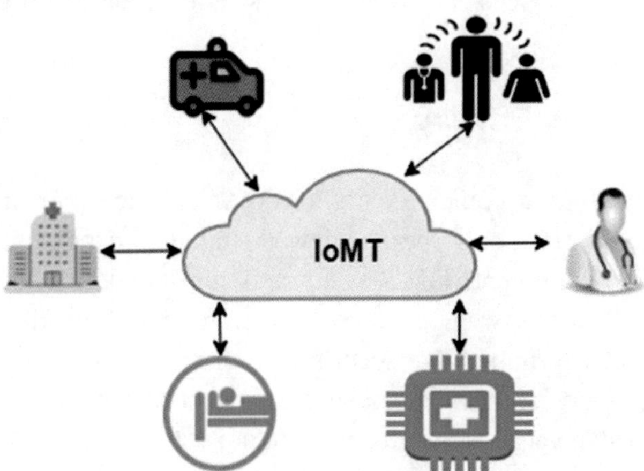

Figure 2. Remote health monitoring

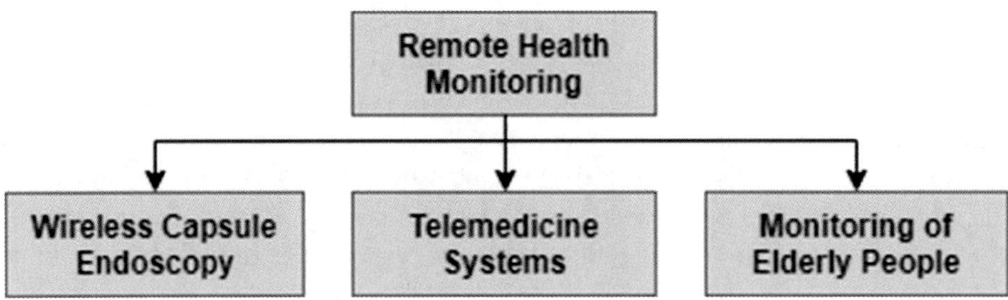

Wireless Capsule Endoscopy (WCE): Imaging technology that uses a capsule-shaped, microscopic camera to take photos of the digestive tract is a subset of Telemonitoring. In this capsule, high-resolution and clear ruptures sent by high-quality video sensors show the inside of the patient's intestines.

Telemedicine systems: Quality healthcare may be delivered to faraway regions thanks to telemedicine, an IoMT medical technology that is currently in development. Visiting a doctor in person or going to the emergency department is no longer necessary thanks to modern technology that enables the ability to treat patients from any location at any time.

Monitoring of aged patients: Elderly patients' care and monitoring are currently a hot topic in scientific research. A health monitoring system is required to keep track of the well-being of the elderly who are afflicted with diseases like Alzheimer's, dementia, linguistic impairment, and hearing loss (among others). Monitoring of the elderly is provided through sensors and wearable devices attached to the patients' bodies through the Internet of Things (IoT). IoMT-based health monitoring applications at these healthcare centers get information from these sensors, and these centers use these applications to help older people keep track of their own health. The centers' services can be received by elderly patients from the comfort of their own homes.

IoMT Security and Privacy

In this section, we'll take a quick look at IoMT system security and privacy. Kaur et al. (2020) used data from 35 peer-reviewed studies to examine the difficulties of IoT healthcare equipment. IoMT safety and confidentiality, the network, the data, the hardware and software, etc., problems were identified within the scope of this article. It was determined that security and privacy were the most major and serious difficulties among the other challenges they faced. Healthcare providers and information security experts should take care to protect users' personal information, according to the authors. According to the evaluation Joyia G. J. et al (2020) 30 papers on healthcare security and privacy were reviewed. A bar chart was used to compare various forms of security threats. These threats include misuse of resources, conspiracy, information leakage, information leakage, data theft, etc. According to the authors, security breaches and data breaches are the primary threats to IoMT applications. In addition, they pointed out that fake data and modifications of data are severe dangers to the security and privacy of IoMT applications. They believe that greater research into access restrictions is necessary. The Survey Parvathy V. S (2021) showed various tiers of healthcare systems and then explored security and privacy for each level separately.

Data Level: Confidentiality, authenticity, and accessibility all fall within the purview of this level. In order to maintain patient data confidentiality, the information that is collected, stored, and exchanged should be correct and up-to-date. Patients should be able to access their data as soon as the security measures are updated.

Sensor Level: Lightweight processing and communication are required for the security approaches used at the sensor level. In order to protect IoMT devices from an intruder, sensors must be tamperproof. An additional requirement is the provision of a real-time intrusion detection system for sensors that depart and return to the environment in which patients are situated. After a network attack, sensors should be able to self-heal, i.e., recover from the damage they sustained. It is possible to employ over-the-air programming to provide self-healing methods, such as altering the network's security policies to thwart malicious attacks. Finally, techniques for bringing new users into (and removing them from) a network are required. Those who join the network can't see the previous messages, and those who leave the network can't see the future ones.

Medical Server Level: Effective access control measures must be established in order to gain access to the patient's data. These approaches should be able

Figure 3. IoMT security and privacy

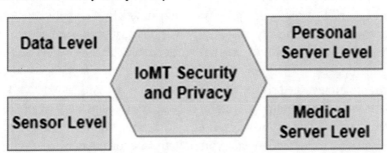

to keep policy sets current in an efficient manner. For IoMT applications, it is critical to have a reliable mechanism for managing keys and distributing them. Because symmetric key cryptography is more appropriate for resource-constrained IoMT devices, these mechanisms typically use it.

As a potential future study direction, the Majumder et al. (2017) mention blockchain technology. They use MedRec as an example of how blockchain can be used to secure electronic health records, permission management, and access to medical records.

As stated in Dias D. et al. (2018), IoMT systems can be vulnerable to assaults that cause genuine physical injury and endanger the lives of patients due to a lack of security awareness on the part of patients, doctors, medical personnel, etc. Because of this, the authors devised the IoMT Security Assessment Framework, or IoMT-SAF, a web-based tool that recommends a comprehensive set of assessment attributes, or 260 questions, to help organizations analyses their IoMT security. Among the various types of these queries and attributes are web security, software security, personal privacy, and physical security. Depending on the situation, this aids IoMT users in enforcing security according to their own security goals. The Poll asks about many privacy and security issues such as data encryption, access control, third-party audits you can trust, data search, etc.

Encryption of Data: Due to the limited resources of sensors in IoMT applications, lightweight cryptographic techniques must be used to ensure confidentiality while not compromising real-time and uninterrupted monitoring systems. This can be accomplished by using algorithms with a smaller memory footprint. Protocols for managing keys are also an important part of these kinds of programs.

Access Control: It is possible to restrict access to certain resources, such as those belonging to a patient's doctor or a medical staff member's computer, to those who are permitted to do so. The authors talked about attribute-based encryption, symmetric encryption, and asymmetric encryption as ways to use encryption for access control Islam et al. (2020).

There is a risk of data corruption in cloud-based IoMT applications because cloud servers aren't completely trustworthy. Various unsupervised machine learning approaches allow service providers to be held accountable using supervised machine learning methods.

In order to protect the privacy of the users, sensitive healthcare data is typically encrypted before being sent to a cloud server. As a result, users can search for encrypted data in a variety of ways. Some of these methods are advanced search data encryption and public-key encryption with keyword search.

Figure 4. Challenges in IoMT security and privacy

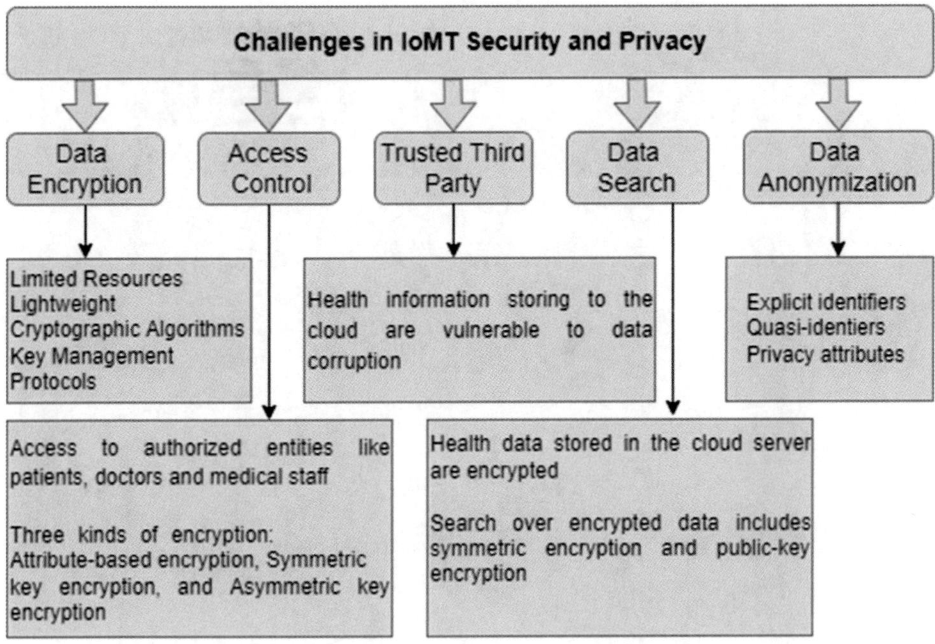

The following categories apply to the private medical data of patients: Patient identifiers include the patient's name, identification number, and phone number. A patient's name, date of birth, address, and age are all examples of quasi-identifiers. Income and illness are examples of sensitive information that falls under the category of "privacy attributes."

IoMT Systems Framework Development Methods

Cloud-based and blockchain-based frameworks can be used to build and implement IoMT systems, respectively. There have been a number of studies on cloud-based IoMT systems, including Dian (2020), Islam et al. (2020), and Sainadh et al. (2021). On the other hand, IoMT systems that run in the cloud have some problems, such as a centralized architecture and a lack of services.

Blockchain technology has the potential to benefit many industries, including finance, notary services, personal data management, and insurance. The technology can also be used in the medical, academic, administration, technology, Internet of Things (IoT), and sharing economy. There have been a number of studies on blockchain-based healthcare applications. Healthcare management, supply chain

Figure 5. IoMT framework based on cloud

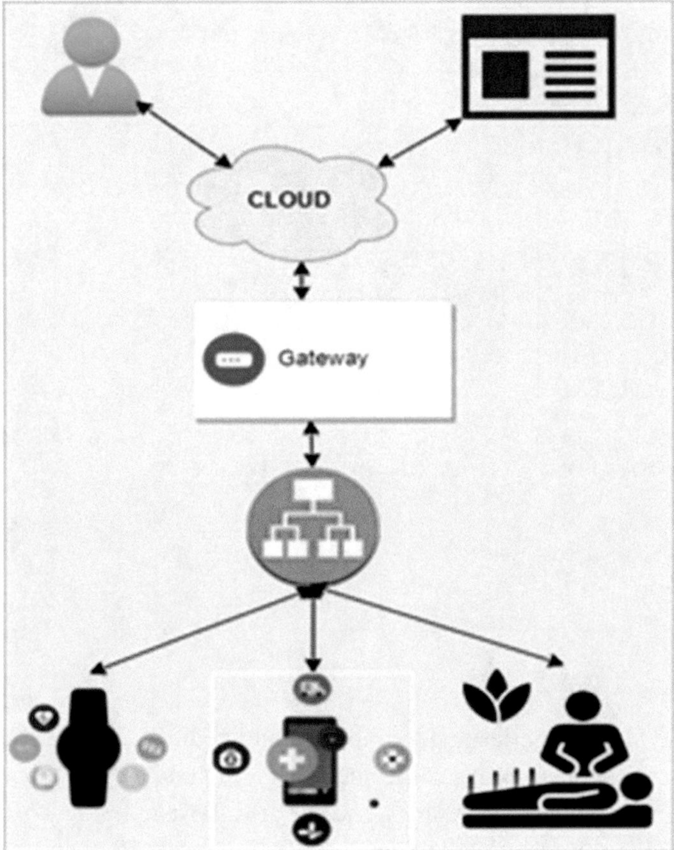

management, health care big data, and IoMT applications were all covered in these studies.

The authors of the study Quintana et al. (2018) developed a concise outline of the process of implementing healthcare systems that are based on blockchain technology. The authors emphasized that consideration should be given to the scalability, security, and privacy of data when developing these systems. The blockchain-based IoMT work, on the other hand, is not looked at in their paper, and there are no systematic ways to lower the scalability limits.

The Internet of Medical Things (IoMT) domain itself comprises major applications such as remote health monitoring, emergency medical care, wireless pill endoscopes, telehealth systems, and monitoring of elderly patients. In addition, a number of research studies and surveys have been carried out in reference to the IoMT applications in terms of the privacy and security point of view. As a result, we found that none of these studies investigated blockchain technology as a future alternative for benefits such as decentralized reliability, integrity, transparency, accountability, and other such things. The present top-of-the-line survey Majumder et al. (2019)

examined the impact of several types of technology on IoMT. Big data, software-defined networks, edge/fog computing, machine learning, and blockchain all come into this area. The quality of service offered by IoMT systems could also benefit from the application of these technologies, according to the authors. However, this survey does not primarily focus on blockchain-based Internet of Things (IoMT) platforms. In contrast to these systems, our research addresses the durability of blockchain-based IoMT systems in full. As the survey emphasized, despite its briefness, blockchain technology is a promising direction for future research that has the potential to provide substantial security for users' sensitive information and security.

There are systems in which sensors and wearable devices are constrained in terms of computational power, communication bandwidth, and storage capacity. Instead of requiring only a small amount of computation and storage capacity, blockchain technology demands an enormous quantity of both of these types of resources. In addition, the number of entities taking part in IoMT systems is increasing. In addition to sensors, wearable medical devices, private clinics and healthcare centers, enterprise research organizations and insurance firms are also included in this group of enterprises. There is a growing demand for extremely large IoMT systems, but centralized communication is unable to meet this demand. Because of this, substantial and exhaustive research is needed on the blockchain-based IoMT software. This study should be about scalability, which is the most important part, and it should also give advice about this.

SMART MEDICAL KIT SYSTEM ARCHITECTURE

The Smart Medical Kit (SMK) should have a smart medicine box with sophisticated deep learning algorithms to achieve cognitive sentimental cognition and medication monitoring in the health care system. Medical cloud resources can be managed remotely via edge computing, which provides low latency and a secure infrastructure Zhang et al. (2020). As an optional piece of hardware, the health assistant system now includes smart clothing for the purpose of gathering physiological data from depression patients. The MEMO-system, which are a smart medical carrier, an application interface that can be used to talk to users, an edge-computing device, medical cloud computing, and a wearable device that is not required but can be used.

Smart Medicine Box

A smart medicine box is designed to collect and transmit data on patients' behavior and environmental conditions. It is the heart of the system's hardware processing and the foundation for a patient health management program Tabei et al. (2020). To help depression sufferers get the most out of their treatment, this study presents a multi-purpose electronic medicine box that also improves the brain's ability to perceive the environment. The Medicine-Box has two more modules besides the medicine module and the environment module. These are the medication module and the environment module.

Intuitive Software Interface

A crucial interface to realize connection with patients, an intuitive software interface most commonly referred to as an API, matches a medicine kit. The intuitive software interface is actually the software application of the SMK. Patients are provided with tasks such as prescription plans, drug reminders, activity data, and individualized health suggestions through the SMK system, which is comprised of both hardware and software that work together to provide these services. This application programming interface mostly displays the patient's previous drug record, the mobility status, and so on. In addition to making it possible to record data, the application programming interface (API) also makes use of a number of lightweight, clever algorithms. This allows the API to offer individualized therapy recommendations and counselling to patients suffering from depression. The medicine box is linked to an app that reminds people with depression to take their medicine at the right times. This helps people develop good medication habits and move toward a full recovery.

Edge-Computing Phase

The proximity computing paradigm of the edge computing terminal relies on the local medical centers in the neighborhood to give services to patients. Local edge computing sites have the potential to alleviate the pressure that is placed on medical services as a result of the widespread distribution of medical resources. In addition, these sites can make it easier for physicians to access the information of their patients in order to make prudent medical decisions that could mean the difference between life and death. Edge nodes perform some of the more straightforward processing of data during cloud transmission. This helps to reduce the amount of data that must be sent from the device to the cloud. Through the use of edge computing, fundamental patient care and health detection can be maintained even in the event of a provisional collapse of the information center or an internal network Le et al. (2021).

Medical Cloud Engine

The MEMO system's regulating and storage functions are centralized within the medical cloud engine. The storage and processing capabilities offered by Medical Cloud Engine are made possible by leveraging cloud computing technology. Users will have access to a resource management environment that can be configured thanks to the virtualization of computing resources, which will also make the delivery of on-demand resources possible. As a result, virtual storage technology enables huge amounts of data to be transferred simultaneously. In order to provide patients with emotion recognition, disease warnings, health advice, and other services, our system relies on an intelligent medical cloud engine (API). The API analyses patient data in depth by using a wide range of algorithms that are based on artificial intelligence.

Wearable Device

Patients' psychological responses, as well as their physical data, are important indicators that help to reflect the illness state of depressed patients. The medication behavior of depressive patients is one important indicator that helps to reflect the health status of depressive patients. Smart clothing is an excellent option for collecting physiological data from patients. Micro-sensors are sewn into the fabric of the clothing, and the benefits of wearing smart clothing include data collection that is unaffected by interference, accurate physiological detection, and a comfortable wearing experience. The patient's physiological health is monitored and the patient's physiological data is gathered via "smart clothing," which is an optional form of wearable technology. The above physical data will be used as extra information in an investigation of the health status of patients who are suffering from depression Karmore et al. (2020).

The smart garments contain a number of different microsensors, each of which sends its own unique signal to a data processing module. This module is responsible for collecting and processing the information collected by the sensors.

When the system is in the connectionless state, the processed data remains in the local storage module. When the communication module becomes available, data will be transmitted to the cloud storage. In addition to this, the module that is being charged will supply power to all of the modules that are now being used. In the final stage, the data about the patients is uploaded to a cloud storage service in order to facilitate additional analysis and storage.

VIRTUAL HEALTHCARE SERVICES

Multiple emerging technologies need to be integrated into existing healthcare systems in order to construct resilient and robust healthcare systems. This will make it possible to give care that is everywhere and personal, care that is centered on the patient, intelligent disease identification and estimation, and monitoring of patients from afar.

Virtual Clinics and Remote Monitoring of Patients

Using various communications channels and digital health technologies, remote-patient monitoring and tracking can be used to provide healthcare services to patients in remote locations. This objective can be reached by the utilization of intelligent wearables, intelligent devices based on sensors, and intelligent health applications. For instance, sensor-based wearable technology devices have been utilized in order to monitor the detecting features of COVID-19. Currently on the market, there is a wide selection of remote patient monitoring systems to choose from. Some of these systems are responsible for monitoring the patient's vital indicators, such as their heart rate and the amount of oxygen that is present in their blood, while others are responsible for monitoring the patient's temperature and the rate at which they breathe. It is possible to notify patients if changes in their physiological state become concerning, so avoiding the need for hospitalization. Patients and healthcare professionals can communicate virtually via phone, video connection, or other web-based platforms in virtual clinics. Virtual clinics have the potential to reduce the spread of highly contagious diseases, decrease the amount of time that patients are required to wait, and improve the quality of medical care by decreasing the amount of direct patient engagement Cacovean et al. (2020).

Emotive eHealth

The practice of diagnosing and treating patients through the benefits of information and telecommunications systems is known as telemedicine. Telemedicine has a wide range of cutting-edge technical tools that can improve healthcare service delivery. Services like tele-consultation, remote patient monitoring, and tele-expertise are only some of the many telemedicine services available Cacovean et al. (2020). Patients who need therapy as an integral component of their treatment or for their overall well-being might receive post-diagnosis rehabilitation through tele-rehabilitation services. In the event of a patient's physical injury or damage, smart virtual treatment is frequently applied. Therapeutic communication, audiology, and neurophysiology are examples of non-physical services. Technology-based interventions for the elderly need to be accessible, low-cost, and simple to use. Additionally, the necessity of in-depth training and instruction for those who are engaged cannot be emphasized enough. Many diseases, both contagious and non-contagious, can now be treated with telemedicine. This frees up healthcare resources and improves access to high-quality care. According to the findings of empirical research, the implementation of telemedicine is hampered by a variety of variables, including those that are technological, organizational, legal, regulatory, individual, economic, and cultural. It's possible that many underdeveloped countries face a setback due to infrastructural development and finance as well as a lack of computing equipment and internet connectivity for patients. The lack of emotional qualities in existing telemedicine services is a major drawback.

Ambient Assisted Living

The detection and management of illness, as well as patient monitoring, have become more sophisticated as a result of the implementation of technologies such as artificial intelligence, surgical robots, and nanotechnology. When a patient of any age or medical condition can use technology to aid them with their everyday activities and monitor their health, we say they are living an AAL-enabled life. In AAL, the utilization of a home automation assistance method for the purpose of regulating the health status of patients and getting prescriptions from physicians in a remote location has proven to be beneficial. Even though AAL systems are most commonly used for elderly patients, autistic health care workers, convalescent patients, and patients dealing with disabilities, Ali et al. (2020) were able to successfully construct a smart home platform for ambient assisted living (AAL) for people with dementia. The technology that AAL offers includes, among other things, smart sensors, wireless body area networks, wearable devices that can communicate with significant medical information systems, and monitoring sensors.

Smart Wellness Self-Management

When it comes to self-management, it's an ongoing process that requires constant attention to one's self-identified requirements. Patient self-monitoring in real time, quick observation of health data, and early interference in medical behavior are all becoming increasingly important in healthcare 5.0. Wearable sensors and Internet of Things (IoT) and Bluetooth/wireless-enabled devices have been developed to help meet the demand for intelligent wellness monitoring. Using data from apps that have been shut down to guide self-management or self-treatment has serious consequences.

Reminders for Treatment, Compliance, and Adherence

The term “smart treatment” relates to online prescriptions and medicine delivery. With the use of interconnected smart technology, E-Health systems and smart wearables can be used to track treatment compliance and adherence. For example, research by Deperlioglu et al. (2020) used a sensor-based drug dispenser to remotely monitor treatment adherence. As soon as a patient opens the dispenser, the dispenser will broadcast adherence data to healthcare experts, including the time, number of pills, and date. Emails are sent to both patients and healthcare professionals if a patient misses a dose.

Connected and Personalized Healthcare

Medical practitioners can remotely access, interpret, and analyze biosensor and smart wearable device health data to provide tailored and linked healthcare from anywhere. Patients’ specific healthcare demands will be met by incorporating new technology into smart digital health. It is common practice for medical service providers, healthcare specialists, and patients to engage in the real-time sharing and presentation of patient health data. Therefore, the new technologies that are part of Healthcare 5.0 will lead to the development of a healthcare model that is proactive and episodic. This model will be quite different from the more traditional paradigm.

SIGNIFICANT EMERGING TECHNOLOGIES AND THEIR RESPECTIVE FUNCTIONS IN HEALTHCARE 5.0

Nanotechnology, 5G technology, drone technology, blockchain, robots, big data, IoT, AI, and cloud computing can all be used in healthcare 5.0.

Nanotechnology

The applications of nanotechnology will be of tremendous help to Healthcare 5.0. The delivery of medical care could experience a revolutionary shift because of the application of nanotechnology. Nanotechnology plays an important part in the process of developing new types of protective equipment as well as vaccines. Nanotechnology encompasses not only the manipulation and production of nanodevices but also their materials, processes, and applications as well. This technology is being used in a variety of medical fields, including gene therapy with non-viral nanostructures, targeted drug delivery, disease prevention and treatment, and more. Evidence of this may be seen in the application of nanotechnology in medical care, which has resulted in the creation of new nanomaterials and nanodevices, as well as in the utilization of nano-implants, nano-biosensors, and the Internet of Nano Things (IoNT). Through the application of IoNT concepts in the medical field, improvements have been made toward more personalized, fast, and convenient health monitoring and treatment. In the field of medicine, the term "nano things" refers to the nanoscale miniaturization of biosensing and intelligent health implants that make use of nanobiosensors and nanosensors. The use of this technology has allowed for the performance of nanoscale operations as well as the intelligent administration of drugs. Because of the biochemical and biophysical signals they pick up, nanobiosensors are able to identify diseases at an early stage at the level of a single cell or molecule. Several different types of nanosensors, such as optical/colorimetric, electrochemical, and chiral sensors, have been utilised in the process of detecting COVID-19. As a consequence of this, the combination of the IoNT and nanosensors will result in the development of a wide range of nano-based health monitoring applications. Some examples of these applications are a glucose sensor, a cholesterol sensor, and a sodium sensor.

IoT

The Internet of Things (IoT) has seen widespread adoption in the healthcare industry as a means to connect various medical devices and share patient information Khan M A et al. (2020). Emerging in the field of healthcare are a variety of sensor-based Internet of Things versions, each with their own set of distinguishing qualities. Because of the Internet of Things, it is now feasible to connect health-related gadgets, wearables, cognitive medical devices, and the internet of medical things via the internet of things. The Internet of Things (IoT) serves as the link between nanoscale items and preexisting communication networks, allowing for the execution of activities such as sensing, actuation, and transfer via electromagnetic radiation. Because of this, the varieties of the Internet of Things make networked healthcare possible. Networked healthcare makes it easier to integrate intelligent medical devices and to share extensive amounts of health data remotely. Smart devices, for instance, make it possible to do remote monitoring of health-care services, thus transforming traditionally practiced medicine into "smart" medicine. As a consequence of this, healthcare staff now have the ability to remotely access, process, and analyze data from biosensors and intelligent wearable devices in order to improve the delivery of healthcare services. In addition to these changes, the Internet of Medical Things (IoMT), the Internet of Things (IoT), and the Internet of Health Things (IoHT) all make it possible to get access to a wide range of medical information and services that can be tailored to each patient's needs Rghioui et al. (2021).

Artificial Intelligence

The next generation of healthcare, which will be known as healthcare 5.0, will be created when AI and automation are incorporated into the delivery of medical treatment. Using highly integrated sensor-based AI embedded systems like smart wearables, it is feasible to monitor, gather, and diagnose diseases by using the symptoms retrieved from sensory data. This can be done in real time. The use of sensors gives intelligent systems the ability to recognize and react to their environments. Medical AI 5.0 encompasses many different concepts, such as the design of emotional sensor-based AI smart devices, the automated and accurate detection and diagnosis of diseases, as well as the development of smart drugs and the effective remote monitoring of patients. Patients with post-traumatic stress disorder can't be monitored by smart wearables since they don't have the cognitive ability to do it. Sensor-based artificial intelligence systems in healthcare 5.0 will have the ability to think, interact with humans through the use of sensors, and respond to input from the surrounding environment in a manner that is consistent with human behavior. This is such a powerful sensation Punitha Ponmalar et al. (2019). Emotion modelling and high-level reasoning will eventually be integrated into AI systems that are extremely modular, bio-inspired, and hybrid in nature. Cognitive artificial intelligence systems that are built on sensors have the potential to alter the delivery of healthcare in a variety of different ways. Sensor-based cognitive AI systems can be useful in a variety of mental health monitoring applications. One such application is one that monitors a person's mental health by listening to their cellphone calls and analyzing the speaker's speech in order to identify signs of anxiety and fluctuations in mood. Wearable devices that are capable of monitoring a patient's mood, tension, anxiety, and even pain could be developed utilizing emotion-aware artificial intelligence as part of the next generation of healthcare, known as healthcare 5.0 (AI). This can be used to help individuals with chronic conditions estimate their risk behavior in order to reduce readmissions and personalize the care that they get. Research and clinical trials are not the only areas that stand to benefit from artificial intelligence and other growing technologies. Medical imaging diagnostics, drug development and production, clinical trials, and autonomous robotic surgery all stand to see improvements.

5G Technology

New global wireless standards are required in order to ensure the successful digital integration of smart devices into healthcare 5.0. These standards must have high data transfer rates and capacity, and they must be organized in a multiple-in-multiple-out architecture. The only way to swiftly and reliably obtain health data is if it can be retrieved at a high and consistent data rate. This is a requirement for developing technologies such as robots and artificial intelligence, as well as for cloud computing Marques et al. (2019). The high user data rate and extensive network signal coverage both contribute to the fact that 5G is an important and necessary technology. It has the capacity to manage one thousand times the normal amount of traffic in the transmission channel. Utilizing this technology allowed for the development of a method of data transfer that features extremely low latency, high levels of security, and a low cost. A sea change from the mobile networks of today is signaled by the introduction of 5G, which will provide high-speed access everywhere and an integrated user experience. Intelligent sensor systems with high data transfer rates can be used to provide remote clinical services, like healthcare delivery and diagnosis, to patients who live a long way from a provider's office. These patients can be diagnosed and treated using the communication infrastructure.

Robotics

There has been an abrupt shift toward practices driven by technology, which has pushed the limits of technology in nearly every business, including health care. This has caused a number of problems for those industries. The implementation of robots will undoubtedly have a significant impact on Healthcare 5.0 Syed et al. (2019). This includes sending medical supplies to health institutions and medication to patients who have COVID-19; offering medical advice and virtual rehabilitation utilizing robots and drones; and delivering medical supplies and medication to patients who have COVID-19. The performance of everyday tasks has also been made easier for healthcare personnel thanks to the introduction of automated systems. Recent advancements in digital automation and robotics technology continue to serve as a driving force behind the creation of many types of robots, including telerobots, collaborative robots, autonomous robots, social robots, and wearable robots. The provision of medical services has seen significant advancements as a result of the use of robots to carry out surgical procedures, make diagnoses of medical conditions, and manufacture immunizations. It is still necessary to overcome a great number of obstacles in the field of robots, particularly in healthcare 5.0. This is due to the lack of emotional recognition as well as the absence of individualized treatment and applications that are ubiquitous throughout the body.

Drone Technology

The medical field is changing all over the world because of new technologies like robots, drones, and other self-operating equipment. In point of fact, evidence of this can be found in the growth in their usage during the COVID-19 pandemic. The use of drones by regulatory authorities to monitor compliance with COVID-19 procedures like lockout and mobility restrictions is an excellent example of this. These authorities want to make sure that the processes are followed as specified. There are a variety of potential applications for drone technology in the future, including medical and food supplies, surveillance, the screening of infectious symptoms, and the promotion of public awareness. In COVID-19 high-risk areas, contaminated surfaces are being cleaned up with the help of drones.

Big Data

The ever-increasing quantities of health data made available by digital technologies have been a driving force behind recent scientific advancements in the field of medicine. Because of advancements in digital health technologies such as telemedicine, electronic medical records, electronic health records, personal health records, and other digital health platforms, there has been a significant improvement in both the cost-effectiveness and efficiency of medical care, as well as a reduction in the number of errors made by medical professionals. As a result of the interconnection of intelligent sensors, smart devices, and various other digital health technologies, there will be an increase in the use of big data in healthcare 5.0. This kind of data will be extremely helpful to researchers in terms of both the identification and prevention of diseases, as well as the delivery of tailored medical care in the near future. As a direct consequence of this, patients and healthcare professionals are on the cusp of enormous prospects, and it is anticipated that big data will have an impact on health systems that is unparalleled. For instance, in the context of COVID-19, artificial intelligence models analyzed health data in the form of big data to detect COVID-19 from X-ray chest images, effective contact tracking through intelligent mobile applications, and clustering and mapping COVID-19 hotspots, among other things. This was accomplished by analyzing symptoms, patient care data, X-ray reports, and case history.

Cloud Computing

Cloud computing makes use of the Internet and remote servers to supply computing resources and data to computer systems so that programs and data can be managed. It improves productivity while simultaneously cutting costs associated with storing, processing, analyzing, and managing the medical records of patients. Because of the one-of-a-kind procedures and adaptability of this technology, accessing the resources stored in the cloud is now simpler and more efficient than ever before. Cloud service providers take advantage of the Internet's underlying infrastructure in order to link patients and medical professionals through the use of cloud-based health applications.

An example of this would be the development of a cloud-based, sensor-equipped smart helmet for miners, which would monitor the wearer's levels of worry, fatigue, and attention. The improvement of these many kinds of interventions paves the way for personalized healthcare to be offered. The concept of cloud computing has the potential to support a range of other operations connected to healthcare, such as the remote monitoring of patients, the sharing and updating of medical records, and perhaps most importantly, the provision of online therapeutic and diagnostic services. This is an extremely important point because of the integration of smart devices and smart applications. As a consequence of this, new digital health technologies need to be developed. These new technologies need to have powerful application programming interfaces and a substantial shift in communication protocols.

Blockchain

The financial services sector has taken note of blockchain because of its capacity to enable peer-to-peer electronic coin transactions between users without the need for a third-party escrow service. The data that is required to be stored is put into chronological order and made public using the blocks that make up a blockchain. Transactions are stored in an append-only data structure, which means that they are unable to keep up with the continual influx of new information. The non-reputability and immutability of the blockchain are two of its most valuable characteristics. Because they are immutable and cannot be updated computationally, transactions on the blockchain cannot be changed or manipulated in any way. A blockchain stores many versions of each transaction, which helps to ensure that it cannot be disputed. As a direct consequence of this, healthcare organizations are increasingly looking to blockchain technology as a means to allow the safe sharing of patient data Stavrotheodoros et al. (2022). For this reason, for instance, it has been hypothesized that the implementation of blockchain technology within the healthcare sector will improve digital access rules in addition to data aggregation and liquidity (secure transmission of health data across multiple entities). Other applications of blockchain technology include electronic medical records, claims made to health insurance companies, remote patient monitoring, and the supply chain for pharmaceuticals. In the near future, version 5.0 of blockchain applications in the healthcare industry may be able to offer scalability and patient-driven semantic interoperability by building strong API links between a wide range of digital health systems.

REFERENCES

Ali, F., El-Sappagh, S., Islam, S. R., Kwak, D., Ali, A., Imran, M., & Kwak, K. S. (2020). A smart healthcare monitoring system for heart disease prediction based on ensemble deep learning and feature fusion. *Information Fusion*, *63*, 208–222. doi:10.1016/j.inffus.2020.06.008

Ali, O., Shrestha, A., Soar, J., & Wamba, S. F. (2018). Cloud computing-enabled healthcare opportunities, issues, and applications: A systematic review. *International Journal of Information Management*, *43*, 146–158. doi:10.1016/j.ijinfomgt.2018.07.009

Bahri, S., Zoghlami, N., Abed, M., & Tavares, J. M. R. (2018). Big data for healthcare: A survey. *IEEE Access : Practical Innovations, Open Solutions*, *7*, 7397–7408. doi:10.1109/ACCESS.2018.2889180

Baker, S. B., Xiang, W., & Atkinson, I. (2017). Internet of things for smart healthcare: Technologies, challenges, and opportunities. *IEEE Access : Practical Innovations, Open Solutions*, *5*, 26521–26544. doi:10.1109/ACCESS.2017.2775180

Cacovean, D., Ioana, I., & Nitulescu, G. (2020). IoT system in diagnosis of Covid-19 patients. *Informações Econômicas*, *24*(2), 75–89. doi:10.24818/issn14531305/24.2.2020.07

Calvaresi, D., Cesarini, D., Sernani, P., Marinoni, M., Dragoni, A. F., & Sturm, A. (2017). Exploring the ambient assisted living domain: A systematic review. *Journal of Ambient Intelligence and Humanized Computing*, *8*(2), 239–257. doi:10.100712652-016-0374-3

Charulatha, A. R., & Sujatha, R. (2020). Smart healthcare use cases and applications. In *Internet of Things Use Cases for the Healthcare Industry* (pp. 185–203). Springer. doi:10.1007/978-3-030-37526-3_8

Dash, S., Shakyawar, S. K., Sharma, M., & Kaushik, S. (2019). Big data in healthcare: Management, analysis and future prospects. *Journal of Big Data*, *6*(1), 1–25. doi:10.118640537-019-0217-0

Deperlioglu, O., Kose, U., Gupta, D., Khanna, A., & Sangaiah, A. K. (2020). Diagnosis of heart diseases by a secure internet of health things system based on autoencoder deep neural network. *Computer Communications*, *162*, 31–50. doi:10.1016/j.comcom.2020.08.011 PMID:32843778

Dian, F. J., Vahidnia, R., & Rahmati, A. (2020). Wearables and the Internet of Things (IoT), applications, opportunities, and challenges: A Survey. *IEEE Access : Practical Innovations, Open Solutions*, *8*, 69200–69211. doi:10.1109/ACCESS.2020.2986329

Dias, D., & Paulo Silva Cunha, J. (2018). Wearable health devices—Vital sign monitoring, systems and technologies. *Sensors (Basel)*, *18*(8), 2414. doi:10.339018082414 PMID:30044415

Islam, M., Mahmud, S., Muhammad, L. J., Nooruddin, S., & Ayon, S. I. (2020). Wearable technology to assist the patients infected with novel coronavirus (COVID-19). *SN Computer Science*, *1*(6), 1–9. doi:10.100742979-020-00335-4 PMID:33063058

Islam, M., Rahaman, A., & Islam, M. R. (2020). Development of smart healthcare monitoring system in IoT environment. *SN Computer Science*, *1*(3), 1–11. doi:10.100742979-020-00195-y PMID:33063046

Joyia, G. J., Liaqat, R. M., Farooq, A., & Rehman, S. (2017). Internet of medical things (IoMT): Applications, benefits and future challenges in healthcare domain. *Journal of Communication*, *12*(4), 240–247.

Karmore, S., Bodhe, R., Al-Turjman, F., Kumar, R. L., & Pillai, S. (2020). IoT based humanoid software for identification and diagnosis of Covid-19 suspects. *IEEE Sensors Journal*. PMID:36346089

Kaur, H., Atif, M., & Chauhan, R. (2020). An internet of healthcare things (IoHT)-based healthcare monitoring system. In *Advances in intelligent computing and communication* (pp. 475–482). Springer. doi:10.1007/978-981-15-2774-6_56

Khan, M. A., & Algarni, F. (2020). A healthcare monitoring system for the diagnosis of heart disease in the IoMT cloud environment using MSSO-ANFIS. *IEEE Access : Practical Innovations, Open Solutions*, *8*, 122259–122269. doi:10.1109/ACCESS.2020.3006424

Le, D. N., Parvathy, V. S., Gupta, D., Khanna, A., Rodrigues, J. J., & Shankar, K. (2021). IoT enabled depthwise separable convolution neural network with deep support vector machine for COVID-19 diagnosis and classification. *International Journal of Machine Learning and Cybernetics*, *12*(11), 3235–3248. doi:10.100713042-020-01248-7 PMID:33727984

Majumder, S., & Deen, M. J. (2019). Smartphone sensors for health monitoring and diagnosis. *Sensors (Basel)*, *19*(9), 2164. doi:10.339019092164 PMID:31075985

Majumder, S., Mondal, T., & Deen, M. J. (2017). Wearable sensors for remote health monitoring. *Sensors (Basel)*, *17*(1), 130. doi:10.339017010130 PMID:28085085

Marques, G., Pires, I. M., Miranda, N., & Pitarma, R. (2019). Air quality monitoring using assistive robots for ambient assisted living and enhanced living environments through internet of things. *Electronics (Basel)*, *8*(12), 1375. doi:10.3390/electronics8121375

Nasr, M., Islam, M. M., Shehata, S., Karray, F., & Quintana, Y. (2021). Smart healthcare in the age of AI: Recent advances, challenges, and future prospects. *IEEE Access : Practical Innovations, Open Solutions*, *9*, 145248–145270. doi:10.1109/ACCESS.2021.3118960

Parvathy, V. S., Pothiraj, S., & Sampson, J. (2021). Automated internet of medical things (iomt) based healthcare monitoring system. In *Cognitive Internet of Medical Things for Smart Healthcare* (pp. 117–128). Springer. doi:10.1007/978-3-030-55833-8_7

Patton, M. (2015). *US health care costs rise faster than inflation.* Retrieved from Forbes: https://scholar. google. com/scholar

Punitha Ponmalar, P., & Vijayalakshmi, C. R. (2019, December). Aggregation in IoT for Prediction of Diabetics with Machine Learning Techniques. In *International conference on Computer Networks, Big data and IoT* (pp. 789-798). Springer.

Quintana, Y., Darren, F. A. H. Y., Crotty, B., Ruchira, J. A. I. N., Kaldany, E., Gorenberg, M., ... Safran, C. (2018). Infosage: Supporting elders and families through online family networks. *AMIA ... Annual Symposium Proceedings - AMIA Symposium. AMIA Symposium*, *2018*, 932. PMID:30815136

Rghioui, A., Naja, A., Mauri, J. L., & Oumnad, A. (2021). An IOT based diabetic patient monitoring system using machine learning and node MCU. *Journal of Physics: Conference Series*, *1743*(1), 012035. doi:10.1088/1742-6596/1743/1/012035

. Rghioui, A., & Oumnad, A. (2018). Challenges and Opportunities of Internet of Things in Healthcare. *International Journal of Electrical & Computer Engineering, 8*(5).

Sainadh, A. V. M. S., Mohanty, J. S., Teja, G. V., & Bhogal, R. K. (2021, May). IoT Enabled Real-Time Remote Health Monitoring System. In *2021 5th International Conference on Intelligent Computing and Control Systems (ICICCS)* (pp. 428-433). IEEE. 10.1109/ICICCS51141.2021.9432103

Stavrotheodoros, S., Kaklanis, N., Votis, K., Tzovaras, D., & Astell, A. (2022). A hybrid matchmaking approach in the ambient assisted living domain. *Universal Access in the Information Society*, *21*(1), 53–70. doi:10.100710209-020-00756-1

Syed, L., Jabeen, S., Manimala, S., & Alsaeedi, A. (2019). Smart healthcare framework for ambient assisted living using IoMT and big data analytics techniques. *Future Generation Computer Systems*, *101*, 136–151. doi:10.1016/j.future.2019.06.004

Tabei, F., Gresham, J. M., Askarian, B., Jung, K., & Chong, J. W. (2020). Cuff-less blood pressure monitoring system using smartphones. *IEEE Access : Practical Innovations, Open Solutions*, *8*, 11534–11545. doi:10.1109/ACCESS.2020.2965082

Wood, E., Mohamedally, D., Sebire, N. J., & Visram, S. (2020). *44 Internet of healthcare things (IoHT) handheld device for secure patient data retrieval*. Academic Press.

Zhang, G., Mei, Z., Zhang, Y., Ma, X., Lo, B., Chen, D., & Zhang, Y. (2020). A noninvasive blood glucose monitoring system based on smartphone PPG signal processing and machine learning. *IEEE Transactions on Industrial Informatics*, *16*(11), 7209–7218. doi:10.1109/TII.2020.2975222

Zhu, H., Wu, C. K., Koo, C. H., Tsang, Y. T., Liu, Y., Chi, H. R., & Tsang, K. F. (2019). Smart healthcare in the era of internet-of-things. *IEEE Consumer Electronics Magazine*, *8*(5), 26–30. doi:10.1109/MCE.2019.2923929

Chapter 10
Securing Healthcare Systems Integrated With IoT:
Fundamentals, Applications, and Future Trends

S. Boopathi
Muthayammal Engineering College, India

ABSTRACT

This chapter provides an overview of healthcare security systems integrated with IoT, discussing fundamentals, applications, benefits, challenges, and considerations for implementation. Secure data transmission, access control, authentication mechanisms, and privacy preservation techniques are needed to ensure a secure ecosystem. The chapter discusses methods for detecting and responding to security threats, such as intrusion detection systems, security information and event management systems and user training and awareness programs. It emphasizes the importance of compliance with relevant regulations and standards to ensure legal and ethical handling of patient data. The study explores future trends and emerging technologies, such as blockchain, artificial intelligence, and 5G, and their potential impact on healthcare security. By implementing the recommendations, healthcare organizations can enhance security, safeguard patient privacy, and promote trust in the healthcare ecosystem.

INTRODUCTION

Healthcare security systems play a crucial role in safeguarding patient data, protecting medical devices, and ensuring the overall security of healthcare environments. With the rapid advancement of technology, the integration of Internet of Things (IoT)

DOI: 10.4018/978-1-6684-6894-4.ch010

into healthcare security systems has emerged as a promising solution to enhance efficiency, connectivity, and security in the healthcare sector. The IoT refers to a network of interconnected physical devices, sensors, and software that can collect, exchange, and analyze data. In the healthcare context, IoT offers immense potential for improving patient care, streamlining operations, and enabling remote monitoring and management of medical devices. However, the integration of IoT into healthcare security systems introduces new challenges and considerations that need to be addressed to ensure the confidentiality, integrity, and availability of sensitive healthcare information. One of the primary advantages of integrating IoT into healthcare security systems is improved connectivity and communication. IoT-enabled devices can gather real-time data from various sources, such as patient monitors, wearable devices, and environmental sensors. This data can be transmitted securely to healthcare providers, allowing them to monitor patients remotely, track vital signs, and provide timely interventions. The seamless connectivity offered by IoT enhances care coordination, reduces response times, and improves patient outcomes. However, the integration of IoT devices into healthcare environments introduces security risks and vulnerabilities. The sheer number of interconnected devices increases the attack surface and potential entry points for cyber threats. Data privacy and protection become paramount concerns, as healthcare IoT devices collect and transmit sensitive patient information. Unauthorized access, data breaches, and malicious attacks on IoT devices pose significant risks to patient confidentiality and the overall integrity of healthcare systems. To address these challenges, healthcare organizations must implement robust security measures in their IoT deployments (Thibaud et al., 2018; Xu, 2020). Device authentication and access control mechanisms are essential to ensure that only authorized personnel can access and interact with IoT devices. Encryption and secure communication channels should be employed to protect the confidentiality and integrity of data transmitted between IoT devices and healthcare networks.

In addition, network security plays a crucial role in healthcare IoT integration. Segmentation and isolation of IoT devices from critical healthcare systems can help contain potential security breaches and limit the impact of attacks. Vulnerability management, including regular updates and patches for IoT devices, is critical to address newly discovered security vulnerabilities and protect against emerging threats. Compliance with regulatory requirements, such as the Health Insurance Portability and Accountability Act (HIPAA), is also crucial when integrating IoT into healthcare security systems. Healthcare organizations must ensure that their IoT deployments adhere to privacy regulations and data protection laws, including proper consent management and privacy-aware data sharing practices. As the field continues to evolve, ongoing research and innovation are needed to address emerging challenges and leverage the full potential of IoT in healthcare security systems.

Technologies such as blockchain, artificial intelligence (AI)-driven security, and edge computing show promise in enhancing the security and resilience of healthcare IoT deployments (Thibaud et al., 2018).

Hence, the integration of IoT into healthcare security systems offers transformative benefits but also introduces new security challenges. By implementing robust security measures, including authentication, encryption, network segmentation, and vulnerability management, healthcare organizations can leverage the power of IoT while ensuring the confidentiality, integrity, and availability of sensitive healthcare information. Compliance with regulatory requirements and continued research in emerging technologies will be crucial in shaping the future of secure healthcare IoT integration. The applications, benefits and challenges for implementation of IoT with Health care field are explored below (Darshan & Anandakumar, 2015; Thibaud et al., 2018; Xu, 2020).

IoT Applications in the Healthcare Sector

- **Remote Patient Monitoring:** IoT devices, such as wearable sensors, can continuously monitor patient vitals and transmit data to healthcare providers. This enables remote monitoring of patients with chronic conditions, early detection of abnormalities, and timely interventions.
- **Smart Medical Devices:** IoT integration allows medical devices to collect and share data in real-time. For example, smart insulin pumps can monitor glucose levels and automatically deliver insulin doses, improving diabetes management. Smart pill dispensers can track medication adherence and send reminders to patients.
- **Asset and Inventory Management:** IoT enables healthcare facilities to track and manage medical equipment, supplies, and medication inventory more efficiently. RFID tags and sensors can provide real-time location and status information, reducing inventory waste and improving resource allocation.
- **Smart Healthcare Facilities:** IoT can optimize energy consumption, security, and patient flow within healthcare facilities. Automated lighting and temperature control systems, occupancy sensors, and real-time location systems enhance patient comfort, safety, and operational efficiency.

Benefits of IoT in Healthcare

- **Improved Patient Outcomes:** Remote monitoring, timely interventions, and personalized care enabled by IoT can lead to better patient outcomes, reduced hospital readmissions, and improved quality of life for patients.

- **Enhanced Operational Efficiency:** IoT streamlines processes, reduces manual tasks, and optimizes resource allocation. This improves workflow efficiency, reduces healthcare staff workload, and ultimately leads to cost savings.
- **Cost Reduction:** IoT devices can help prevent equipment failures through predictive maintenance, reducing downtime and costly repairs. Efficient inventory management minimizes waste and inventory carrying costs.
- **Patient Empowerment:** IoT enables patients to actively participate in their healthcare by accessing real-time data, setting health goals, and receiving personalized feedback. This fosters patient engagement and promotes self-management of chronic conditions.

Challenges and Considerations for Implementing IoT in Healthcare

Implementing IoT in healthcare comes with its own set of challenges and considerations:

- **Data Privacy and Security:** The vast amount of sensitive patient data collected by IoT devices raises concerns about data privacy, security breaches, and unauthorized access. Robust security measures, encryption, and compliance with privacy regulations are essential.
- **Interoperability:** Healthcare organizations often use various devices and systems from different manufacturers, which may not be compatible or interoperable. Ensuring seamless integration and data exchange between these systems is a significant challenge.
- **Infrastructure and Network Complexity:** Implementing IoT requires a reliable and secure network infrastructure capable of handling the volume of data generated by IoT devices. Scalability, bandwidth, and network stability must be considered during implementation.
- **Regulatory Compliance:** Healthcare IoT must comply with regulations and standards, such as HIPAA (Health Insurance Portability and Accountability Act) in the United States, to ensure the privacy and security of patient data. Compliance with these regulations adds complexity to IoT implementation.
- **Standardization:** The lack of universal standards and protocols for IoT devices and systems poses interoperability challenges. Establishing industry-wide standards and protocols is crucial for seamless integration and data exchange.

HEALTHCARE IOT ARCHITECTURE AND INFRASTRUCTURE

Healthcare IoT architecture and infrastructure refer to the underlying structure and components required to implement a secure and reliable Internet of Things (IoT) system in the healthcare industry (Figure 1). A well-designed architecture and infrastructure are essential to support the connectivity, data transmission, and integration of IoT devices in healthcare environments (Jabbar et al., 2017; Verma et al., 2019). Here are the key aspects of healthcare IoT architecture and infrastructure:

- **Edge Devices:** These are the IoT devices deployed at the edge of the network, such as wearable sensors, medical devices, and environmental sensors. They collect and transmit data to the central system or cloud for processing and analysis.
- **Network Connectivity:** Robust and secure network connectivity is crucial for healthcare IoT. This includes Wi-Fi, cellular, or specialized IoT networks (e.g., LoRaWAN) that enable seamless communication between edge devices, gateways, and the central system.
- **Gateways:** Gateways act as intermediaries between edge devices and the central system. They aggregate and preprocess data from multiple devices, perform protocol translations, and ensure secure transmission to the central system.
- **Cloud or Central System:** The central system or cloud platform receives, stores, and processes data from IoT devices. It can be hosted on-premises or in a cloud environment. The central system provides data storage, analytics capabilities, and interfaces for healthcare providers to access and analyze the collected data.
- **Data Storage and Management:** Healthcare IoT systems generate a vast amount of data. Robust data storage solutions are required to efficiently store and manage this data. This may involve databases, data lakes, or cloud storage systems with appropriate security and access controls.
- **Data Processing and Analytics:** The central system should have capabilities to process and analyze the collected data in real-time or batch processing modes. This includes data normalization, filtering, aggregation, and applying analytics algorithms to derive meaningful insights.
- **Security Measures:** Healthcare IoT systems must implement strong security measures to protect patient data and ensure the integrity of the system. This includes encryption of data during transmission and storage, access controls, device authentication mechanisms, and regular security updates and patches.
- **Integration With Existing Systems:** Healthcare IoT systems need to seamlessly integrate with existing healthcare IT infrastructure, such as

electronic health records (EHR) systems, hospital information systems (HIS), and clinical decision support systems (CDSS). Integration enables data exchange and interoperability, supporting comprehensive patient care.

- **Scalability and Flexibility:** Healthcare IoT architecture and infrastructure should be designed with scalability and flexibility in mind. The system should accommodate the growing number of IoT devices, support future technological advancements, and adapt to changing healthcare needs and regulations.
- **Regulatory Compliance:** Healthcare IoT systems must comply with relevant regulatory requirements, such as HIPAA (in the United States) or GDPR (in the European Union). Compliance ensures the privacy and security of patient data and protects against legal and reputational risks.

Developing a robust healthcare IoT architecture and infrastructure requires careful planning, collaboration between stakeholders, and a comprehensive understanding of the healthcare environment. By addressing connectivity, data management, security, and integration aspects, healthcare organizations can deploy a reliable and secure IoT system that enhances patient care, improves operational efficiency, and enables data-driven insights.'

Components and Interconnections of a Secure IoT System in Healthcare

A secure IoT system in healthcare consists of several components and their interconnections. Here are the key components and their interconnections (Raghuvanshi et al., 2022; Sultana & Tamanna, 2021):

Edge Devices: IoT devices such as wearable sensors, medical devices, and environmental sensors. Connected to gateways or directly to the network. Collect and transmit data to the central system for processing and analysis.

Gateways: Act as intermediaries between edge devices and the central system. Aggregate and preprocess data from multiple edge devices. Ensure secure transmission of data to the central system. Perform protocol translations if necessary.

Network Infrastructure: Provides the connectivity between edge devices, gateways, and the central system. Can include Wi-Fi, cellular, or specialized IoT networks (e.g., LoRaWAN).

Ensures reliable and secure communication between devices and the central system.

Central System: Receives, stores, and processes data from edge devices. Can be hosted on-premises or in a cloud environment. Provides data storage, analytics capabilities, and user interfaces for accessing and analyzing data.

Figure 1. Architecture: IoT integrated health care system

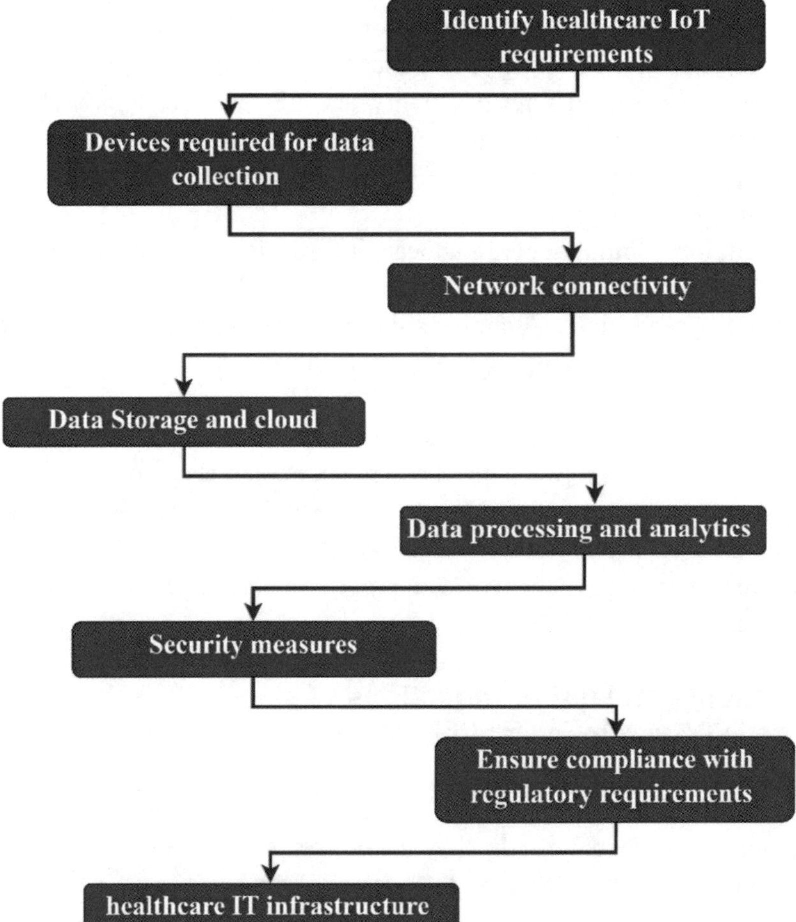

Data Storage and Management: Databases, data lakes, or cloud storage systems store and manage the collected data. Ensure efficient and secure storage of sensitive patient information. Implement appropriate access controls and data encryption to protect data integrity and privacy.

Data Processing and Analytics: Central system processes and analyzes the collected data. Performs tasks such as data normalization, filtering, aggregation, and applying analytics algorithms. Derives meaningful insights from the data for decision-making and healthcare interventions.

Security Measures: Encryption of data during transmission and storage to protect against unauthorized access. Implement authentication mechanisms to ensure only authorized devices and users can access the system. Regular security updates and patches to address vulnerabilities. Monitoring and detection systems to identify and respond to security threats.

Integration With Existing Systems: Integration with existing healthcare IT infrastructure, such as EHR, HIS, and CDSS. Enables seamless data exchange and interoperability between IoT systems and existing healthcare systems. Supports comprehensive patient care and ensures continuity across different healthcare applications.

Scalability and Flexibility: Design the system to accommodate the growing number of IoT devices and changing healthcare needs. Ensure the system can scale up to handle increased data volume and user demands. Allow for future technological advancements and the integration of new devices and applications.

Regulatory Compliance: Adhere to relevant regulations and standards such as HIPAA (in the United States) or GDPR (in the European Union). Ensure the system complies with privacy and security requirements to protect patient data.

These components are interconnected through network connections, data flows, and APIs to create a secure and efficient IoT system in healthcare. Each component plays a crucial role in ensuring the integrity, confidentiality, and availability of data, as well as supporting effective healthcare delivery.

SECURE DATA TRANSMISSION

Secure data transmission is a critical aspect of healthcare IoT systems to protect the confidentiality and integrity of patient data. Encryption and secure communication channels are used to ensure that data transmitted between IoT devices, gateways, and the central system remains secure and protected from unauthorized access or tampering (Jabbar et al., 2017). Here's an overview of encryption and secure communication channels for healthcare IoT:

Encryption

Encryption transforms data into a coded form using cryptographic algorithms, making it unreadable to unauthorized individuals.

Two main types of encryption commonly used in healthcare IoT are:

- **Symmetric Encryption:** Involves using the same key to encrypt and decrypt data. It provides fast processing but requires securely sharing the key between devices.
- **Asymmetric Encryption (Public-Key Encryption):** Utilizes a pair of keys, a public key for encryption and a private key for decryption. It eliminates the

need to share a secret key but has slower processing compared to symmetric encryption.

Secure Communication Channels

- **Transport Layer Security (TLS)/Secure Sockets Layer (SSL):** Widely used protocols for secure communication over the internet. TLS/SSL protocols establish encrypted connections between devices, ensuring data confidentiality and integrity during transmission.
- **Virtual Private Network (VPN):** Creates a secure and encrypted connection between devices or networks over a public network (e.g., the internet). VPNs provide a secure tunnel for transmitting data, protecting it from eavesdropping or unauthorized access.
- **IPsec (Internet Protocol Security):** A suite of protocols that provide secure communication at the IP (Internet Protocol) level. IPsec can be used to encrypt and authenticate data packets to ensure secure transmission between devices.

Certificate-Based Authentication

Certificates are used to authenticate the identity of devices or systems in a healthcare IoT network. Public Key Infrastructure (PKI) is commonly used to issue and manage digital certificates. Each device has a unique certificate, containing its public key, which is used for authentication and establishing secure connections.

Data Integrity Measures

Hashing algorithms, such as SHA-256 (Secure Hash Algorithm 256-bit), can be applied to data to create a unique digital fingerprint, or hash. Hashes are used to verify data integrity during transmission. If the received data does not match the calculated hash, it indicates tampering or data corruption.

Access Controls and Authorization

Access controls should be implemented to ensure that only authorized devices or users can access the IoT system and transmit/receive data. User authentication mechanisms, such as usernames, passwords, or biometric authentication, can be employed to restrict access to sensitive data.

Implementing encryption and secure communication channels requires careful configuration, adherence to security best practices, and the use of reliable cryptographic algorithms. Additionally, regular updates and patches to address vulnerabilities in encryption protocols are essential to maintain a secure healthcare IoT environment.

ACCESS CONTROL AND AUTHENTICATION

Access control and authentication are crucial security measures in healthcare IoT systems to ensure that only authorized individuals or devices can access sensitive data and resources. These measures help protect patient privacy, prevent unauthorized access, and maintain the integrity of the system (Aghili et al., 2019; Verma et al., 2019). Here's an overview of access control and authentication in healthcare IoT:

User Authentication

User authentication verifies the identity of individuals accessing the system. Common authentication methods include passwords, PINs, biometrics (e.g., fingerprints, facial recognition), smart cards, or two-factor authentication (combining multiple authentication factors for enhanced security). Strong password policies and regular password updates should be enforced to prevent unauthorized access.

Device Authentication

Device authentication validates the identity of IoT devices connecting to the system. Each device is assigned a unique identifier or certificate, which is used to authenticate and authorize its access. Public Key Infrastructure (PKI) can be used to issue and manage digital certificates for device authentication.

Role-Based Access Control (RBAC)

RBAC assigns access permissions based on predefined roles within the healthcare IoT system. Each user or device is assigned a specific role that determines their level of access to resources and data. RBAC simplifies access management by granting permissions based on job responsibilities or organizational hierarchies.

Access Control Lists (ACLs)

ACLs define specific rules that determine which users or devices are allowed or denied access to specific resources. ACLs can be based on various criteria such as user/device identity, time of access, or location.

Privilege Management

Privilege management ensures that users or devices only have access to the resources and data they require to perform their authorized tasks. Privileges should be assigned on a need-to-know basis, minimizing the risk of unauthorized access to sensitive information.

Auditing and Logging

Auditing and logging mechanisms track and record access attempts, changes to access control settings, and system activities. Logs provide an audit trail for monitoring and investigating potential security incidents or policy violations.

Regular Security Assessments and Updates

Regular security assessments help identify vulnerabilities in the access control and authentication mechanisms. Patch management ensures that the system is up to date with the latest security updates and fixes.

Training and Awareness

Training and awareness programs educate users and administrators about security best practices, the importance of strong authentication, and the potential risks associated with unauthorized access.

Implementing effective access control and authentication requires a layered approach, combining user authentication, device authentication, and fine-grained access controls. It is essential to regularly review and update access control policies, monitor access logs, and stay informed about emerging security threats to maintain a secure healthcare IoT environment.

Mechanisms to Control Access and Authenticate Users in Healthcare IoT

In healthcare IoT systems, several mechanisms are used to control access and authenticate users, ensuring that only authorized individuals or devices can access sensitive data and resources. Here are some common mechanisms used in healthcare IoT for access control and user authentication:

- **Usernames and Passwords:** Users are assigned unique usernames and passwords to authenticate their identity. Password policies, such as minimum length, complexity requirements, and regular password updates, enhance security. Two-factor authentication (2FA) can be implemented, requiring users to provide an additional verification factor, such as a temporary code sent to their mobile device.

- **Biometric Authentication:** Biometric characteristics, such as fingerprints, facial recognition, or iris scans, can be used to authenticate users. Biometric data is unique to individuals and difficult to forge, enhancing the security of the authentication process.
- **Smart Cards or Tokens:** Users are provided with physical smart cards or tokens containing digital certificates or secure elements. These cards or tokens are used for authentication and can be used in conjunction with PINs or biometric verification.
- **Role-Based Access Control (RBAC):** RBAC assigns access permissions based on predefined roles. Each user is assigned a specific role (e.g., doctor, nurse, administrator), and their access privileges are determined by their role. RBAC simplifies access management by granting permissions based on job responsibilities or organizational hierarchies.
- **Access Control Lists (ACLs):** ACLs define specific rules that determine which users or devices are allowed or denied access to specific resources. ACLs can be based on criteria such as user/device identity, time of access, or location.
- **Certificates and Public Key Infrastructure (PKI): C**ertificates are used to authenticate the identity of devices or systems in a healthcare IoT network. PKI provides a framework for issuing, distributing, and managing digital certificates. Each device or user is assigned a unique certificate containing a public key for authentication and establishing secure connections.
- **Multi-Factor Authentication (MFA):** MFA combines multiple authentication factors, such as something the user knows (e.g., password), something the user has (e.g., smart card), or something the user is (e.g., biometrics). MFA enhances security by requiring users to provide multiple pieces of evidence to authenticate their identity.
- **Access Auditing and Logging:** Auditing and logging mechanisms track and record access attempts, changes to access control settings, and system activities. Logs provide an audit trail for monitoring and investigating potential security incidents or policy violations.
- **Regular Security Assessments and Updates:** Regular security assessments help identify vulnerabilities in the access control and authentication mechanisms. Patch management ensures that the system is up to date with the latest security updates and fixes.

These mechanisms work together to control access and authenticate users in healthcare IoT systems, safeguarding sensitive data and ensuring the integrity of the system. It is important to select and implement appropriate mechanisms based on the specific security requirements and risk profile of the healthcare environment.

TECHNIQUES FOR PRESERVING PRIVACY IN HEALTHCARE IOT SYSTEMS

Preserving privacy in healthcare IoT systems involves implementing various techniques and measures to protect the confidentiality and integrity of patient information (Abouelmehdi et al., 2018; Yamin et al., 2019). Here are some key techniques used for privacy preservation in healthcare IoT (Figure 2):

Data Encryption: Encryption is employed to transform sensitive data into an unreadable form using cryptographic algorithms. Both data at rest and data in transit should be encrypted to prevent unauthorized access. Strong encryption algorithms and secure key management practices should be implemented.

Anonymization and Pseudonymization: Anonymization involves removing or altering personally identifiable information (PII) from data to prevent the identification of individuals. Pseudonymization replaces identifiable information with pseudonyms or codes, making it difficult to link the data to specific individuals.

These techniques minimize the risk of reidentification while still allowing for data analysis and research.

Differential Privacy: Differential privacy adds noise or randomness to query responses or datasets to protect individual privacy. It ensures that the privacy of individuals cannot be compromised even if an adversary has access to the majority of the dataset.

Access Control and Authorization: Access control mechanisms are used to restrict access to sensitive data and resources. Role-based access control (RBAC) assigns access privileges based on predefined roles and responsibilities. Fine-grained access controls and permission settings ensure that only authorized individuals can access specific data.

Data Minimization: Data minimization involves collecting and retaining only the minimum necessary data for a specific purpose. Unnecessary or sensitive

Figure 2. Techniques for preserving privacy in healthcare IOT systems

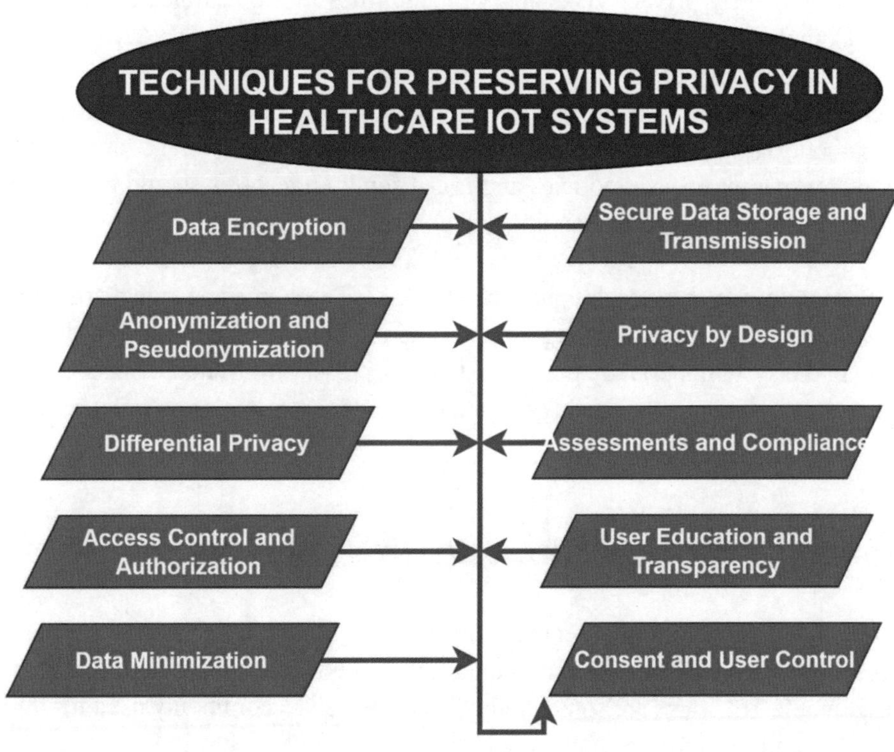

data that is not relevant to the healthcare IoT system's functionality should be avoided or anonymized.

Consent and User Control: Users should have control over the sharing and use of their personal health information. Consent mechanisms should be implemented to ensure that individuals provide informed consent for data collection and usage. Users should have the ability to revoke or modify consent preferences at any time.

Secure Data Storage and Transmission: Robust security measures, including secure cloud storage, encryption, access controls, and secure communication channels, should be employed to protect data. Data should be protected against unauthorized access, data breaches, and interception during transmission.

Privacy by Design: Privacy should be considered and integrated into the design and development of healthcare IoT systems from the beginning. Privacy-enhancing technologies and practices should be implemented by default rather than as an afterthought.

Regular Privacy Assessments and Compliance: Regular privacy assessments help identify privacy risks and vulnerabilities in the healthcare IoT system. Compliance with relevant privacy regulations, such as HIPAA or GDPR, should be ensured.

User Education and Transparency: Users should be provided with clear information about data practices, including data collection, usage, storage, and sharing. Transparent privacy policies and user-friendly interfaces should be provided to promote user understanding and control over their data.

By employing these techniques, healthcare IoT systems can safeguard patient privacy, comply with privacy regulations, and maintain the trust and confidence of users in the system's privacy practices. Privacy preservation should be an ongoing effort, with continuous monitoring and updates to address emerging privacy challenges and evolving regulations.

THREAT DETECTION AND INCIDENT RESPONSE

Detecting and responding to security threats in healthcare IoT systems is crucial to protect sensitive patient data and maintain the integrity of the system (Sanzgiri & Dasgupta, 2016). Here are some methods and strategies commonly used for threat detection and response in healthcare IoT:

Intrusion Detection Systems (IDS) and Intrusion Prevention Systems (IPS): IDS monitors network traffic and system logs to detect potential security breaches or malicious activities.

IPS goes a step further by actively blocking or mitigating identified threats to prevent further damage. These systems use rule-based or behavior-based analysis to identify anomalies and raise alerts.

Security Information and Event Management (SIEM) Systems: SIEM systems collect and analyze log data from various sources to identify security incidents and patterns. They provide real-time monitoring, event correlation, and reporting capabilities to detect and respond to security threats promptly.

Endpoint Protection: Endpoint protection solutions include antivirus, anti-malware, and host intrusion detection/prevention systems installed on IoT devices. These solutions monitor and protect endpoints from malicious software, unauthorized access, and other threats.

Network Segmentation and Segregated IoT Networks: Network segmentation divides the network into separate segments to isolate IoT devices and critical healthcare systems from each other. Segregated IoT networks restrict access to IoT devices and limit their connectivity to necessary services, reducing the attack surface.

Anomaly Detection and Behavioral Analytics: Anomaly detection techniques analyze patterns and behaviors to identify deviations from normal operation. Behavioral analytics leverage machine learning algorithms to establish baseline behavior and detect anomalies that may indicate security threats.

Threat Intelligence and Information Sharing: Organizations can subscribe to threat intelligence services to stay updated on the latest security threats and vulnerabilities. Sharing information and collaborating with other healthcare providers or security communities can help in identifying and mitigating emerging threats.

Incident Response and Preparedness: Developing an incident response plan with predefined procedures and roles ensures a timely and effective response to security incidents. Regular drills and simulations help test the response capabilities and identify areas for improvement.

Security Patching and Updates: Regularly applying security patches and updates to IoT devices, operating systems, and software is crucial to address known vulnerabilities.

User Training and Awareness: Training healthcare staff and IoT system users about security best practices, phishing awareness, and password hygiene helps prevent security incidents caused by human error or social engineering.

Continuous Monitoring and Auditing: Continuous monitoring of network traffic, system logs, and user activities helps identify suspicious behavior or unauthorized access. Regular audits of security controls, configurations, and access privileges ensure compliance and highlight potential weaknesses.

By implementing these methods, healthcare organizations can enhance their ability to detect and respond to security threats in IoT systems promptly, minimizing potential damage and protecting patient data. It is essential to regularly update security measures and stay informed about emerging threats to maintain a strong security posture.

COMPLIANCE AND REGULATORY CONSIDERATIONS

Healthcare IoT systems are subject to compliance requirements and regulations to ensure the privacy, security, and integrity of patient data (Charles et al., 2019; Slama et al., 2015). Here are some of the key compliance requirements and regulations applicable to healthcare IoT systems:

Health Insurance Portability and Accountability Act (HIPAA)

HIPAA sets standards for the privacy and security of protected health information (PHI) in the United States. Healthcare organizations and their business associates must comply with HIPAA's Security Rule and Privacy Rule, which outline requirements for safeguarding PHI and controlling access to it.

General Data Protection Regulation (GDPR)

GDPR is a comprehensive data protection regulation applicable to European Union (EU) member states. It applies to healthcare IoT systems that process personal data of EU residents. GDPR establishes strict requirements for consent, data minimization, data transfers, security, breach notification, and individual rights.

Medical Device Regulations (MDR)

Medical Device Regulations govern the design, manufacturing, and use of medical devices in various regions, such as the European Union (EU) and the United States. Healthcare IoT devices that are considered medical devices must comply with relevant regulations, such as the EU Medical Device Regulation (MDR) or the US Food and Drug Administration (FDA) regulations.

Cybersecurity Frameworks and Standards

Healthcare IoT systems may be required to comply with cybersecurity frameworks and standards, such as the National Institute of Standards and Technology (NIST) Cybersecurity Framework or ISO 27001. These frameworks provide guidelines and best practices for managing cybersecurity risks and protecting sensitive data.

Data Breach Notification Laws

Many countries and regions have data breach notification laws that require organizations to notify individuals and authorities in the event of a data breach. Healthcare IoT systems must have processes in place to detect, respond to, and report data breaches promptly and appropriately.

Ethical Guidelines and Principles

Ethical considerations are increasingly important in healthcare IoT systems to address issues such as data privacy, consent, fairness, transparency, and accountability. Ethical guidelines and principles, such as those outlined by the European Commission's Ethics Guidelines for Trustworthy AI or professional organizations like the American Medical Association (AMA), provide guidance on responsible and ethical use of healthcare IoT technologies.

National and Regional Regulations

In addition to the aforementioned regulations, healthcare IoT systems must comply with national or regional laws and regulations specific to the jurisdiction where they are deployed. These may include data protection laws, health information exchange regulations, and sector-specific requirements.

Compliance with these regulations and requirements is essential for healthcare IoT systems to protect patient privacy, maintain data security, and meet legal and ethical obligations. It is important for organizations to understand and adhere to the specific regulations applicable to their jurisdiction and ensure ongoing compliance through risk assessments, audits, and adherence to industry best practices.

CASE STUDIES AND BEST PRACTICES

The implementation, factors and outcomes of Some case studies are explained as below (Hsiao et al., 2019; Slama et al., 2015).

Case Study: Remote Patient Monitoring (RPM) System

- **Implementation:** A healthcare provider deployed an RPM system using IoT devices to remotely monitor patients with chronic conditions.
- **Success Factors:** The system enabled continuous monitoring of vital signs, allowing early detection of deteriorating conditions and proactive interventions.
- **Outcome:** Effective data integration and analysis were crucial for deriving actionable insights. Interoperability between IoT devices and existing healthcare systems played a significant role in the success of the deployment.

Case Study: Smart Medication Management System

- **Implementation:** A hospital implemented an IoT-based smart medication management system to improve medication safety and reduce errors.
- **Success Factors:** The system utilized IoT devices, barcode scanning, and real-time data capture to ensure accurate medication administration and documentation.
- **Outcome:** Robust data security measures were essential to protect patient information. Comprehensive training and workflow redesign were necessary to ensure smooth adoption by healthcare staff.

Case Study: Asset Tracking and Inventory Management

- **Implementation:** A healthcare facility deployed an IoT-based asset tracking and inventory management system to improve efficiency and reduce costs.
- **Success Factors:** The system utilized RFID or Bluetooth-enabled tags to track medical equipment, supplies, and medication inventory in real-time.
- **Lessons Learned:** Proper planning and mapping of IoT infrastructure, including network coverage and tag placement, were critical for accurate tracking. Regular maintenance and calibration of IoT devices were necessary to maintain data accuracy.

Case Study: Fall Detection and Prevention System

- **Implementation:** A nursing home implemented an IoT-based fall detection and prevention system to enhance resident safety.
- **Success Factors:** The system utilized wearable IoT devices with built-in sensors to detect falls and send alerts to caregivers.
- **Lessons Learned:** Careful consideration of device usability, comfort, and battery life was crucial to ensure acceptance and adoption by elderly residents. False alarms and accuracy of fall detection algorithms required continuous refinement and fine-tuning.

Case Study: Remote Consultation and Telemedicine

- **Implementation:** A healthcare organization implemented an IoT-enabled remote consultation and telemedicine system to provide virtual healthcare services.
- **Success Factors:** The system incorporated IoT devices such as video conferencing tools, remote examination tools, and secure data transmission protocols.

- **Lessons Learned:** Ensuring reliable network connectivity and high-quality audio and video communication were vital for effective telemedicine. Adequate privacy and security measures were essential to protect patient data during remote consultations.

Outcomes from these case studies include the importance of interoperability, data security, user training and acceptance, usability, and continuous monitoring and refinement of IoT systems. It is crucial for organizations to consider these factors and adapt best practices to their specific healthcare IoT deployments to ensure successful implementation and achieve desired outcomes.

FUTURE TRENDS AND EMERGING TECHNOLOGIES

Future trends and emerging technologies have the potential to revolutionize healthcare security and address existing challenges. Here are some key areas of exploration and their potential impact:

Blockchain Technology: Blockchain offers decentralized and secure data storage and sharing, enabling enhanced privacy and integrity of healthcare records. It can facilitate secure patient data exchange, streamline consent management, and ensure auditability of data access and modifications.

Artificial Intelligence (AI) and Machine Learning (ML): AI and ML algorithms can analyze vast amounts of healthcare data to identify patterns, detect anomalies, and predict security threats. They can enhance threat detection, automate security monitoring, and provide real-time incident response.

Edge Computing: Edge computing brings computation and data storage closer to IoT devices, reducing latency and enhancing data security and privacy. It enables faster data processing, local decision-making, and reduced dependence on cloud services, improving overall system performance and security.

5G and Enhanced Connectivity: The deployment of 5G networks will provide high-speed, low-latency connectivity, enabling real-time data transmission and remote monitoring. It will support the growth of telemedicine, remote patient monitoring, and other healthcare IoT applications while ensuring secure and reliable data transmission.

Biometric Authentication: Biometric authentication methods such as fingerprint, iris, and facial recognition can enhance user authentication in healthcare IoT systems. They provide a higher level of security compared to traditional authentication methods and reduce the risk of unauthorized access.

Threat Intelligence and Analytics: Advanced threat intelligence platforms and analytics tools can provide real-time insights into emerging security threats and vulnerabilities. They enable proactive threat hunting, rapid incident response, and informed decision-making to mitigate risks effectively.

Privacy-Preserving Technologies: Emerging techniques such as federated learning, homomorphic encryption, and secure multi-party computation can enable data analysis while preserving privacy. They allow collaborative analysis of sensitive healthcare data without exposing individual patient information.

Quantum Computing: Quantum computing has the potential to break current cryptographic algorithms, posing new challenges to healthcare security. However, it also offers opportunities for developing quantum-resistant encryption algorithms and enhancing data security in the long term.

These emerging technologies hold promise for enhancing healthcare security by addressing current limitations and introducing new capabilities. However, along with their benefits, it is crucial to consider the potential risks and ethical implications associated with their implementation. As these technologies mature, healthcare organizations need to stay informed, evaluate their applicability, and adapt their security strategies to leverage their benefits effectively while ensuring patient privacy and data protection.

CONCLUSION AND RECOMMENDATIONS

Based on the topics discussed, here are some recommendations to strengthen the security of healthcare IoT systems:

- **Implement a Robust Healthcare IoT Architecture:** Design a secure and scalable architecture that encompasses all necessary components and interconnections while considering factors such as data flow, device management, and interoperability.
- **Secure Data Transmission:** Utilize encryption and secure communication channels, such as Transport Layer Security (TLS), to protect data during transmission between IoT devices, gateways, and backend systems.
- **Access Control and Authentication:** Implement strong access control mechanisms, such as multi-factor authentication and role-based access control, to ensure only authorized users can access healthcare IoT systems and sensitive patient data (Anitha et al., 2023; Subha et al., 2023).
- **Privacy Preservation:** Employ privacy-preserving techniques like anonymization, pseudonymization, and differential privacy to protect patient privacy while still allowing for valuable data analysis and insights.
- **Continuous Monitoring and Threat Detection:** Deploy robust intrusion detection and prevention systems, leverage behavioral analytics and anomaly

detection, and regularly monitor network traffic, system logs, and user activities to detect and respond to security threats in a timely manner.

- **Regular Security Assessments and Updates:** Conduct regular security assessments, penetration testing, and vulnerability scanning to identify and address any weaknesses or vulnerabilities in healthcare IoT systems. Keep devices and software up to date with security patches and updates.
- **Compliance With Regulations:** Stay abreast of relevant compliance requirements and regulations, such as HIPAA, GDPR, and medical device regulations, and ensure healthcare IoT systems adhere to these standards.
- **User Training and Awareness:** Educate healthcare staff, users, and patients about the importance of security best practices, phishing awareness, and maintaining strong passwords to minimize the risk of security incidents caused by human error or social engineering attacks.
- **Collaboration and Information Sharing:** Foster collaboration among healthcare organizations, regulatory bodies, and security communities to share knowledge, exchange threat intelligence, and stay informed about emerging security threats and mitigation strategies.

REFERENCES

Abouelmehdi, K., Beni-Hessane, A., & Khaloufi, H. (2018). Big healthcare data: Preserving security and privacy. *Journal of Big Data*, *5*(1), 1–18. doi:10.118640537-017-0110-7

Aghili, S. F., Mala, H., Shojafar, M., & Peris-Lopez, P. (2019). LACO: Lightweight three-factor authentication, access control and ownership transfer scheme for e-health systems in IoT. *Future Generation Computer Systems*, *96*, 410–424. doi:10.1016/j.future.2019.02.020

Anitha, C., R, K. C., Vivekanand, C. V., Lalitha, S. D., Boopathi, S., & R, R. (2023, February). Artificial Intelligence driven security model for Internet of Medical Things ({IoMT}). *IEEE Explore*. doi:10.1109/ICIPTM57143.2023.10117713

Charles, W., Marler, N., Long, L., & Manion, S. (2019). Blockchain compliance by design: Regulatory considerations for blockchain in clinical research. *Frontiers in Blockchain*, *2*, 18. doi:10.3389/fbloc.2019.00018

Darshan, K. R., & Anandakumar, K. R. (2015). A comprehensive review on usage of Internet of Things (IoT) in healthcare system. *2015 International Conference on Emerging Research in Electronics, Computer Science and Technology (ICERECT)*, 132–136. 10.1109/ERECT.2015.7499001

Hsiao, Y.-C., Wu, M.-H., & Li, S. C. (2019). Elevated performance of the smart city—A case study of the IoT by innovation mode. *IEEE Transactions on Engineering Management*, *68*(5), 1461–1475. doi:10.1109/TEM.2019.2908962

Jabbar, S., Ullah, F., Khalid, S., Khan, M., & Han, K. (2017). Semantic interoperability in heterogeneous IoT infrastructure for healthcare. *Wireless Communications and Mobile Computing*, *2017*, 2017. doi:10.1155/2017/9731806

Raghuvanshi, A., Singh, U. K., & Joshi, C. (2022). A review of various security and privacy innovations for IoT applications in healthcare. *Advanced Healthcare Systems: Empowering Physicians with IoT-Enabled Technologies*, 43–58.

Sanzgiri, A., & Dasgupta, D. (2016). Classification of insider threat detection techniques. *Proceedings of the 11th Annual Cyber and Information Security Research Conference*, 1–4.

Slama, D., Puhlmann, F., Morrish, J., & Bhatnagar, R. M. (2015). *Enterprise IoT: Strategies and Best practices for connected products and services*. O'Reilly Media, Inc.

Subha, S., Inbamalar, T. M., R, K. C., Suresh, L. R., Boopathi, S., & Alaskar, K. (2023, February). A Remote Health Care Monitoring system using internet of medical things ({IoMT}). *IEEE Explore*. doi:10.1109/ICIPTM57143.2023.10118103

Sultana, N., & Tamanna, M. (2021). Exploring the benefits and challenges of Internet of Things (IoT) during Covid-19: A case study of Bangladesh. *Discover Internet of Things*, *1*(1), 20. doi:10.100743926-021-00020-9

Thibaud, M., Chi, H., Zhou, W., & Piramuthu, S. (2018). Internet of Things (IoT) in high-risk Environment, Health and Safety (EHS) industries: A comprehensive review. *Decision Support Systems*, *108*, 79–95. doi:10.1016/j.dss.2018.02.005

Verma, A., Prakash, S., Srivastava, V., Kumar, A., & Mukhopadhyay, S. C. (2019). Sensing, controlling, and IoT infrastructure in smart building: A review. *IEEE Sensors Journal*, *19*(20), 9036–9046. doi:10.1109/JSEN.2019.2922409

Xu, G. (2020). IoT-Assisted ECG Monitoring Framework with Secure Data Transmission for Health Care Applications. *IEEE Access : Practical Innovations, Open Solutions*, *8*, 74586–74594. doi:10.1109/ACCESS.2020.2988059

Yamin, M., Alsaawy, Y., & Alkhodre, B., A., & Abi Sen, A. A. (. (2019). An innovative method for preserving privacy in Internet of Things. *Sensors (Basel)*, *19*(15), 3355. doi:10.339019153355 PMID:31370150

Chapter 11
A Blockchain IoT Hybrid Framework for Security and Privacy in a Healthcare Database Network

Puneeta Singh
KIET Group of Institutions, India

Pritish Sinha
Galgotias University, India

Abhinav Raghav
Chandigarh University, India

ABSTRACT

Deep concern is rising in healthcare systems regarding medical data and computing medical customary. With advancement in blockchain technology, an advanced and more secure way of medical data management, sharing, and other services can be implemented with simple innovations in IoT and blockchain. This technology relies on grouping data into block and hold sets of information that once filled are closed and linked to other blocks of data creating a chain of data. This innovation grants high fidelity and a secure way of storing data without any involvement of third-party systems. In this research, the authors harness opportunity and trends that blockchain provides in advanced healthcare systems and how integration of other technologies can lead one of most secure and automatic systems in the health sector and medicine, records serving.

BACKGROUND

Digitization in the modern world has led to many. Every part of our lives is becoming more technical, from educational methods to internet transactions (Azaria et al., 2016;

DOI: 10.4018/978-1-6684-6894-4.ch011

Barry et al., 2020; Bergmann et al., 2017; Chen et al., 2019; Xie et al., 2021). In this situation, "money" is also not left behind. The concept of crypto-currency itself is an innovation of blockchain technology. Bitcoin is the most efficient crypto-currency in digital currency history. Bitcoin is a decentralized kind of online currency that is widely accepted for internet transactions all over the world, obviating the need for any third party to oversee the cash flow (Castro & Liskov, 1999; Dubovitskaya et al., 2017; Ekblaw et al., 2016; Li et al., 2020; Ratta et al., 2021).

Blockchain preserves data in decentralized way, thus independent of any consistent body where all data or transactions occur at Centre of organization (Wang et al., 2018).

Blockchain can be usefully described in other aspects too including tamper proof quality of data stored i.e., data is immutable once accepted in chain structure (Nakamoto, 2008).

Ethereum is one of blockchain structure that has allowed many innovations and decentralized applications by young developers.

Rapid growth in hardware technologies came up with IoT infrastructure evolving connectivity of sensors to Information and Communication Technologies, devices, objects, and services. IoT devices in daily life with smart object is a huge challenge as its implementation is directly based on collection and distribution of information (WHO, 2016).

Privacy by policy and privacy by design is at potential risk in stand-alone IoT system for a work system. Combining Blockchain IoT hybrid is a simple solution in solving each approach disadvantage (Labs, 2019). Our research is concerned about decentralization in blockchain technologies in public access control while limiting data distribution in multi authority sections using consortium approach.

METHODS

Problem Statement and Research

Statement

Boost in population and more need of medical assistance day by day is upscaling deep issue regarding data management, security, and privacy of medical records. Any records from past can be required during medical emergencies and traditional paperback system can fail sometimes due to unnecessary conditions. Ordinary options avail data storage in hard drives or Cloud spaces but there's limitation in storing and types of data that can be saved. Moreover, health institutes are unable to keep these data saved for long time so tends to clear and store new data. Thus, a new way of data management with low storage and high security options is required.

Expected Solution

Blockchain innovation has pulled in various researchers, associations particularly within the use of digital cryptocurrency. A blockchain is termed as decentralized record that can securely store exchanges made in a peer to peer arrange. Additionally, it makes transactions more reliable. Blockchain technology has allowed two parties to conduct exchanges securely without any middle person party mediation ().

Healthcare system has openly accepted role of Artificial Intelligence, Augmented / Virtual Reality and IoT aside of blockchain.

Case Studies

Table 1. Top cited researches on blockchain healthcare system

Citation No.	Title	Blockchain type	Service
(Azaria et al., 2016)	Using blockchain for medical data access and permission management	Private	Data Security
(Chen et al., 2019)	Blockchain based medical records secure storage and medical service framework.	Public	Storage
(Xie et al., 2021)	Applications of Blockchain in the Medical Field	Public	Case Study
(Dubovitskaya et al., 2017)	Secure and trustable electronic medical records sharing using blockchain	Consortium	Data Sharing
(Ratta et al., 2021)	Application of blockchain and internet of things in healthcare and medical sector	Ethereum	IoT service
(Ekblaw et al., 2016)	"MedRec" prototype for electronic health records	Ethereum	Record management

Decentralization in Blockchain

What Is Decentralisation?

Decentralization in blockchain is exchange of control and decision-making from a centralized entity (person, organization, or gather thereof) to a conveyed network. Decentralized systems are a self-system that reliefs trust level over an organization and its participant to be pressed upon each other's and prevent any data misleads or corruption with full force.

Blockchain as a Solution

Decentralized data access control (DDAC) over consortium blockchain is defined below:

Consortium network N = (P, C, T) follows ACC constraints-

- **Atomicity:** Nodes per applied for *with permission* participants
- **Consensus:** Owner consented execution or multi organization vote right system for an order to be placed.
- **Confidentiality:** Participant read access to data objects

Access Control

Access Control (AC) is system that maintains authentication and resource communication right to its participants according to security defined guidelines and policies in AC.

An optimal model of AC to IoT devices been a challenge task in early stage pof full defined system to implement. Various levels of AC mechanism been developed like-

i. Role Based Access Control (RBAC)
ii. Access Control List (ACL)
iii. Capability-Based Access Control (Capac)

These ACL strategies still not fully appropriate for IT infrastructure but a solution involving blockchain system is better administration service for tracking activities in data crystal.

Blockchain Access Control Infrastructure

Public Blockchain

All blockchains refers to decentralized data storing ability only differences are in nature and allowance to public or organization (A Decentralized Privacy-Preserving Healthcare Blockchain for IoT Sensors, 2019; Ancile, n.d.).

Table 2. Various AC model limitation

Access Control Models	Limitation in IoT System
ACL	Slow scalability and granularity Centralized infrastructure
RBAC	Non user driven Policy management turns crucial issue
Capac	Cannot consider contexts

Public blockchains are majorly used in cryptocurrency mining and exchanges. This blockchains have network based cryptographic equations to validate transactions also referred as mining (Blockchain-based Secure Data Storage Protocol for Sensors in the Industrial Internet of Things, 2021). This process involves human work and so all public blockchains allow any individual to join and equal right access given to all example creating, validating blocks, etc. (Blockchain-based secure storage and access scheme for electronic medical records, 2020; Chakraborty et al., 2019; Dorri et al., 2017).

Private Blockchain

Private blockchain are usually owned by one organization and all right access are concentrated to them only. This restriction has however devolved the storage method a bit to low centralization since data blocks are only within the organization hold (Azbeg et al., 2018; Ethereum, 2019a; Ethereum, 2019b).

Majorly playing a toll on business virtual currency example Ripple, Simple etc. However still there's chances of rigging private blockchain to overcome this consortium blockchain was developed.

Consortium Blockchain

Consortium blockchains are bit same as private blockchain but only difference is it is in hold of more than one organization so data is more decentralized and fraud will face high number of logistical obstacles since data of these many organizations in jumbled manner is almost hard to crack and isolate (Sinha, Singh, Roy, & Singh, 2022; Szabo, n.d.).

R3 is most famous consortium blockchain with leading of Cargo Smart, Global shipping Business Network that has digitized shipping system and tracking (Singh et al., 2021; Singh et al., 2019; Sinha, Singh, Roy, & Singh, 2022).

Hybrid Blockchain

Hybrid Blockchains uses concept of multi-level permission in a single-handed organization (Kumar & Marchang, 2020; Miyachi & Mackey, 2021). Also, even public blockchain operation can be done on this network with insight of owning organization.

IBM networks for food supply chain is an example of hybrid blockchain.

As medical data privacy, drug transactions and other details which relied on paperback system is important and considered as competitive these system values most of should exist on private, consortium and hybrid blockchain for best security and privacy purpose

Challenges Faced Without Blockchain in AC for IoT Environments

Adaption Into Integrated System

AC mechanisms once developed which involves intensive studies and research cannot be directly deployed on any IoT infrastructure. Each model takes start from scratch technique to implement and deploy consuming much data, time, and work force team.

Scalability

Workload is an issue in IoT environment as more the devices are connected it directly affects speed of working or data transmit. A decentralized and distributed access control however solves issue of scalability in high end infrastructure with many IoT devised environment.

Figure 1. Types of blockchain

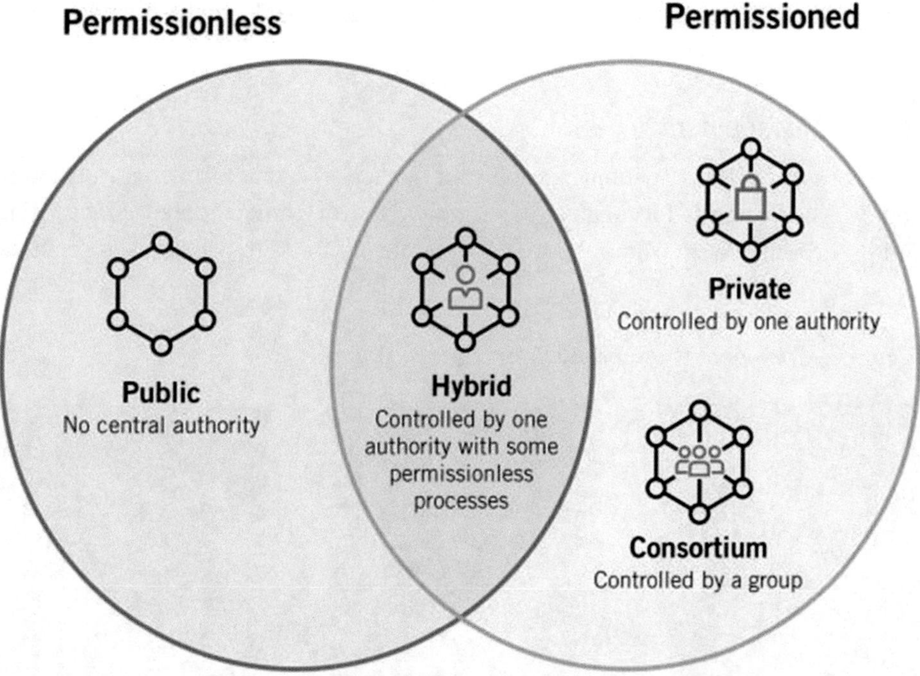

Centralization

Solution is a centralized system as already proven the most in effective way of data management due to high risk of failure in complete network due to a single point issue. In order to limit the risk and failure administrative services are using no AC model that is works on high-risk chances of data corruption and use due to low privacy.

A distributed system ensures no third-party involvement in management and high privacy policy grants to a system

Building Blocks and Functionality

Distributed ledger with link list blocks secured by cryptographic hashes is basic idea of blockchain. Each transaction is converted into hash values of preceding block with timestamp that verifies creation of order. Duplicated stored value in distributed manner prevents any data change in block.

Medicine Tracking

Blockchain can be efficient avoidance of various medical extortion like illegal drug stocking or sales. According to various supply chain reviews many cases of subsiding setups sold 10-30% of fake drugs all over world (Gligoroski, 2020; Wang et al., 2018). Blockchain exchanges implemented on sales of drugs through manufacture to medical services ensures stock details preservation and proper time stamping guarantees data impossible to rig.

Record Management

In most case scenarios a patient can apply for medical assistance from many different bodies. Thus, records for medical community is a very crucial detail. Local filing and paperback system cannot be trusted completely for both privacy and security.

Figure 2. Components of architecture of blockchain

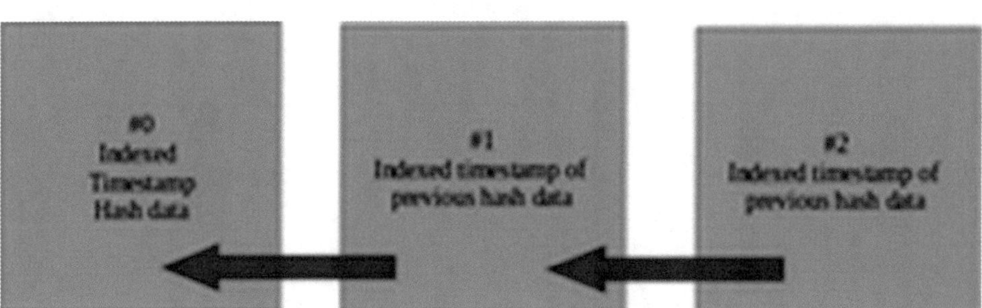

Also, patient cannot be given a complete access to records because they too can rig the process by editing or modifying records. But blockchain gives an option for peer to peer sharing data with decentralized filing system to other bodies over internet easily.

Security Measures

Healthcare professionals tends to have an access to patient data all time. However, if permission granting is rigged this can pose a direct danger to patient life. Blockchain provides cryptographic keys to gain access controls.

Billing System

Local filing and billing system can be exposed to many rigging methods and frauds. Payment system through upi and banks are dangerous and even subject to human error, costing individuals a lot. Combing payment gateway to billing system makes process easier and less cases of delays occur in processing also limiting data dispensing in any transaction.

Background and Definitions

Decentralization

Blockchain spreads data to arrangement point instead of at a single central point to avoid a single point of security disappointment. This system permits for decentralized possession of information, thus providing data management to healthcare sector with consistent, secure, and instant get to information. This approach moreover permits the control of medical data to be transmitted and taken care by various input output operations.

Transparency

Blockchain uses concept of multilateral connection point which provides accuracy in data transparency. Medical information is very sensitive to patient and doctor, while current filing system is not optimal to these issues and 90% of times the data cannot be encapsulated to parties that require only certain portion of data. Blockchain contributes in data sharing with best trusted method and only useful required data is shared among two parties.

Immutability

Centralized healthcare filing system tends to be a threat as they are inclined to hacking and information robbery. Permanence is another striking highlight of blockchain

Figure 3. Conventional record keeping and blockchain

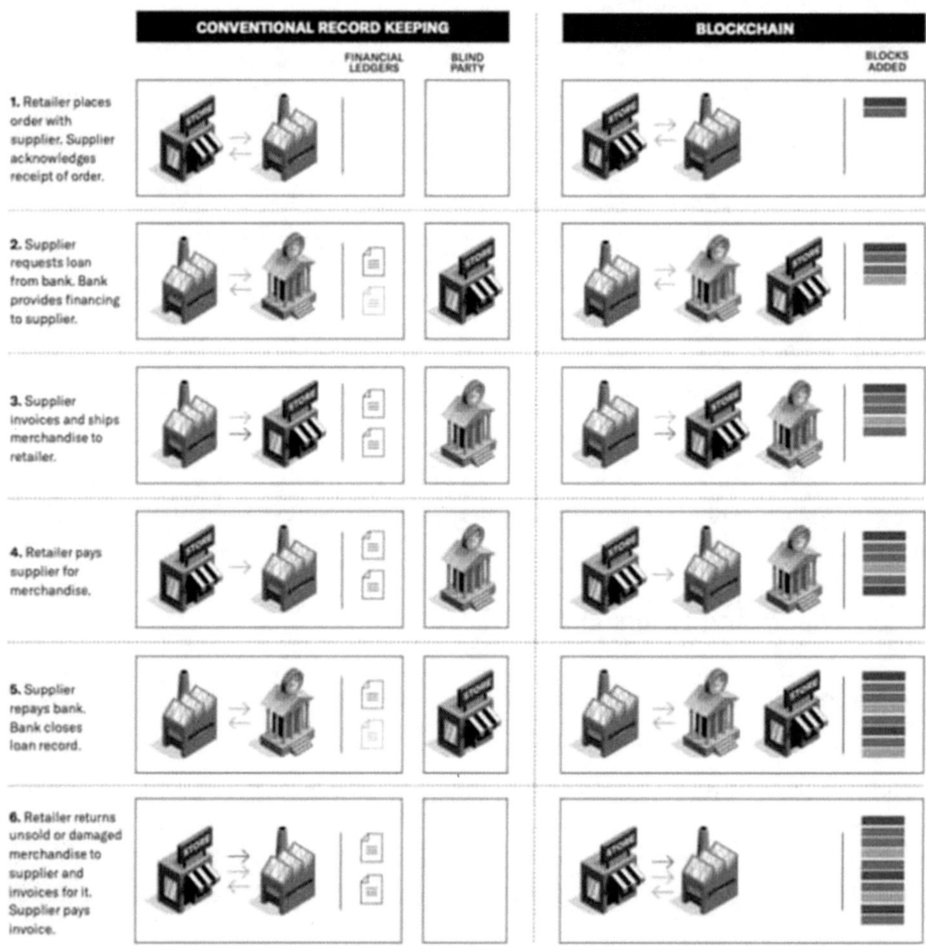

innovation. It refers to the capacity of a blockchain record to stay unaltered and untameably. This striking include has the potential to reshape and change the examining handle into a fast, efficient, and cost-effective strategy.

Moreover, it can enforce more believe and give judgment of the wellbeing information, which is used and shared by therapeutic teach. Blockchain achieves permanence through cryptographic hashing. All transactions are enlisted on computerized squares, wherein each blockchain contains a hash, which is based on hashing the blocks for data preservation.

Data Dispensing

Information provenance is basic for healthcare to set up a certain level of believe in wellbeing information by giving complete information around its creation, get to, and exchange. Blockchain service also involves time stamping services avails more promised data preservation. Storing chronicled wellbeing records on blockchain can enhance trustworthiness for information approval and review purposes. Blockchain can give secure wellbeing information provenance by preventing healthcare frameworks from unauthorized access and change. Too, it empowers trusted traceability in healthcare businesses. Blockchain employments a timestamping process that includes computing hash values of the provenance record, which are exchanged to consensus nodes that guarantee keeping a steady record of all valid transactions.

Privacy and Security

Blockchain grants all its service publicly but with complete anonymity and programmability.

It uses hashed provides to contract communication thus identity of senders and receivers participating in any communication or transaction While programmability offers various features for automation in transaction like billing, access grant etc.

Figure 4. Representation of decentralized storing and authentication process

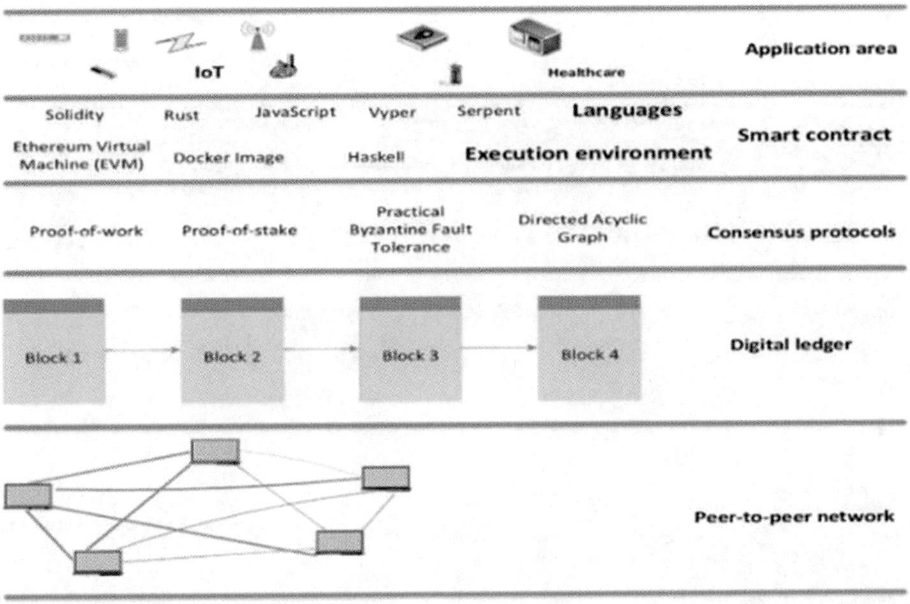

Result and Discussion

The purpose of this study is to discuss blockchain utilization for data management and healthcare. Additionally, integration with IoT is strategized. Moreover, use of blockchain in smart drug dispensing.

Blockchain and IoT

Blockchain adoption is beneficial as it supports variety of applications.

Healthcare where IoT has already made a deep impact in health sector. Use of both technologies benefits and expands the effectiveness of smart automated technology. 3 phases of integration involve light use of blockchain with IoT for model making. Then heavy data is stored decentralized using blockchain application into hybrid model. Most heavy data relate to radiology reports and one

of issue solved is smooth bandwidth in storing files. This hybrid integration handles situations of high latency with ace and easiest hardware implementation sensors.

Data Management in Healthcare IoT

Blockchain ensures data privacy, preservation, and variety of other benefits in application domain. IoT network is heterogeneous in nature and able to generate larger

Figure 5. Components in channel

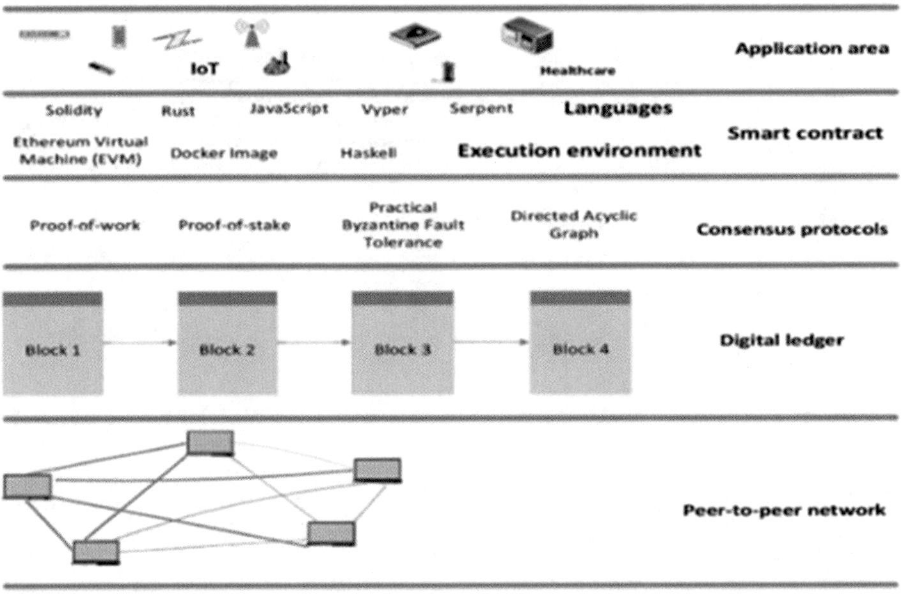

data in both offline and online mode. Thus, a database system of IoT, Blockchain hybrid can compensate critical situations in case of latency or network issues. This has enabled a complete control over accessibility in data tracking and integrity. This blockchain based data management demonstrates autonomous identification of person or object, various authentication systems including voice recognition, biometric or traditional password sets by Hyperledger and NEM access control. Above encryption considered for better data integrity and privacy in single system. Additionally, XOR public encryption also implemented to accomplish above goals.

A side chain system runs back forth to ensure hierarchy in blockchain at global or local level. This clustering also minimizes illegal transactions outside the cluster thus in case of medical supplement everything is count checked and no stealing or trafficking possible.

CONCLUSION

In this book chapter it has been proofed that modern healthcare sector is now accepting high range of disputable technologies one of them can be blockchain in designing a rig free secure system that can provide wide range of features like billing system, automatic form fill that can be highly usable for insurances and accidental cases. Each profile doing transaction in case of patient to health facility is hashed and privacy of individual in preserved. Many hospitals, clinics and practitioner are using different EHR system and paperback reporting system. EHR sharing becomes

Figure 6. Relation between usage and determination factor

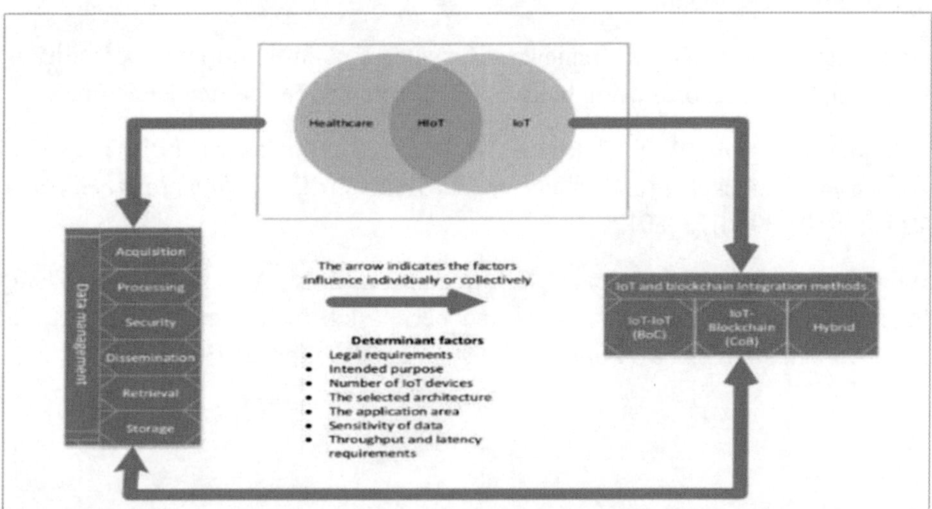

a higher threat for patient in case of data leaks or data manipulation by criminals thus an effective secure process is needed and fulfilled by blockchain and it's services. In case of medical data sharing between different parties due to change in medical facility of patient there are risks of human error or data manipulation by hackers or the process can take time due to high data retention in networking thus traditional EHR system can be life threatening to individuals. Blockchain can be integrated with other latest technologies for more feature like IoT that can be helpful in automatic medicine and report dispensing, AI for easy diagnosis of diseases. Insurance and Accident filing system turns to be an easy task when blockchain mitigates patient whole details to required party without any human error.

a. Blockchain and Artificial Intelligence integration care one of pallet with new efficient data revolutions
b. IoT-based health systems has evolved extensively with blockchain and benefits in real time monitoring of medical tests. Trusted by many health systems bodies one of taken instance by Estonian's.
c. ERP system can be easily implemented on blockchains for more efficient and reliable systems.
d. Blockchain can be established over widespread connection with low data redency in a restrictive manner securing your privacy and data integrity.

REFERENCES

A Decentralized Privacy-Preserving Healthcare Blockchain for IoT Sensors. (2019). doi:10.3390/s19020326

Ancile: Privacy-preserving framework for access control and interoperability of electronic health records using blockchain technology. (n.d.). Academic Press.

Araujo, R. P., Qiang, W. Y., & Rhodes, B. D. (2020). Challenges of PBFT-inspired consensus for blockchain and enhancements over Neo dBFT. *Future Internet*, *12*(8), 129. doi:10.3390/fi12080129

Azaria, A., Ekblaw, A., Vieira, T., & Lippman, A. (2016, August). Medrec: Using blockchain for medical data access and permission management. In *2016 2nd international conference on open and big data (OBD)* (pp. 25-30). IEEE.

Azbeg, Ouchetto, Andaloussi, Fetjah, & Sekkaki. (2018). Blockchain and IoT for Security and Privacy: A Platform for Diabetes Self-management. In *2018 4th International Conference on Cloud Computing Technologies and Applications (Cloudtech).* IEEE. doi:10.1109/CloudTech.2018.8713343

Barry, L., Holloway, J., & McMahon, J. (2020). A scoping review of the barriers and facilitators to the implementation of interventions in autism education. *Research in Autism Spectrum Disorders*, *78*, 101617. doi:10.1016/j.rasd.2020.101617

Bergmann, T., Camatta, R., Birkner, J., & Sappok, T. (2017, January). Vision, Concretism, Repetitism: Typical Artistic Design Features in Drawings by Adults With Autism and Intellectual Disability. Journal of Mental Health Research in Intellectual Disabilities, 10, 96-96.

Blockchain-based Secure Data Storage Protocol for Sensors in the Industrial Internet of Things. (2021). *IEEE Trans Ind Inf, 1*. doi:10.1109/TII.2021.3112601

Blockchain-based secure storage and access scheme for electronic medical records. (2020). *IPFS Access, 8*, 59389-59401. doi:10.1109/ACCESS.2020.2982964

Castro & Liskov. (1999). Practical Byzantine fault tolerance. *OSDI, 99*, 173–186,

Chakraborty, S., Aich, S., & Kim, H.-C. (2019). A Secure Healthcare System Design Framework using Blockchain Technology. In *2019 21st International Conference on Advanced Communication Technology (ICACT).* IEEE. 10.23919/ICACT.2019.8701983

Chen, Y., Ding, S., Xu, Z., Zheng, H., & Yang, S. (2019). Blockchain-based medical records secure storage and medical service framework. *Journal of Medical Systems*, *43*(1), 1–9. doi:10.100710916-018-1121-4 PMID:30467604

Dorri, A., Kanhere, S. S., & Jurdak, R. (2017). Towards an Optimized BlockChain for IoT. In *Proceedings of the Second International Conference on Internet-of-Things Design and Implementation – IoTDI '17*. ACM Press. Doi:10.1145/3054977.3055003

Dubovitskaya, A., Xu, Z., Ryu, S., Schumacher, M., & Wang, F. (2017). Secure and trustable electronic medical records sharing using blockchain. *AMIA ... Annual Symposium Proceedings - AMIA Symposium. AMIA Symposium*, *2017*, 650. PMID:29854130

Ekblaw, A., Azaria, A., Halamka, J. D., & Lippman, A. (2016, August). A Case Study for Blockchain in Healthcare: "MedRec" prototype for electronic health records and medical research data. In *Proceedings of IEEE open & big data conference* (Vol. 13, p. 13). IEEE.

Ethereum. (2019a). *Ethereum/wiki, online*. https://github.com/ethereum/wiki/Light-client-protocol

Ethereum. (2019b). *Go Ethereum*. https://geth.ethereum.org/

Gligoroski, S. A. (2020). Pedersen, A. Faxvaag, Blockchain in healthcare and health sciences—A scoping review. *International Journal of Medical Informatics*, *134*, 104040. doi:10.1016/j.ijmedinf.2019.104040 PMID:31865055

Kumar, R., & Marchang, N. R. (2020). Distributed Off-Chain Storage of Patient Diagnostic Reports in Healthcare System Using IPFS and Blockchain. In *2020 International Conference on COMmunication Systems & NETworkS (COMSNETS)*. IEEE. 10.1109/COMSNETS48256.2020.9027313

Labs, P. (2019). *IPFS Powers the Distributed Web*. https://ipfs.io/

Li, A., Wei, X., & He, Z. (2020). Robust proof of stake: A new consensus protocol for sustainable blockchain systems. *Sustainability (Basel)*, *12*(7), 2824. doi:10.3390u12072824

Mettler, M. (2016). Blockchain technology in healthcare: The revolution starts here. *Proceedings of the IEEE 18th International Conference on e-Health Networking, Applications and Services (Healthcom)*.

Miyachi, K., & Mackey, T. K. (2021). hOCBS: A privacy-preserving blockchain framework for healthcare data leveraging an on-chain and off-chain system design. *Information Processing & Management*, *102535*(3), 102535. doi:10.1016/j.ipm.2021.102535

Nakamoto, S. (2008). *Bitcoin: A Peer-to-Peer Electronic Cash System*. BN Publishing.

Ratta, P., Kaur, A., Sharma, S., Shabaz, M., & Dhiman, G. (2021). Application of blockchain and internet of things in healthcare and medical sector: Applications, challenges, and future perspectives. *Journal of Food Quality*. doi:10.1155/2021/7608296

Reisman, M. (2017). EHRs: The challenge of making electronic data usable and interoperable. *Pharm Ther*, *42*(9), 572. PMID:28890644

Ricci, S. (2018). Lightweight Ring Signatures for Decentralized Privacy-preserving Transactions. *Proceedings of the 15th International Joint Conference on e- Business and Telecommunications*, 526–531.

Singh, P., Singh, A. P., & Gupta, A. (2021). Design Strategies for Mobile Ad-hoc Network to Prevent from Attack. In *Proceedings of the 3rd International Conference on Advanced Computing and Software Engineering*. SCITEPRESS - Science and Technology Publications. 10.5220/0010566800003161

Singh, P., Verma, S., & Kavita. (2019). Analysis on Different Strategies Used in Blockchain Technology. *Journal of Computational and Theoretical Nanoscience, 16*(10), 4350–4355. doi:10.1166/jctn.2019.8524

Sinha, P., Singh, R., Roy, R., & Singh, P. (2022). Education and Analysis of Autistic Patients Using Machine Learning. *2022 International Conference on Emerging Smart Computing and Informatics (ESCI),* 1-6. 10.1109/ESCI53509.2022.9758322

Sinha, P., Singh, R., Roy, R., & Singh, P. (2022, March). Education and Analysis of Autistic Patients Using Machine Learning. In *2022 International Conference on Emerging Smart Computing and Informatics (ESCI)* (pp. 1-6). IEEE. 10.1109/ESCI53509.2022.9758322

Szabo, N. (n.d.). Formalizing and Securing Relationships on Public Networks. *First Monday, 2*(9). https://journals.uic.edu/ojs/index.php/fm/article/view/548 doi:10.5210/fm.v2i9.548

Wang, S., Wang, J., Wang, X., Qiu, T., Yuan, Y., Ouyang, L., Guo, Y., & Wang, F.-Y. (2018). Blockchain-powered parallel healthcare systems based on the ACP approach. *IEEE Transactions on Computational Social Systems, 5*(4), 942–950. doi:10.1109/TCSS.2018.2865526

WHO. (2016). *Technical package for cardiovascular disease management in primary health care.* https://apps.who.int/iris/handle/10665/252661

WHO. (2022). *Integrated chronic disease prevention and control.* https://www.who.int/chp/about/integrated_cd/en/

Xie, Y., Zhang, J., Wang, H., Liu, P., Liu, S., Huo, T., Duan, Y.-Y., Dong, Z., Lu, L., & Ye, Z. (2021). Applications of Blockchain in the Medical Field: Narrative Review. *Journal of Medical Internet Research, 23*(10), e28613. doi:10.2196/28613 PMID:34533470

Chapter 12
Categorical Data Clustering Using Meta Heuristic Link-Based Ensemble Method:
Data Clustering Using Soft Computing Techniques

Kousik Nalliyanna Goundar Veerappan
Arden University, UK

Yuvaraj Natarajan
Sri Shakthi Institute of Engineering and Technology, Coimbatore, India

Arshath Raja
B.S. Abdur Rahman Crescent Institute of Science and Technology, Chennai, India

Jeyaprabhavathi Perumal
Arden University, UK

S Jerald Nirmal Kumar
Sharda University, India

ABSTRACT

Conventional ensemble clustering is a consensus function that fails to produce final clusters. Such poor clusters partitioning creates poor stability with reduced clustering accuracy. This motivates to improve the final clustering quality using a hybrid ensemble-based model. In this study, an optimized link-based ensemble clustering approach is proposed to refine the incomplete datasets and to refine unknown entries in categorical dataset. The proposed work uses link-based similarity measure to find the availability of unknown datasets from link network of clusters.

DOI: 10.4018/978-1-6684-6894-4.ch012

The ensemble clustering generates a refined cluster-association matrix in the form of weighted graphs. The final cluster partitioning acquires the final clustering partitions with a refined matrix as its input that decomposes the graph into clusters. The comparison with conventional methods is made against performance metrics to evaluate the model efficacy.

INTRODUCTION

The problem of partitioning a set of objects into groups is defined informally by data clustering so that objects in one group are similar, while objects in various groups are different (Rhmann et al., 2022). Category data clustering refers to the case of categorical attributes where data objects are defined (Bai & Liang, 2022). An attribute that has a categorical domain is a set of discrete, inherently unparalleled values (Singh et al., 2021).

Substantial research in several domains has for decades concentrated on a clustering problem of high practical importance. As the volume of data collected increases, it becomes essential to measure and understand the data. In this process, clustering plays a major role. Due to the growth in research activities in recent years, new clustering algorithms can be developed that handle large quantities of data and produce high-quality results (Saha et al., 2022).

Compared to clustering numerical information, categorical information is comparatively demanding. The inherent geometric possessions can be separated from the data facts in numeric information in significant distance functions. A distance or distinction can never be defined unambiguously in the case of categorical facts (Mahjour et al., 2021).

The grouping of categorical information appears to be more complex than numerical information, because the higher possessions of specific attributes have. Insufficient procedures for grouping categorical information have been anticipated in recent years. It is sufficient to supplement that the similarity measurement of those accessible algorithms covers all attribute standards uniformly (Priya et al., 2021). In other words, unusual value attributes have the same amount as the recurring attributes in parallel calculations.

However, the cluster ensemble technology, which is considered as an effective solution for clustering algorithms, uses categorical data sets, does avoid those limitations. The solidity and clustering quality is well improved (Vega-Márquez et al., 2021). In the information or binary clustering ensemble matrix, the data points are related, which leave many zero entries unknown, thus reducing the quality of the data partition. A linked approach using refined cluster association matrix is presented to this degeneration in the quality of the data partition (Dasari et al., 2021;

Gharehchopogh et al., 2022; Mohd Ali et al., 1955; Panja et al., 2022; Rezaee et al., 2021; Suryanarayana & Prakash, 2022).

The study aims at improving the quality of clustering the categorical datasets using a link-based ensemble. The objectives specific to the present study is given below: To combine or aggregate the decisions of a various individual clustering algorithm for increased accuracy and eminence of ensemble clustering method over categorical datasets with incomplete information. To improve the quality, robustness, and stability of link-based ensemble clustering algorithms than ensemble clustering and individual clustering algorithms over categorical datasets. To improve the cluster partitioning using feature-based or spectral graph-based partitioning to increase the stability inside the system with improved clustering accuracy. To increase the accuracy in finding similarity between the categorical data based on uniqueness present in the data and grouping related data objects into clusters. To reduce the complexity associated with data dimensionality, since it prominently affects the clustering at each stage, i.e. base clustering, intermediate clustering, and final clustering.

PROBLEM FORMULATION

To design clustering algorithms, the study needs to formulate a mathematical notations, in which "similar objects are grouped and similar subjects grouped separately".

- A measurement between two data objects.
- A similarity or distance measurement between a Data Object and an Object Cluster.
- A data object cluster quality measurement.

PROPOSED METHOD

The research work bridges the gap between link-based ensemble and data clustering over categorical datasets. The research work eliminates the incomplete dataset or unknown entries using link-based ensemble technique.

This section proposes a link-based technique to refine the incomplete datasets that filter unknown entries in the dataset. The proposed work uses link-based similarity measure to find the availability of unknown datasets from link network of clusters. It also bridges the gap between link analysis and data clustering. It improves the clustering ability in three stages of clustering that includes base clustering, ensemble clustering and final data partitioning over categorical data. The base clustering generates base clusters that form a cluster ensemble, namely direct or indirect (fixed and random) types. The ensemble clustering generates a refined cluster-association matrix in the form of weighted graphs. At the third stage, the final cluster partitioning acquires the final clustering partitions with a refined matrix as its input that decomposes the graph into clusters.

To achieve these aims, the present study proposes an improved ensemble framework to cluster the categorical datasets. The study uses two different methods to achieve this aim. These methods include (i) Hybrid Firefly algorithm based link-based clustering ensemble with Bipartite Graph Partitioning (HFALCE) and (ii) modified k-means centroid clustering algorithm based Link-based Clustering Ensemble with Featured-Based Partitioning (MKLCE).

Initially, the base clusters are formed using Hybrid Firefly algorithm and Modified k-means centroid clustering algorithm. It then uses a cluster ensemble to categorise the categorical datasets. At the next stage, a redefined matrix is generated using a Weighted Triple quality link-based Similarity Algorithm. Finally, the cluster partitions are generated using Bipartite Graph Partitioning Consensus Function and Featured-Based Partitioning Consensus Function. The architecture of the proposed system is given in Figure 1.

The HFALCE method uses link-based clustering to avoid degradation in clustering at the time of partitioning the categorical data. In the three stages of clustering, HFALCE method proposes firefly algorithm for initial clustering, link-based ensemble clustering using multi-viewpoint and Entropy-based Weighted Triple Quality measurements at the second stage that ensembles the categorical data points into clusters. The second stage is carried out to avoid the optimum local problem, and further, it avoids the issues related to a high dimensional dataset (incomplete data items). This improves the quality of categorical data clustering at the middle stage. Finally, the data partitioning or third level clustering is carried out using bipartite spectral graph consensus clustering.

Base Clustering Using Firefly Algorithm

The firefly algorithm is used in the proposed system to generate the base clusters. It segregates the data clusters as different categories that include direct and indirect (fixed and random) clusters. The Firefly Algorithm is a stochastic global optimisation problem that uses a distance metric to cluster the data points. The objective function in the firefly algorithm is designed by finding a difference between the data points in a centroid, and it chooses the obtained best data point. The firefly searches for the best location of a data point inside a cluster. The selection of an optimal data point is chosen based on dataset categories. Finally, it finds the best data point using a new location and best centroid value. This helps to obtain the base clusters without degrading the quality of clusters.

Figure 1. Architecture of proposed study

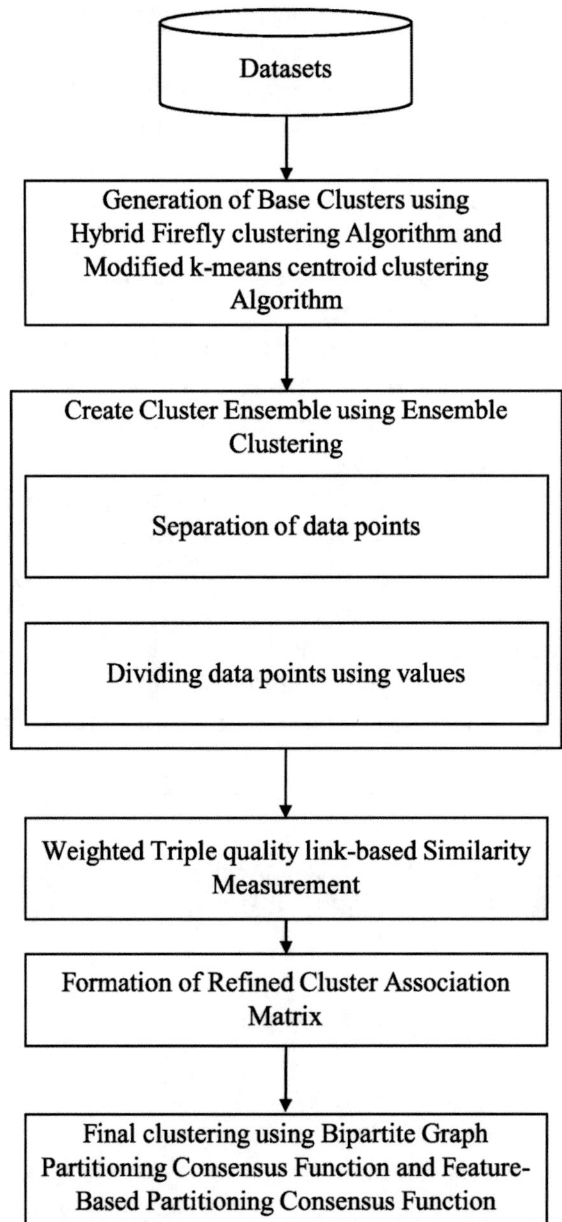

The inter-cluster and intra-cluster of data samples are collected using the clustering process. Clustering is used to reduce the volume of data and pre-processing dimensions and to analyze similarity or discrepancies. Many standards are taken into consideration to resolve clustering problems, which is given in Equation (1).

$$d\left(X,c_j\right)=\sqrt{\sum_{i=1}^{m}\left(x_i-c_j\right)^2} \tag{1}$$

Where
m is regarded as the total number of data,
X is regarded as the data vector, and
c_j is regarded as the cluster center.

Consider a sample with n-dimensional space points and these are assigned with Euclidean distance standards in each cluster. The main objective of the firefly algorithm is to find a cluster centre to achieve an optimal local solution. However, because of its dependence on the final output on the start value of the centres and on new convergence and because of its local optimum, it fails to resolve the clustering problem.

Base Clustering Using a K-Means Centroid Clustering Algorithm

The k-means centroid clustering algorithm method generates the base clusters using k means variance clustering algorithm with centroid selection technique. The centroid selection is carried out using mean distance measurement. This method finds the pairwise distance between the data points, and it then sorts the data points using Euclidean distance measurement between the data point pairs. Finally, it uses the average from the mean values. This method is intended to handle both the categorical and numeric data points. In this study, the initial base clustering is performed using a modified k-means centroid clustering algorithm that clusters the given raw dataset into different data types. The clustered datasets are given as inputs to link-based clustering ensemble algorithm, and then the similarity measurement is carried out using a recursive C-Rank formula to find the similarity between the clusters. Once the refined matrix is obtained from the link-based ensemble method. The feature-based partitioning is used to generate the final clusters. This method improves the clustering quality and solves the initial centroid problem. The accuracy of clustering is improved to acquire the task of clustering with improved quality.

Link-Based Cluster Ensemble

At the second stage, the MKLCE method uses link-based clustering ensemble approach similar to HFALCE approach. It generates a refined matrix that clusters well the categorical data based on different ensemble base clusters. This stage determines the quality of obtained clusters using the rarity of links connected with adjacent clusters.

Multi-Viewpoint-Based Similarity Measure

The multi-viewpoint-based similarity measurement is used for improving the quality of clustering. The quality in clustering is improved using the processes shown in the following sections. This method uses an optimal partitioning method, which estimates the similarity measurement between the clusters. Since the clustering efficiency is purely determined using similarity measurement between the clusters.

This method creates a candidate ensemble at the time of each iteration over M clusters. The data point is considered as a different ensemble model during the formation of clusters. The cluster is chosen finally using a maximum average distance. The cluster association or refined matrix is then found between the data point pairs using an association degree. The similarity between two different clusters is found using binary cluster co-association matrix.

Final Clustering Using Feature-Based Partitioning

At the third stage, the MKLCE method uses Feature-based partitioning that uses feature-based partitioning to decomposition the RM to clusters at the third stage. This method transforms the clusters from ensembles to categorical data using cluster label as a new feature that describes the data points. This helps to formulate the final solution using k-means numerical clustering algorithm. This feature-based method combines a clustering approach with numerical ensemble matrix. This method clusters categorical data using cluster labels using a weighted similarity partitioning algorithm. This method considers only the high-level data matrix using similarity, despite the presence of refined binary association matrix. It is to be noted that the dissimilar matrix is used as concepts for this method. Further, the consensus function is designed using a cosine measure that finds pairwise similarity between the clustered points and then it is transformed to a similarity graph.

Final Clustering Using Spectral Graph Bi-Partitioning

The spectral graph-partitioning technique is applied to clusters obtained from ensemble approach in order to avoid the ensemble problem. This method initially applies a bipartite graph that provides a new solution transformed from Refined Matrix. It creates a weighted bipartite graph that is applied over consensus function. Further, it enriches the Refined Matrix using a weighted distance metric, and this is accomplished using similarity measurement between the clusters. This method generates final clusters using complete information ensemble. This clusters the ensemble datasets with improved quality.

RESULTS AND DISCUSSIONS

This section presents the performance analysis of the proposed ensemble methods namely HFALCE and MKLCE. The testing and evaluation are carried out using a benchmark datasets on proposed and existing methods. The proposed method is tested in terms of various ensemble types, which is discussed below. Various performance metrics are used to test the performance of the proposed system and to check the quality of clustering than the existing methods.

Simulation Settings

This simulation for the proposed system is carried out using a 3.00 GHz Intel(R) i7-6950X CPU running Windows 10 and the coding is made available in Java environment.

Performance Evaluation

The base clustering in proposed and other methods is through k-mode clustering technique, which is given by

- **Link-Based Cluster Ensemble (LCE) Algorithm (Iam-On et al., 2010):** LCE focuses on refinement of the BA matrix that is less costly to build as a parallel similarity alternative to enhance the efficiency of previous link-based methods (CTS and SRS) to the cluster ensemble problem. Here, HBGF method is extended based on information in the conventional BA matrix, in which every entry BA is a crisp degree of association between cluster and sample. Like the case with the CO matrix, the BA contains a large number of 0 entries. These cluster similarities found in a link network of clusters can be estimated by these hidden or unknown associations
- **Cluster-based Similarity Partitioning Algorithm (CSPA):** CO matrix similarity graph is created with CSPA method. The graph is subsequently

Table 1. Description of datasets

Dataset	Data Points (N)	Attributes (D)	Attribute Values (AV)	Classes (K)
Zoo	96	14	34	6
Lymphography	143	15	57	5
Primary Tumor	345	16	40	21
Breast Cancer	680	8	85	3
20 Newsgroup	999	6078	12178	2

divided into clusters with the same size using a multilevel K-way graph partitioning and manages multi-screen graph partitioning in 3 different phases: coarsened phase, successively decreased graph size, initial divided phase, computed a little k- way partition of the smaller graph, and phase, subsequently improved partitioning as the larger graphs is projected.

- **Hyper-Graph Partitioning (HGPA) Algorithm:** HGPA builds the binary cluster-association (BA) matrix and a hypergraph with vertical data points and identical weighted clusters in the ensemble. BA is the basis for a hyper-graphic structure. The underlying HMETIS division into K parts with roughly the same size shall be used by HMETIS.

Performance Metrics

For comparison, the proposed method is evaluated against various performance metrics with some existing methods.

Results and Evaluation

This section first discusses the performance evaluation of between HFALCE and other existing methods and then it discusses the performance between MKLCE and other existing methods. Finally, the comparison between HFALCE with MKLCE.

Finally, we compare the accuracy, cohesion clustering, variance, precision and recall rate between the proposed HFALCE and MKLCE and other existing methods. The results are evident from Figures 1-5, where the proposed HFALCE achieves

Figure 2. Accuracy

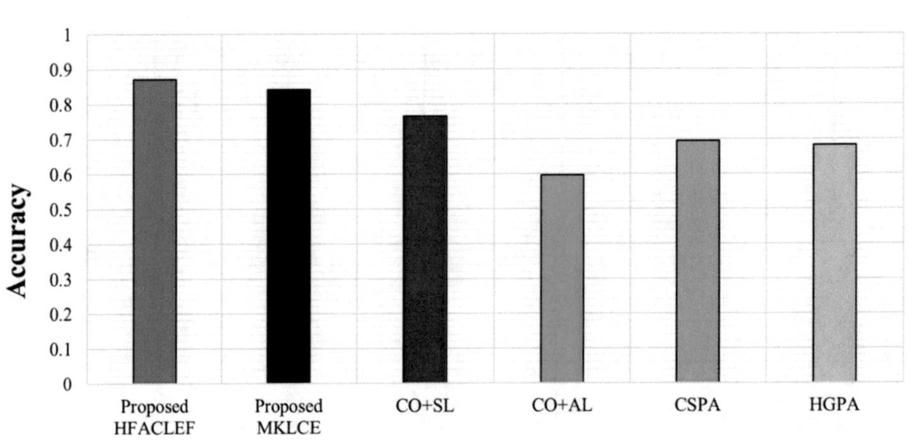

Figure 3. Cohesion

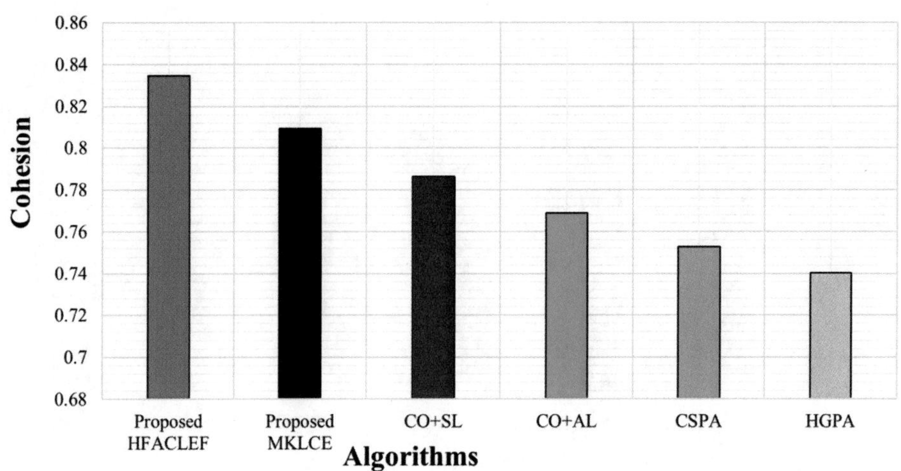

Figure 4. Variance

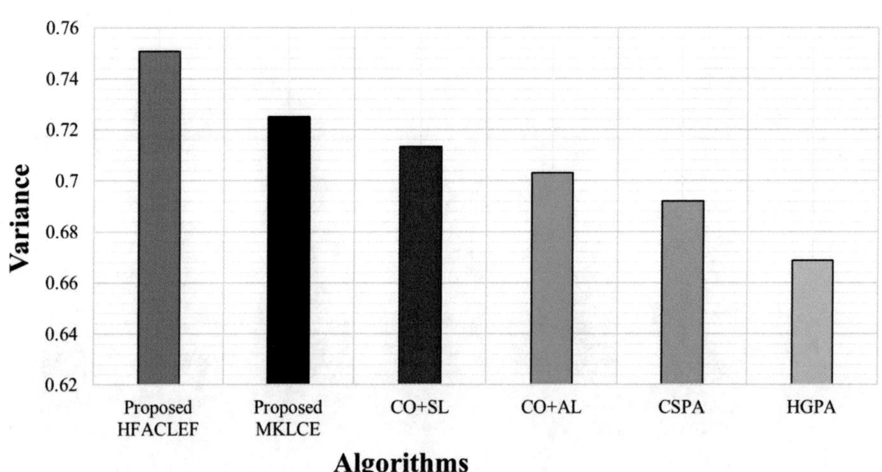

improved accuracy, cohesion clustering, variance, precision and recall rate than MKLCE and other existing methods.

CONCLUSION

In this chapter, categorical data clustering is achieved effectively using two different methods namely proposed HFALCE and proposed MKLCE. The simulation result shows

Figure 5. Precision

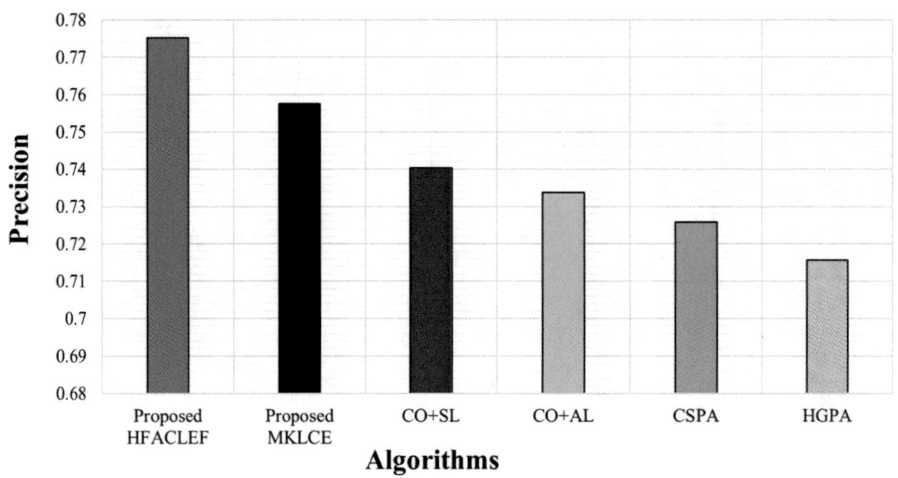

Figure 6. Recall

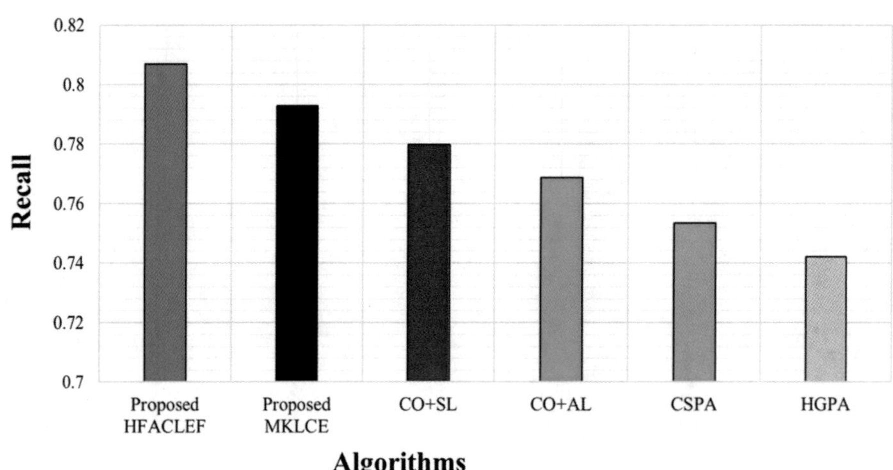

that the proposed HFALCE achieves higher performance than the proposed MKLCE and other existing methods. It is inferred from the results that the use of firefly algorithm at the initial clustering stage produces effective clustering ensembles in proposed HFALCE than in proposed MKLCE method with improved k-means algorithm.

REFERENCES

Bai, L., & Liang, J. (2022). A categorical data clustering framework on graph representation. *Pattern Recognition*, *128*, 108694. doi:10.1016/j.patcog.2022.108694

Dasari, D. B., Edamadaka, G., Chowdary, C., & Sobhana, M. (2021). Anomaly-based network intrusion detection with ensemble classifiers and meta-heuristic scale (ECMHS) in traffic flow streams. *Journal of Ambient Intelligence and Humanized Computing*, *12*(10), 9241–9268. doi:10.100712652-020-02628-1

Gharehchopogh, F. S., Maleki, I., & Dizaji, Z. A. (2022). Chaotic vortex search algorithm: Metaheuristic algorithm for feature selection. *Evolutionary Intelligence*, *15*(3), 1777–1808. doi:10.100712065-021-00590-1

Mahjour, S. K., Santos, A. A. S., Correia, M. G., & Schiozer, D. J. (2021). Scenario reduction methodologies under uncertainties for reservoir development purposes: Distance-based clustering and metaheuristic algorithm. *Journal of Petroleum Exploration and Production Technology*, *11*(7), 3079–3102. doi:10.100713202-021-01210-5

Mohd Ali, N., Besar, R., & Aziz, A. (1955). N. A. (2022). Hybrid Feature Selection of Breast Cancer Gene Expression Microarray Data Based on Metaheuristic Methods: A Comprehensive Review. *Symmetry*, *14*(10). Advance online publication. doi:10.3390ym14101955

Panja, A. K., Karim, S. F., Neogy, S., & Chowdhury, C. (2022). A novel feature based ensemble learning model for indoor localization of smartphone users. *Engineering Applications of Artificial Intelligence*, *107*, 104538. doi:10.1016/j.engappai.2021.104538

Priya, S., Selvakumar, S., & Velusamy, R. L. (2021). Evidential theoretic deep radial and probabilistic neural ensemble approach for detecting phishing attacks. *Journal of Ambient Intelligence and Humanized Computing*, 1–25.

Rezaee, M. J., Eshkevari, M., Saberi, M., & Hussain, O. (2021). GBK-means clustering algorithm: An improvement to the K-means algorithm based on the bargaining game. *Knowledge-Based Systems*, *213*, 106672. doi:10.1016/j.knosys.2020.106672

Rhmann, W., Pandey, B., & Ansari, G. A. (2022). Software effort estimation using ensemble of hybrid search-based algorithms based on metaheuristic algorithms. *Innovations in Systems and Software Engineering*, *18*(2), 309–319. doi:10.100711334-020-00377-0

Saha, A., Rajak, S., Saha, J., & Chowdhury, C. (2022). A Survey of Machine Learning and Meta-heuristics Approaches for Sensor-based Human Activity Recognition Systems. *Journal of Ambient Intelligence and Humanized Computing*, 1–28. doi:10.100712652-022-03870-5

Singh, I., Kumar, N., Srinivasa, K. G., Maini, S., Ahuja, U., & Jain, S. (2021). A multi-level classification and modified PSO clustering based ensemble approach for credit scoring. *Applied Soft Computing*, *111*, 107687. doi:10.1016/j.asoc.2021.107687

Suryanarayana, G., & Prakash, K. (2022). Novel dynamic k-modes clustering of categorical and non categorical dataset with optimized genetic algorithm based feature selection. *Multimedia Tools and Applications*, *81*(17), 1–20. doi:10.100711042-022-12126-5

Vega-Márquez, B., Nepomuceno-Chamorro, I. A., Rubio-Escudero, C., & Riquelme, J. C. (2021). OCEAn: Ordinal classification with an ensemble approach. *Information Sciences*, *580*, 221–242. doi:10.1016/j.ins.2021.08.081

Compilation of References

. Rghioui, A., & Oumnad, A. (2018). Challenges and Opportunities of Internet of Things in Healthcare. *International Journal of Electrical & Computer Engineering, 8*(5).

A Decentralized Privacy-Preserving Healthcare Blockchain for IoT Sensors. (2019). doi:10.3390/s19020326

Abawajy, J. H., & Hassan, M. M. (2017). Federated Internet of Things and Cloud Computing Pervasive Patient Health Monitoring System. *IEEE Communications Magazine*, *55*(1), 48–53. doi:10.1109/MCOM.2017.1600374CM

Abolfaz Mehbodiya, Kumar, Rane, Bhatia, & Singh. (2021). Smartphone-Based mHealth and Internet of Things for Diabetes Control and Self-Management. *Journal of Healthcare Engineering*. doi:10.1155/2021/2116647

Abouelmehdi, K., Beni-Hessane, A., & Khaloufi, H. (2018). Big healthcare data: Preserving security and privacy. *Journal of Big Data*, *5*(1), 1–18. doi:10.118640537-017-0110-7

Abraham, A., Das, S., & Konar, A. (2006). Document clustering using differential evolution. *Proceedings of the 2006 IEEE Congress on Evolutionary Computations (CEC 2006),* 1784-1791. 10.1109/CEC.2006.1688523

Abualigah, L. M., Khader, A. T., & Hanandeh, E. S. (2018). A new feature selection method to improve the document clustering using particle swarm optimization algorithm. *Journal of Computational Science*, *25*, 456–466. doi:10.1016/j.jocs.2017.07.018

Aceto, G., Persico, V., & Pescapé, A. (2020). Industry 4.0 and health: Internet of things, big data, and cloud computing for healthcare 4.0. *Journal of Industrial Information Integration*, *18*, 100129. doi:10.1016/j.jii.2020.100129

Afolayan, J. O., Adebiyi, M. O., Arowolo, M. O., Chakraborty, C., & Adebiyi, A. A. (2022). Breast Cancer Detection Using Particle Swarm Optimization and Decision Tree Machine Learning Technique. In C. Chakraborty & M. R. Khosravi (Eds.), *Intelligent Healthcare*. Springer. doi:10.1007/978-981-16-8150-9_4

Aghdam, M. H., Tanha, J., Naghsh-Nilchi, A. R., & Basiri, M. E. (2009). Combination of ant colony optimization and Bayesian classification for feature selection in a bioinformatics dataset. *Journal of Computer Science and Systems Biology*, *2*(3), 186–199. doi:10.4172/jcsb.1000031

Aghili, S. F., Mala, H., Shojafar, M., & Peris-Lopez, P. (2019). LACO: Lightweight three-factor authentication, access control and ownership transfer scheme for e-health systems in IoT. *Future Generation Computer Systems*, *96*, 410–424. doi:10.1016/j.future.2019.02.020

Ahmadi, A., Karray, F., & Kamel, M. (2007). Multiple cooperating swarms for data clustering. *Proceedings of the 2007 IEEE Swarm Intelligence Symposium (SIS 2007),* 206-212. 10.1109/SIS.2007.368047

Ahmad, P., Qamar, S., & Rizvi, S. Q. A. (2015). Techniques of data mining in healthcare: A review. *International Journal of Computer Applications*, *120*(15), 38–50. doi:10.5120/21307-4126

Al-Abassi, Karimipour, HaddadPajouh, Dehghantanha, & Parizi. (n.d.). Industrial Big Data Analytics: Challenges and Opportunities. In *Handbook of Big data Privacy*. Academic Press.

Al-Andoli, M. N., Tan, S. C., & Cheah, W. P. (2022). Distributed parallel deep learning with a hybrid backpropagation-particle swarm optimization for community detection in large complex networks. *Information Sciences*, *600*, 94–117. doi:10.1016/j.ins.2022.03.053

Alexander, F. J., Hoisie, A., & Szalay, A. (2011). Big data. *Computing in Science & Engineering*, *13*(6), 10–13. doi:10.1109/MCSE.2011.99

AlGhatrif, M., & Lindsay, J. (2012). A brief review: History to understand fundamentals of electrocardiography. *Journal of Community Hospital Internal Medicine Perspectives*, *2*(1), 14383. doi:10.3402/jchimp.v2i1.14383 PMID:23882360

Ali, F., El-Sappagh, S., Islam, S. R., Kwak, D., Ali, A., Imran, M., & Kwak, K. S. (2020). A smart healthcare monitoring system for heart disease prediction based on ensemble deep learning and feature fusion. *Information Fusion*, *63*, 208–222. doi:10.1016/j.inffus.2020.06.008

Ali, O., Shrestha, A., Soar, J., & Wamba, S. F. (2018). Cloud computing-enabled healthcare opportunities, issues, and applications: A systematic review. *International Journal of Information Management*, *43*, 146–158. doi:10.1016/j.ijinfomgt.2018.07.009

Aly, R. H. M., Rahouma, K. H., & Hamed, H. F. (2019). Brain Tumors Diagnosis and Prediction Based on Applying the Learning Metaheuristic Optimization Techniques of Particle Swarm, Ant Colony and Bee Colony. *Procedia Computer Science*, *163*, 165–179. doi:10.1016/j.procs.2019.12.098

Ameryan, M. (2014). Clustering Based on Cuckoo Optimization Algorithm. Academic Press.

Ancile: Privacy-preserving framework for access control and interoperability of electronic health records using blockchain technology. (n.d.). Academic Press.

Anitha, C., R, K. C., Vivekanand, C. V., Lalitha, S. D., Boopathi, S., & R, R. (2023, February). Artificial Intelligence driven security model for Internet of Medical Things ({IoMT}). *IEEE Explore*. doi:10.1109/ICIPTM57143.2023.10117713

Anter, A. M., Bhattacharyya, S., & Zhang, Z. (2020). Multi-stage fuzzy swarm intelligence for automatic hepatic lesion segmentation from CT scans. *Applied Soft Computing*, *96*, 106677. doi:10.1016/j.asoc.2020.106677

Araujo, R. P., Qiang, W. Y., & Rhodes, B. D. (2020). Challenges of PBFT-inspired consensus for blockchain and enhancements over Neo dBFT. *Future Internet*, *12*(8), 129. doi:10.3390/fi12080129

Ari, A. A. A., Gueroui, A., Titouna, C., Thiare, O., & Aliouat, Z. (2019). Resource allocation scheme for 5G C-RAN: A swarm intelligence based approach. *Computer Networks*, *165*, 106957. doi:10.1016/j.comnet.2019.106957

Arora & Chana. (2014). A Survey of Clustering Techniques for Big Data Analysis. Academic Press.

Azaria, A., Ekblaw, A., Vieira, T., & Lippman, A. (2016, August). Medrec: Using blockchain for medical data access and permission management. In *2016 2nd international conference on open and big data (OBD)* (pp. 25-30). IEEE.

Azbeg, Ouchetto, Andaloussi, Fetjah, & Sekkaki. (2018). Blockchain and IoT for Security and Privacy: A Platform for Diabetes Self-management. In *2018 4th International Conference on Cloud Computing Technologies and Applications (Cloudtech)*. IEEE. doi:10.1109/CloudTech.2018.8713343

Babu, B. S., Kamalakannan, J., Meenatchi, N., M, S. K. S., S, K., & Boopathi, S. (2023). Economic impacts and reliability evaluation of battery by adopting Electric Vehicle. *IEEE Explore*, 1–6. doi:10.1109/ICPECTS56089.2022.10046786

Bahri, S., Zoghlami, N., Abed, M., & Tavares, J. M. R. (2018). Big data for healthcare: A survey. *IEEE Access : Practical Innovations, Open Solutions*, *7*, 7397–7408. doi:10.1109/ACCESS.2018.2889180

Bai, L., & Liang, J. (2022). A categorical data clustering framework on graph representation. *Pattern Recognition*, *128*, 108694. doi:10.1016/j.patcog.2022.108694

Baker, S. B., Xiang, W., & Atkinson, I. (2017). Internet of things for smart healthcare: Technologies, challenges, and opportunities. *IEEE Access : Practical Innovations, Open Solutions*, *5*, 26521–26544. doi:10.1109/ACCESS.2017.2775180

Balaji, S., Nathani, K., & Santhakumar, R. (2019). IoT technology, applications and challenges: A contemporary survey. *Wireless Personal Communications*, *108*(1), 363–388. doi:10.100711277-019-06407-w

Barry, L., Holloway, J., & McMahon, J. (2020). A scoping review of the barriers and facilitators to the implementation of interventions in autism education. *Research in Autism Spectrum Disorders*, *78*, 101617. doi:10.1016/j.rasd.2020.101617

Bayoumi, A., & McCaslin, R. (2016). Internet of Things – A Predictive Maintenance Tool forGeneralMachinery, Petrochemicals and Water Treatment. Sustainable Vital Technologies in Engineering &. *Informatics (MDPI).*

Becker, D. E. (2006). Fundamentals of electrocardiography interpretation. *Anesthesia Progress, 53*(2), 53–64. doi:10.2344/0003-3006(2006)53[53:FOEI]2.0.CO;2 PMID:16863387

Bénézit, F., Turnier, P. L., & Declerck, C. (2020). Utility of hyposmia and hypogeusia for the diagnosis of COVID-19. *The Lancet. Infectious Diseases, 20*(9), 1014–1015. doi:10.1016/S1473-3099(20)30297-8 PMID:32304632

Bergmann, T., Camatta, R., Birkner, J., & Sappok, T. (2017, January). Vision, Concretism, Repetitism: Typical Artistic Design Features in Drawings by Adults With Autism and Intellectual Disability. Journal of Mental Health Research in Intellectual Disabilities, 10, 96-96.

Bharne, P. K., Gulhane, V. S., & Yewale, S. K. (2011). Data clustering algorithms based on Swarm Intelligence. *2011 3rd International Conference on Electronics Computer Technology*, 407-411. 10.1109/ICECTECH.2011.5941931

Bida, I., & Aouat, S. (2019). A new approach based on bat algorithm for inducing optimal decision trees classifiers. In A. Rocha & M. Serrhini (Eds.), *EMENA-ISTL 2018.SIST* (Vol. 111, pp. 631–640). Springer. doi:10.1007/978-3-030-03577-8_69

Bing, X., Youwei, Z., Xueyan, Z., & Xuekai, S. (2021). An Improved Artificial Bee Colony Algorithm Based on Faster Convergence. *2021 IEEE International Conference on Artificial Intelligence and Computer Applications (ICAICA)*, 776-779. 10.1109/ICAICA52286.2021.9498254

Blockchain-based Secure Data Storage Protocol for Sensors in the Industrial Internet of Things. (2021). *IEEE Trans Ind Inf, 1*. doi:10.1109/TII.2021.3112601

Blockchain-based secure storage and access scheme for electronic medical records. (2020). *IPFS Access, 8*, 59389-59401. doi:10.1109/ACCESS.2020.2982964

Boopathi, S. (2021). Improving of Green Sand-Mould Quality using Taguchi Technique. *Journal of Engineering Research*. doi:10.36909/jer.14079

Boopathi, S., Arigela, S. H., Raman, R., Indhumathi, C., Kavitha, V., & Bhatt, B. C. (2023). Prominent Rule Control-based Internet of Things: Poultry Farm Management System. *IEEE Explore*, 1–6. doi:10.1109/ICPECTS56089.2022.10047039

Boopathi, S., Khare, R., Jaya Christiyan, K. G., Muni, T. V., & Khare, S. (2023). Additive manufacturing developments in the medical engineering field. In Development, Properties, and Industrial Applications of 3D Printed Polymer Composites (pp. 86–106). IGI Global. doi:10.4018/978-1-6684-6009-2.ch006

Boopathi, S., Siva Kumar, P. K., & Meena, R. S. J., S. I., P., S. K., & Sudhakar, M. (2023). Sustainable Developments of Modern Soil-Less Agro-Cultivation Systems. In Human Agro-Energy Optimization for Business and Industry (pp. 69–87). IGI Global. doi:10.4018/978-1-6684-4118-3.ch004

Boopathi, S. (2019). Experimental investigation and parameter analysis of LPG refrigeration system using Taguchi method. *SN Applied Sciences*, *1*(8), 892. doi:10.100742452-019-0925-2

Boopathi, S. (2022a). An experimental investigation of Quench Polish Quench (QPQ) coating on AISI 4150 steel. *Engineering Research Express*, *4*(4), 45009. doi:10.1088/2631-8695/ac9ddd

Boopathi, S. (2022b). An Extensive Review on Sustainable Developments of Dry and Near-Dry Electrical Discharge Machining Processes. *Journal of Manufacturing Science and Engineering*, *144*(5), 50801. doi:10.1115/1.4052527

Boopathi, S. (2022c). An investigation on gas emission concentration and relative emission rate of the near-dry wire-cut electrical discharge machining process. *Environmental Science and Pollution Research International*, *29*(57), 86237–86246. doi:10.100711356-021-17658-1 PMID:34837614

Boopathi, S. (2022d). Cryogenically treated and untreated stainless steel grade 317 in sustainable wire electrical discharge machining process: A comparative study. *Environmental Science and Pollution Research International*, 1–10. doi:10.100711356-022-22843-x PMID:36057706

Boopathi, S. (2022e). Experimental investigation and multi-objective optimization of cryogenic Friction-stir-welding of AA2014 and AZ31B alloys using MOORA technique. *Materials Today. Communications*, *33*, 104937. doi:10.1016/j.mtcomm.2022.104937

Boopathi, S. (2022f). Performance Improvement of Eco-Friendly Near-Dry Wire-Cut Electrical Discharge Machining Process Using Coconut Oil-Mist Dielectric Fluid. *Journal of Advanced Manufacturing Systems*, 1–20. Advance online publication. doi:10.1142/S0219686723500178

Boopathi, S., Balasubramani, V., Kumar, R. S., & Singh, G. R. (2021). The influence of human hair on kenaf and Grewia fiber-based hybrid natural composite material: An experimental study. *Functional Composites and Structures*, *3*(4), 45011. doi:10.1088/2631-6331/ac3afc

Boopathi, S., Balasubramani, V., & Sanjeev Kumar, R. (2023). Influences of various natural fibers on the mechanical and drilling characteristics of coir-fiber-based hybrid epoxy composites. *Engineering Research Express*, *5*(1), 15002. doi:10.1088/2631-8695/acb132

Boopathi, S., Haribalaji, V., Mageswari, M., & Asif, M. M. (2022). Influences of Boron Carbide Particles on the Wear Rate and Tensile Strength of Aa2014 Surface Composite Fabricated By Friction-Stir Processing. *Materiali in Tehnologije*, *56*(3), 263–270. doi:10.17222/mit.2022.409

Boveiri, H. R., Khayami, R., Elhoseny, M., & Gunasekaran, M. (2019). Swarm Intelligence in Data Science: An efficient swarm intelligence approach for task scheduling in cloud-based internet of things applications. *Journal of Ambient Intelligence and Humanized Computing*, *10*(9), 3469–3479. doi:10.100712652-018-1071-1

Breivold, H. P., & Sandström, K. (2015). Internet of Things for Industrial Automation –Challenges and Technical Solutions. In *IEEE International Conference on Data Science and Data Intensive Systems*. Sydney: IEEE. 10.1109/DSDIS.2015.11

Byrd, K., Mansurov, A., & Baysal, O. (2016). O. Baysal Mining Twitter data for influenza detection and surveillance. *Proc. Int. Work. Softw. Eng. Healthc. Syst. - SEHS*, *16*, 43–49. doi:10.1145/2897683.2897693

Cacovean, D., Ioana, I., & Nitulescu, G. (2020). IoT system in diagnosis of Covid-19 patients. *Informações Econômicas*, *24*(2), 75–89. doi:10.24818/issn14531305/24.2.2020.07

Cai, H. (2020). Sex difference and smoking predisposition in patients with COVID-19. *The Lancet. Respiratory Medicine*, *8*(4), e20. doi:10.1016/S2213-2600(20)30117-X PMID:32171067

Cai, J., Sun, W., Huang, J., Gamber, M., Wu, J., & He, G. (2020). Indirect virus transmission in cluster of COVID-19 cases, Wenzhou, China, 2020. *Emerging Infectious Diseases*, *26*(6), 1343–1345. doi:10.3201/eid2606.200412 PMID:32163030

Callaway, E. (2020). The race for coronavirus vaccines: A graphical guide. *Nature*, *580*(7805), 576–577. doi:10.1038/d41586-020-01221-y PMID:32346146

Calvaresi, D., Cesarini, D., Sernani, P., Marinoni, M., Dragoni, A. F., & Sturm, A. (2017). Exploring the ambient assisted living domain: A systematic review. *Journal of Ambient Intelligence and Humanized Computing*, *8*(2), 239–257. doi:10.100712652-016-0374-3

Carter, M. (2014). Medicine and the media: How Twitter may have helped Nigeria contain Ebola. *BMJ (Clinical Research Ed.)*, 349.

Castillejo, Martinez, Rodriguez-Molina, & Cuerva. (2013). Integration of wearable devices in a wireless sensor network for an E-health application. *IEEE Wireless Communications, 20*(4), 38–49. doi:10.1109/MWC.2013.6590049

Castro & Liskov. (1999). Practical Byzantine fault tolerance. *OSDI, 99*, 173–186,

Chakraborty, S., Aich, S., & Kim, H.-C. (2019). A Secure Healthcare System Design Framework using Blockchain Technology. In *2019 21st International Conference on Advanced Communication Technology (ICACT).* IEEE. 10.23919/ICACT.2019.8701983

Chakraborty, T., & Datta, S. K. (2017). Application of swarm intelligence in internet of things. In *2017 IEEE International Symposium on Consumer Electronics (ISCE)* (pp. 67–68). IEEE 10.1109/ISCE.2017.8355550

Chang, Chiang, Wu, & Chang. (2016). A Context-Aware, Interactive M-health system for Diabetics. *IT Professional, 18*(3), 14–22. doi:10.1109/MITP.2016.48

Charles, W., Marler, N., Long, L., & Manion, S. (2019). Blockchain compliance by design: Regulatory considerations for blockchain in clinical research. *Frontiers in Blockchain*, *2*, 18. doi:10.3389/fbloc.2019.00018

Charulatha, A. R., & Sujatha, R. (2020). Smart healthcare use cases and applications. In *Internet of Things Use Cases for the Healthcare Industry* (pp. 185–203). Springer. doi:10.1007/978-3-030-37526-3_8

Chawathe, S. S. (2018). Indoor Localization Using Bluetooth-LE Beacons. *Proc. 9th IEEE Annu. Ubiquitous Computing, Electronics and Mobile Communication Conference (UEMCON)*, 262–268. 10.1109/UEMCON.2018.8796600

Chen, Hossain, Butler, Ramakrishnan, & Prakash. (2014). *Flu Gone Viral: Syndromic Surveillance of Flu on Twitter using Temporal Topic Models.* . doi:10.1109/ICDM.2014.137

Chen, Y., Wang, Y., Cao, L., & Jin, Q. (2018). An Effective Feature Selection Scheme for Healthcare Data Classification Using Binary Particle Swarm Optimization. *2018 9th International Conference on Information Technology in Medicine and Education (ITME)*, 703-707. 10.1109/ITME.2018.00160

Chen, Z., & Meng, Q.-C. (2004). An incremental clustering algorithm based on swarm intelligence theory. *Proceedings of 2004 International Conference on Machine Learning and Cybernetics, 3*, 1768-1772. 10.1109/ICMLC.2004.1382062

Cheng, S., Liu, B., Shi, Y., Jin, Y., & Li, B. (2016). Evolutionary computation and bigdata: key challenges and future directions. In Y. Tan & Y. Shi (Eds.), DMBD. Academic Press.

Cheng, S. (2017). Cloud service resource allocation with particle swarm optimization algorithm. In C. He, H. Mo, L. Pan, & Y. Zhao (Eds.), *BIC-TA 2017. CCIS* (Vol. 791, pp. 523–532). Springer. doi:10.1007/978-981-10-7179-9_41

Cheng, S., Liu, B., Ting, T., Qin, Q., Shi, Y., & Huang, K. (2016). Survey on data sciencewith population-based algorithms. *Big Data Analytics, 1*(1), 3. doi:10.118641044-016-0003-3

Cheng, S., Shi, Y., Qin, Q., & Bai, R. (2013). Swarm intelligence in big data analytics. In *IDEAL 2013. LNCS* (Vol. 8206, pp. 417–426). Springer. doi:10.1007/978-3-642-41278-3 51

Chen, H. L., Yang, B., Wang, G., Wang, S. J., Liu, J., & Liu, D. Y. (2012). Support vector machine based diagnostic system for breast cancer using swarm intelligence. *Journal of Medical Systems, 36*(4), 2505–2519. doi:10.100710916-011-9723-0 PMID:21537848

Chen, Y., Chen, L., Deng, Q., Zhang, G., Wu, K., Ni, L., Yang, Y., Liu, B., Wang, W., Wei, C., Yang, J., Ye, G., & Cheng, Z. (2020). The presence of SARS-CoV-2 RNA in feces of COVID19 patients. *Journal of Medical Virology, 92*(7), 833–840. doi:10.1002/jmv.25825 PMID:32243607

Chen, Y., Ding, S., Xu, Z., Zheng, H., & Yang, S. (2019). Blockchain-based medical records secure storage and medical service framework. *Journal of Medical Systems, 43*(1), 1–9. doi:10.100710916-018-1121-4 PMID:30467604

Chen, Z., & Huang, X. (2017). End-to-end learning for lane keeping of self-driving cars. *IEEE Intelligent Vehicles Symposium (IV).* 10.1109/IVS.2017.7995975

Chu, X., Wu, T., Weir, J. D., Shi, Y., Niu, B., & Li, L. (2018). Learning-interaction diversification framework for swarm intelligence optimizers: A unified perspective. *Neural Computing & Applications, 32*(6), 1–21. doi:10.100700521-018-3657-0

Clerc, M., & Kennedy, J. (2002). The particle swarm-explosion, stability, and convergence in a multi dimensional complex space. *IEEE Transactions on Evolutionary Computation*, *6*(1), 58–73. doi:10.1109/4235.985692

ClinicalTrials.gov. (n.d.). *COVID-19 | Recruiting Studies*. https://clinicaltrials.gov/ct2/results?term=COVID-19&Search=Apply&recrs=a&age_v=&gndr=&type=&rslt=

Costa & Santos. (2019). An Overview of Data Mining Representation Techniques. *2019 7th International Conference on Future Internet of Things and Cloud Workshops (FiCloudW)*, 90-95. 10.1109/FiCloudW.2019.00029

Cui, X., Potok, T. E., & Palathingal, P. (2005). Document clustering using particle swarm optimization. *Proceedings of 2005 IEEE Swarm Intelligence Symposium (SIS 2005)*, 185-191. 10.1109/SIS.2005.1501621

Darshan, K. R., & Anandakumar, K. R. (2015). A comprehensive review on usage of Internet of Things (IoT) in healthcare system. *2015 International Conference on Emerging Research in Electronics, Computer Science and Technology (ICERECT)*, 132–136. 10.1109/ERECT.2015.7499001

Dasari, D. B., Edamadaka, G., Chowdary, C., & Sobhana, M. (2021). Anomaly-based network intrusion detection with ensemble classifiers and meta-heuristic scale (ECMHS) in traffic flow streams. *Journal of Ambient Intelligence and Humanized Computing*, *12*(10), 9241–9268. doi:10.100712652-020-02628-1

Dash, S., Shakyawar, S. K., Sharma, M., & Kaushik, S. (2019). Big data in healthcare: Management, analysis and future prospects. *Journal of Big Data*, *6*(1), 1–25. doi:10.118640537-019-0217-0

Datta, Barua, & Das. (2019). Application of artificial intelligence in modern healthcare system. *Alginates-Recent Uses of This Natural Polymer*.

Deepa, V. K., & Geetha, J. R. R. (2013). Rapid development of applications in data mining. *2013 International Conference on Green High Performance Computing (ICGHPC)*, 1-4. 10.1109/ICGHPC.2013.6533916

Deng, L., & Li, X. (2013). Machine Learning Paradigms for Speech Recognition: An Overview. *IEEE Transactions on Audio, Speech, and Language Processing*, *21*(5), 1060–1089. doi:10.1109/TASL.2013.2244083

Deng, X. (2009). System Identification Based on Particle Swarm Optimization Algorithm. *2009 International Conference on Computational Intelligence and Security*, 259-263. 10.1109/CIS.2009.167

Deperlioglu, O., Kose, U., Gupta, D., Khanna, A., & Sangaiah, A. K. (2020). Diagnosis of heart diseases by a secure internet of health things system based on autoencoder deep neural network. *Computer Communications*, *162*, 31–50. doi:10.1016/j.comcom.2020.08.011 PMID:32843778

Deshpande, U. U., & Kulkarni, M. A. (2017). IoT based Real Time ECG Monitoring System using Cypress WICED. *International Journal of Advanced Research in Electrical*, *6*(2), 710–720.

Dian, F. J., Vahidnia, R., & Rahmati, A. (2020). Wearables and the Internet of Things (IoT), applications, opportunities, and challenges: A Survey. *IEEE Access : Practical Innovations, Open Solutions*, *8*, 69200–69211. doi:10.1109/ACCESS.2020.2986329

Dias, D., & Paulo Silva Cunha, J. (2018). Wearable health devices—Vital sign monitoring, systems and technologies. *Sensors (Basel)*, *18*(8), 2414. doi:10.339018082414 PMID:30044415

Dighriri, Lee, & Baker. (2018). Big Data Environment for Smart Healthcare Applications Over 5G Mobile Network. *Applications of Big Data Analytics Trends, Issues, and Challenges.*

Domakonda, V. K., Farooq, S., Chinthamreddy, S., Puviarasi, R., Sudhakar, M., & Boopathi, S. (2023). Sustainable Developments of Hybrid Floating Solar Power Plants. In *Human Agro-Energy Optimization for Business and Industry* (pp. 148–167). IGI Global. doi:10.4018/978-1-6684-4118-3.ch008

Dorri, A., Kanhere, S. S., & Jurdak, R. (2017). Towards an Optimized BlockChain for IoT. In *Proceedings of the Second International Conference on Internet-of-Things Design and Implementation – IoTDI '17.* ACM Press. Doi:10.1145/3054977.3055003

Du, J., Zhou, J., Li, C., & Yang, L. (2016). An overview of dynamic data mining. *2016 3rd International Conference on Informative and Cybernetics for Computational Social Systems (ICCSS)*, 331-335. 10.1109/ICCSS.2016.7586476

Dubovitskaya, A., Xu, Z., Ryu, S., Schumacher, M., & Wang, F. (2017). Secure and trustable electronic medical records sharing using blockchain. *AMIA ... Annual Symposium Proceedings - AMIA Symposium. AMIA Symposium*, *2017*, 650. PMID:29854130

Du, S.-Y., & Liu, Z.-G. (2017). Diversity based hybrid particle swarm algorithm. *2017 International Symposium on Intelligent Signal Processing and Communication Systems (ISPACS)*, 444-449. 10.1109/ISPACS.2017.8266520

Eberhart, R., & Kennedy, J. (1995). A new optimizer using particle swarm theory. *Proceedings of the Sixth International Symposium on Micro Machine and Human Science*, 39-43. 10.1109/MHS.1995.494215

Ekblaw, A., Azaria, A., Halamka, J. D., & Lippman, A. (2016, August). A Case Study for Blockchain in Healthcare: "MedRec" prototype for electronic health records and medical research data. In *Proceedings of IEEE open & big data conference* (Vol. 13, p. 13). IEEE.

Espina, K., & Regina, M. (2017). J.E. Estuar Infodemiology for Syndromic Surveillance of Dengue and Typhoid Fever in the Philippines Proc. *Procedia Computer Science*, *121*, 554–561. doi:10.1016/j.procs.2017.11.073

Ethereum. (2019a). *Ethereum/wiki, online*. https://github.com/ethereum/wiki/Light-client-protocol

Ethereum. (2019b). *Go Ethereum.* https://geth.ethereum.org/

Exposure Notifications. (n.d.). *Helping fight COVID-19*. https://www.google.com/covid19/exposurenotifications/

Fong, S., Deb, S., Yang, X.-S., & Li, J. (2014, July-August). Feature Selection in Life Science Classification: Metaheuristic Swarm Search. *IT Professional*, *16*(4), 24–29. doi:10.1109/MITP.2014.50

Garnier, S. (2007). *The Biological Principles of Swarm Intelligence - Swarm Intelligence*. SpringerLink. link.springer.com/article/10.1007/s11721-007-0004-y

Gharehchopogh, F. S., Maleki, I., & Dizaji, Z. A. (2022). Chaotic vortex search algorithm: Metaheuristic algorithm for feature selection. *Evolutionary Intelligence*, *15*(3), 1777–1808. doi:10.100712065-021-00590-1

Gligoroski, S. A. (2020). Pedersen, A. Faxvaag, Blockchain in healthcare and health sciences—A scoping review. *International Journal of Medical Informatics*, *134*, 104040. doi:10.1016/j.ijmedinf.2019.104040 PMID:31865055

Gong, X., Liu, L., Fong, S., Xu, Q., Wen, T., & Liu, Z. (2019). Comparative research of swarm intelligence clustering algorithms for analyzing medical data. *IEEE Access : Practical Innovations, Open Solutions*, *7*, 137560–137569. doi:10.1109/ACCESS.2018.2881020

Guan, W., Ni, Z., Hu, Y., Liang, W., Ou, C., He, J., Liu, L., Shan, H., Lei, C., Hui, D. S. C., Du, B., Li, L., Zeng, G., Yuen, K.-Y., Chen, R., Tang, C., Wang, T., Chen, P., Xiang, J., ... Zhong, N. (2020). Clinical characteristics of coronavirus disease 2019 in China. *The New England Journal of Medicine*, *382*(18), 1708–1720. doi:10.1056/NEJMoa2002032 PMID:32109013

Guinard, D., Trifa, V., Karnouskos, S., Spiess, P., & Savio, D. (2010). Interacting with the SOA-based internet of things: Discovery, query, selection, and on-demand provisioning of webservices. *IEEE Transactions on Services Computing*, *3*(3), 223–235. doi:10.1109/TSC.2010.3

Gunasekaran, K., Boopathi, S., & Sureshkumar, M. (2022). Analysis of a Cryogenically Cooled Near-Dry Wedm Process Using Different Dielectrics. *Materiali in Tehnologije*, *56*(2), 179–186. doi:10.17222/mit.2022.397

Guo, X., Wang, C., & Yan, R. (2011). An electromagnetic localization method for medical micro-devices based on adaptive particle swarm optimization with neighborhood search. *Measurement*, *44*(5), 852–858. doi:10.1016/j.measurement.2011.01.022

Gupta. (2020, August). Social media based surveillance systems for healthcare using machine learning: A systematic review. *Journal of Biomedical Informatics*, *108*.

Habib, K., Torjusen, A., & Leister, W. (2015). Security Analysis of a Patient Monitoring System for the Internet of Things in eHealth. *Researchgate. Net, 335*(c), 73–78. https://www.researchgate.net/profile/Wolfgang_Leister/publication/320596844_Security_Analysis_of_a_Patient_Monitoring_System_for_the_Internet_of_Things_in_eHealth/links/59efaa13458515c3cc4369d0/Security-Analysis-of-a-Patient-Monitoring-System-for-the-Inte

Hadoop ecosystem components and its architecture from ProjectPro. (n.d.). https://www.projectpro.io/article/hadoop-ecosystem-components-and-its-architecture/114

Harikaran, M., Boopathi, S., Gokulakannan, S., & Poonguzhali, M. (2023). Study on the Source of E-Waste Management and Disposal Methods. In *Sustainable Approaches and Strategies for E-Waste Management and Utilization* (pp. 39–60). IGI Global. doi:10.4018/978-1-6684-7573-7.ch003

Hawn, C. (2009). Take two aspirin and tweet me in the morning: How Twitter, Facebook, and other social media are reshaping health care. *Health Affairs (Project Hope), 28*(2), 361–368. doi:10.1377/hlthaff.28.2.361 PMID:19275991

He, Jin, Du, Zhuang, & Shi. (2012). *Clustering in extreme learning machine feature space.* Academic Press.

Hepp, M., Siorpaes, K., & Bachlechner, D. (2007). Harvesting Wiki consensus: Using Wikipedia entries as vocabulary for knowledge management. *IEEE Internet Computing, 11*(5), 54–65. doi:10.1109/MIC.2007.110

He, W., Yan, G., & Da Xu, L. (2014). Developing vehicular data cloud services in the IoT environment. *IEEE Transactions on Industrial Informatics, 10*(2), 1587–1595. doi:10.1109/TII.2014.2299233

Hindson, J. (2020). COVID-19: Faecal-oral transmission? *Nature Reviews. Gastroenterology & Hepatology, 17*(5), 259–259. doi:10.103841575-020-0295-7 PMID:32214231

Honghao, C., Zuren, F., & Zhigang, R. (2013). Community detection using ant colony optimization. In *2013 IEEE Congress on Evolutionary Computation* (pp. 3072–3078). IEEE. 10.1109/CEC.2013.6557944

Ho, Y. X., O'Connor, B. H., & Mulvaney, S. A. (2014). Features of online health communities for adolescents with type 1 diabetes. *Western Journal of Nursing Research, 36*(9), 1183–1198. doi:10.1177/0193945913520414 PMID:24473058

Hsiao, Y.-C., Wu, M.-H., & Li, S. C. (2019). Elevated performance of the smart city—A case study of the IoT by innovation mode. *IEEE Transactions on Engineering Management, 68*(5), 1461–1475. doi:10.1109/TEM.2019.2908962

Huang, C. T., Lin, H. H., Ruan, S. Y., Lee, M.-S., Tsai, Y.-J., & Yu, C.-J. (2014). Efficacy and adverse events of high-frequency oscillatory ventilation in adult patients with acute respiratory distress syndrome: A metaanalysis. *Critical Care (London, England), 18*(3), R102. doi:10.1186/cc13880 PMID:24886674

Imran, A., Posokhova, I., Qureshi, H. N., Masood, U., Riaz, M. S., Ali, K., John, C. N., Hussain, M. D. I., & Nabeel, M. (2020). AI4COVID-19: AI enabled preliminary diagnosis for COVID-19 from cough samples via an app. *Informatics in Medicine Unlocked, 100378*, 1–31. doi:10.1016/j.imu.2020.100378 PMID:32839734

Imtyaz Ahmed, M., & Kannan, G. (2022). Secure and lightweight privacy preserving Internet of things integration for remote patient monitoring. *Journal of King Saud University - Computer and Information Sciences, 34*(9), 6895–6908. doi:10.1016/j.jksuci.2021.07.016

Indrakumari, R., Poongodi, T., Thirunavukkarasu, K., & Sreeji, S. (2020). *Algorithms for Big Data Delivery over Internet of Things. In The Internet of Things and Big Data Analytics* (1st ed.). Auerbach Publications.

Islam, M., Mahmud, S., Muhammad, L. J., Nooruddin, S., & Ayon, S. I. (2020). Wearable technology to assist the patients infected with novel coronavirus (COVID-19). *SN Computer Science, 1*(6), 1–9. doi:10.100742979-020-00335-4 PMID:33063058

Islam, M., Rahaman, A., & Islam, M. R. (2020). Development of smart healthcare monitoring system in IoT environment. *SN Computer Science, 1*(3), 1–11. doi:10.100742979-020-00195-y PMID:33063046

Jabbar, S., Ullah, F., Khalid, S., Khan, M., & Han, K. (2017). Semantic interoperability in heterogeneous IoT infrastructure for healthcare. *Wireless Communications and Mobile Computing, 2017*, 2017. doi:10.1155/2017/9731806

Jaidka, H., Sharma, N., & Singh, R. (2020). *Evolution of IoT to IIoT: Applications & Challenges.* Available at SSRN 3603739.

Janardhana, K., Singh, V., Singh, S. N., Babu, T. S. R., Bano, S., & Boopathi, S. (2023). Utilization Process for Electronic Waste in Eco-Friendly Concrete: Experimental Study. In Sustainable Approaches and Strategies for E-Waste Management and Utilization (pp. 204–223). IGI Global.

Janardhana, K., Anushkannan, N. K., Dinakaran, K. P., Puse, R. K., & Boopathi, S. (2023). *Experimental Investigation on Microhardness, Surface Roughness, and White Layer Thickness of Dry EDM*. Engineering Research Express. doi:10.1088/2631-8695/acce8f

Janardhanan, J., & Umamaheswari, S. (2020). Data Analytic Tools an Overview. *2020 International Conference on Smart Innovations in Design, Environment, Management, Planning and Computing (ICSIDEMPC),* 46-50. 10.1109/ICSIDEMPC49020.2020.9299645

Jangra, R., & Kait, R. (2017). Analysis and comparison among Ant System; Ant Colony System and Max-Min Ant System with different parameters setting. *2017 3rd International Conference on Computational Intelligence & Communication Technology (CICT),* 1-4. 10.1109/CIACT.2017.7977376

Jeevanantham, Y. A., A, S., V, V., J, S. I., Boopathi, S., & Kumar, D. P. (2023). Implementation of Internet-of Things (IoT) in Soil Irrigation System. *IEEE Explore*, 1–5. doi:10.1109/ICPECTS56089.2022.10047185

Jemal, H., Kechaou, Z., & Ben Ayed, M. (2014). Swarm intelligence and multi agent system in healthcare. *2014 6th International Conference of Soft Computing and Pattern Recognition (SoCPaR),* 423-427. 10.1109/SOCPAR.2014.7008044

Jevtic & Andina. (n.d.). *Swarm Intelligence and Its Applications in Swarm Robotics*. Academic Press.

Jordan, M. (2007). Statistical Machine Learning and Computational Biology. *IEEE International Conference on Bioinformatics and Biomedicine (BIBM 2007).*

Joshi, G. P., & Kim, S. W. (2008). Survey, nomenclature and comparison of reader anti-collision protocols in RFID. *IETE Technical Review*, *25*(5), 234–243. doi:10.4103/0256-4602.44659

Jothi, N., & Husain, W. (2015). Data mining in healthcare–a review. *Procedia Computer Science*, *72*, 306–313. doi:10.1016/j.procs.2015.12.145

Joyia, G. J., Liaqat, R. M., Farooq, A., & Rehman, S. (2017). Internet of medical things (IoMT): Applications, benefits and future challenges in healthcare domain. *Journal of Communication*, *12*(4), 240–247.

Kang, M., Park, E., Cho, B. H., & Lee, K. S. (2018). Recent patient health monitoring platforms incorporating Internet of Things-enabled smart devices. *International Neurourology Journal*, *22*(Suppl 2), S76–S82. doi:10.5213/inj.1836144.072 PMID:30068069

Karmore, S., Bodhe, R., Al-Turjman, F., Kumar, R. L., & Pillai, S. (2020). IoT based humanoid software for identification and diagnosis of Covid-19 suspects. *IEEE Sensors Journal*. PMID:36346089

Katal, A. (2013). *Big Data: Issues*. Challenges, Tools and Good Practices.

Kaur, H., Atif, M., & Chauhan, R. (2020). An internet of healthcare things (IoHT)-based healthcare monitoring system. In *Advances in intelligent computing and communication* (pp. 475–482). Springer. doi:10.1007/978-981-15-2774-6_56

Kaushik, S. (2016). *Introduction to feature selection methods with an example (or how to lead).* https://www.analyticsvidhya.com/blog/2016/12/introduction-to feature-selection-methods-with-an-example-or-how-to-select-t
he-rightvariables

Kawa, A. (2012). *SMART logistics chain*. Intelligent Information and Database Systems. ACIIDS. doi:10.1007/978-3-642-28487-8_45

Kazadi, S. (2000). *Swarm Engineering* [Ph.D Thesis]. California Institute of Technology.

Kazadi, S. (2005). On the Development of a Swarm Engineering Methodology. *Systems, Man and Cybernetics, 2005 IEEE International Conference on, 2*, 1423-1428. 10.1109/ICSMC.2005.1571346

Kelvin, A. A., & Halperin, S. (2020). COVID-19 in children: The link in the transmission chain. *The Lancet. Infectious Diseases*, *20*(6), 633–634. doi:10.1016/S1473-3099(20)30236-X PMID:32220651

Kennedy, J., & Eberhart, R. (1995). Particle swarm optimization. *Proceedings of IEEE International Conference on Neural Networks (ICNN),* 1942-1948. 10.1109/ICNN.1995.488968

Khailany, R. A., Safdar, M., & Ozaslan, M. (2020). Genomic characterization of a novel SARS-CoV-2. *Gene Reports*, *100682*, 1–6. PMID:32300673

Khan, M. A., & Algarni, F. (2020). A healthcare monitoring system for the diagnosis of heart disease in the IoMT cloud environment using MSSO-ANFIS. *IEEE Access : Practical Innovations, Open Solutions*, *8*, 122259–122269. doi:10.1109/ACCESS.2020.3006424

Khan, S., & Kannapiran, T. (2019). Indexing issues in spatial big data management. In *International Conference on Advances in Engineering Science Management and Technology (ICAESMT)*. Uttaranchal University. 10.2139srn.3387792

Khosla & Aggarwal. (2005). A Framework for Identification of Fuzzy Models through Particle Swarm Optimization Algorithm. *2005 Annual IEEE India Conference - Indicon*, 388-391. 10.1109/INDCON.2005.1590196

Kim, D. S., & Tran-Dang, H. (2019). An Overview on Industrial Internet of Things. In *Industrial Sensors and Controls in Communication Networks* (pp. 207–216). Springer.

Kim, Shim, Kim, & Lee. (2013). *DBCURE-MR: An efficient density-based clustering algorithm for large data using MapReduce.* Academic Press.

Kim, J.-M., Chung, Y.-S., Jo, H. J., Lee, N.-J., Kim, M. S., Woo, S. H., Park, S., Kim, J. W., Kim, H. M., & Han, M.-G. (2020). Identification of coronavirus isolated from a patient in Korea with COVID-19. *Osong Public Health and Research Perspectives*, *11*(1), 3–7. doi:10.24171/j.phrp.2020.11.1.02 PMID:32149036

Kirschenbaum, M., & Palmer, D. W. (2015). *Perceptualization of particle swarm optimization. In 2015 Swarm/Human Blended Intelligence Workshop*. SHBI. doi:10.1109/SHBI.2015.7321681

Kittusamy. (n.d.). Applications of Swarm Based Intelligence Algorithm in Pharmaceutical Industry: A Review. *International Research Journal of Pharmacy, 8*(11), 24-27.

Kononenko, I. (2011). Machine learning for medical diagnosis: History, state of the art and perspective. *Artificial Intelligence in Medicine*, *23*(1), 89–109. doi:10.1016/S0933-3657(01)00077-X PMID:11470218

Kostkova, P., Szomszor, M., & St Luis, C. (2014). #Swineflu: The Use of Twitter as an Early Warning and Risk Communication ACM Trans. *Manag. Inf. Syst.*, *5*, 1–25. doi:10.1145/2597892

Kotronis, C., Minou, G., Dimitrakopoulos, G., Nikolaidou, M., Anagnos, D., Amira, A., Bensaali, F., Baali, H., & Djelouat, H. (2017). Managing Criticalities of e-Health IoT systems. *IEEE 17th International Conference on Ubiquitous Wireless Broadband (ICUWB),* 1–5. 10.1109/ICUWB.2017.8251004

Krishnan, D. S. R., Gupta, S. C., & Choudhury, T. (2018). An IoT based Patient Health Monitoring System. *Proceedings on 2018 International Conference on Advances in Computing and Communication Engineering, ICACCE 2018*, 1–7. 10.1109/ICACCE.2018.8441708

Kumar, Dixit, & Gayathri. (2020). Healthcare data analytics using swarm intelligence. Swarm *Intelligence Optimization: Algorithms and Applications*, 101-121.

Kumar, R., & Marchang, N. R. (2020). Distributed Off-Chain Storage of Patient Diagnostic Reports in Healthcare System Using IPFS and Blockchain. In *2020 International Conference on COMmunication Systems & NETworkS (COMSNETS).* IEEE. 10.1109/COMSNETS48256.2020.9027313

Kumara, V., Mohanaprakash, T. A., Fairooz, S., Jamal, K., Babu, T., & B., S. (2023). Experimental Study on a Reliable Smart Hydroponics System. In *Human Agro-Energy Optimization for Business and Industry* (pp. 27–45). IGI Global. doi:10.4018/978-1-6684-4118-3.ch002

Kurdi, M. (2022). Ant colony optimization with a new exploratory heuristic information approach for open shop scheduling problem. *Knowledge-Based Systems*, *242*, 108323. doi:10.1016/j.knosys.2022.108323

Labs, P. (2019). *IPFS Powers the Distributed Web.* https://ipfs.io/

Lakshmi, N., & Raghunandhan, G. H. (2011). A conceptual overview of data mining. *2011 National Conference on Innovations in Emerging Technology,* 27-32. 10.1109/NCOIET.2011.5738828

Laplante, P. A., & Laplante, N. (2016, May-June). The Internet of Things in healthcare: Potential applications and challenges. *IT Professional*, *2–4*(3), 2–4. Advance online publication. doi:10.1109/MITP.2016.42

Le, D. N., Parvathy, V. S., Gupta, D., Khanna, A., Rodrigues, J. J., & Shankar, K. (2021). IoT enabled depthwise separable convolution neural network with deep support vector machine for COVID-19 diagnosis and classification. *International Journal of Machine Learning and Cybernetics*, *12*(11), 3235–3248. doi:10.100713042-020-01248-7 PMID:33727984

Leminen, S., Rajahonka, M., Wendelin, R., & Westerlund, M. (2020). Industrial internet of things business models in the machine-to-machine context. *Industrial Marketing Management*, *84*, 298–311. doi:10.1016/j.indmarman.2019.08.008

Lewnard, Nathan, & Lo. (2020). Scientific and ethical basis for social distancing interventions against COVID-19. *Lancet Infect Disease, 20*, 631–633. doi:10.1016/S1473-3099(20)30190-0

Li, A., Wei, X., & He, Z. (2020). Robust proof of stake: A new consensus protocol for sustainable blockchain systems. *Sustainability (Basel), 12*(7), 2824. doi:10.3390u12072824

Li, C., & Bernoff, J. (2008). *Groundswell: Winning in a world transformed by social technologies*. Harvard Business School Press.

Lim, S., Kwon, O., & Lee, D. H. (2018). Technology convergence in the Internet of Things (IoT) start up ecosystem: A network analysis. *Telematics and Informatics, 35*(7), 1887–1899. doi:10.1016/j.tele.2018.06.002

Liu, Y., & Liang, F. (2009). An Adaptive Hybrid Particle Swarm Optimization. *2009 Second International Symposium on Computational Intelligence and Design*, 87-90. 10.1109/ISCID.2009.29

Li, X., & Yao, X. (2012). Cooperatively coevolving particle swarms for large scale optimization. *IEEE Transactions on Evolutionary Computation, 16*(2), 210–224. doi:10.1109/TEVC.2011.2112662

Li, Y., Jiao, L., Shang, R., & Stolkin, R. (2015). Dynamic-context cooperative quantum-behaved particle swarm optimization based on multilevel thresholding applied to medical image segmentation. *Information Sciences, 294*, 408–422. doi:10.1016/j.ins.2014.10.005

Lu, R., Zhao, X., Li, J., Niu, P., Yang, B., Wu, H., Wang, W., Song, H., Huang, B., Zhu, N., Bi, Y., Ma, X., Zhan, F., Wang, L., Hu, T., Zhou, H., Hu, Z., Zhou, W., Zhao, L., ... Tan, W. (2020). Genomic characterisation and epidemiology of 2019 novel coronavirus: Implications for virus origins and receptor binding. *Lancet, 395*(10224), 565–574. doi:10.1016/S0140-6736(20)30251-8 PMID:32007145

Madhuri, R., Ramakrishna Murty, M., Murthy, J. V. R., Prasad Reddy, P. V. G. D., & Suresh, C. (2014). Cluster Analysis on Different Data Sets Using K-Modes and K-Prototype Algorithms. Academic Press.

MaghdidH. S.GhafoorK. Z.SadiqA. S.CurranK.RabieK. (2020). A novel AI-enabled framework to diagnose coronavirus covid 19 using smartphone embedded sensors: design study. doi:10.1109/IRI49571.2020.00033

Mahalakshmi, & Velmurugan. (2015, September). Detection of Brain Tumor by Particle Swarm Optimization using Image Segmentation. *Indian Journal of Science and Technology, 8*(22), IPL0246.

Mahjour, S. K., Santos, A. A. S., Correia, M. G., & Schiozer, D. J. (2021). Scenario reduction methodologies under uncertainties for reservoir development purposes: Distance-based clustering and metaheuristic algorithm. *Journal of Petroleum Exploration and Production Technology, 11*(7), 3079–3102. doi:10.100713202-021-01210-5

Majumder, S., & Deen, M. J. (2019). Smartphone sensors for health monitoring and diagnosis. *Sensors (Basel), 19*(9), 2164. doi:10.339019092164 PMID:31075985

Majumder, S., Mondal, T., & Deen, M. J. (2017). Wearable sensors for remote health monitoring. *Sensors (Basel)*, *17*(1), 130. doi:10.339017010130 PMID:28085085

Mandal, D., Chatterjee, A., & Maitra, M. (2014). Robust medical image segmentation using particle swarm optimization aided level set based global fitting energy active contour approach. *Engineering Applications of Artificial Intelligence*, *35*, 199–214. doi:10.1016/j.engappai.2014.07.001

Mangla, M., Sharma, N., Mittal, P., & Wadhwa, V. M. (Eds.). (2021). Emerging Technologies for Healthcare: Internet of Things and Deep Learning Models. Scrivener Publishing LLC.

Marques, G., Pires, I. M., Miranda, N., & Pitarma, R. (2019). Air quality monitoring using assistive robots for ambient assisted living and enhanced living environments through internet of things. *Electronics (Basel)*, *8*(12), 1375. doi:10.3390/electronics8121375

McCaughey, D., Baumgardner, C., Gaudes, A., LaRochelle, D., Jiaxin, K., Wu, K. J., & Raichura, T. (2014). Best practices in social media: Utilizing a value matrix to assess social media's impact on health care. *Social Science Computer Review*, *32*(5), 575–589. doi:10.1177/0894439314525332

Meng, Y. (2006). A Swarm Intelligence Based Algorithm for Proteomic Pattern Detection of Ovarian Cancer. *IEEE Symposium on Computational Intelligence and Bioinformatics and Computational Biology.* 10.1109/CIBCB.2006.331010

MetskyH. C.FreijeC. A.Kosoko-ThoroddsenT. S.SabetiP. C.MyhrvoldC. (2020). *CRISPRbased COVID-19 surveillance using a genomically-comprehensive machine learning approach*. doi:10.1101/2020.02.26.967026

Mettler, M. (2016). Blockchain technology in healthcare: The revolution starts here. *Proceedings of the IEEE 18th International Conference on e-Health Networking, Applications and Services (Healthcom).*

Miri, A., Sharifian, S., Rashidi, S., & Ghods, M. (2018). Medical image denoising based on 2D discrete cosine transform via ant colony optimization. *Optik (Stuttgart)*, *156*, 938–948. doi:10.1016/j.ijleo.2017.12.074

Miyachi, K., & Mackey, T. K. (2021). hOCBS: A privacy-preserving blockchain framework for healthcare data leveraging an on-chain and off-chain system design. *Information Processing & Management*, *102535*(3), 102535. doi:10.1016/j.ipm.2021.102535

Mohammed, J., Lung, C. H., Ocneanu, A., Thakral, A., Jones, C., & Adler, A. (2014). Internet of things: Remote patient monitoring using web services and cloud computing. *Proceedings - 2014 IEEE International Conference on Internet of Things, IThings 2014, 2014 IEEE International Conference on Green Computing and Communications, GreenCom 2014 and 2014 IEEE International Conference on Cyber-Physical-Social Computing, CPS 20*, 256–263. 10.1109/iThings.2014.45

Mohanty, A., Venkateswaran, N., Ranjit, P. S., Tripathi, M. A., & Boopathi, S. (2023). Innovative Strategy for Profitable Automobile Industries: Working Capital Management. In Handbook of Research on Designing Sustainable Supply Chains to Achieve a Circular Economy (pp. 412–428). IGI Global.

Mohd Ali, N., Besar, R., & Aziz, A. (1955). N. A. (2022). Hybrid Feature Selection of Breast Cancer Gene Expression Microarray Data Based on Metaheuristic Methods: A Comprehensive Review. *Symmetry*, *14*(10). Advance online publication. doi:10.3390ym14101955

Monrat, Islam, Hossain, & Andersson. (2018). Challenges and Opportunities of Using Big Data for Assessing Flood Risks. *Applications of Big Data Analytics Trends, Issues, and Challenges.*

Mosavi, Lopez, & Varkonyi-Koczy. (2018). *Industrial Applications of Big Data: State of the Art Survey*. Academic Press.

Mousavizadeh, L., & Ghasemi, S. (2020). Genotype and phenotype of COVID-19: their roles in pathogenesis. *J. Microbiol. Immunol. Infect.* doi:10.1016/j.jmii.2020.03.022

Mudimigh, F. S., & Ullah, Z. (2009). Efficient implementation of data mining: Improve customer's behaviour. *2009 IEEE/ACS International Conference on Computer Systems and Applications*, 7-10. 10.1109/AICCSA.2009.5069289

Nakamoto, S. (2008). *Bitcoin: A Peer-to-Peer Electronic Cash System.* BN Publishing.

Nandy, S., Adhikari, M., Khan, M. A., Menon, V. G., & Verma, S. (2022, May). An Intrusion Detection Mechanism for Secured IoMT Framework Based on Swarm-Neural Network. *IEEE Journal of Biomedical and Health Informatics*, *26*(5), 1969–1976. doi:10.1109/JBHI.2021.3101686 PMID:34357873

Narmatha. (2021). Data Mining and Swarm Intelligence in Healthcare Applications. *Journal of Computational and Theoretical Nanoscience, 18*(3), 1100-1106.

Nasr, M., Islam, M. M., Shehata, S., Karray, F., & Quintana, Y. (2021). Smart healthcare in the age of AI: Recent advances, challenges, and future prospects. *IEEE Access : Practical Innovations, Open Solutions*, *9*, 145248–145270. doi:10.1109/ACCESS.2021.3118960

Nayar. (2019). Swarm intelligence and data mining: a review of literature and applications in healthcare. *Proceedings of the Third International Conference on Advanced Informatics for Computing Research.* 10.1145/3339311.3339323

Nayarw. (n.d.). *Swarm Intelligence and Data Mining: A Review of Literature and Applications in Healthcare.* Academic Press.

Nduka, A., Samual, J., Elango, S., Divakaran, S., Umar, U., & Senthilprabha, R. (2019). Internet of Things Based Remote Health Monitoring System Using Arduino. *Proceedings of the 3rd International Conference on I-SMAC IoT in Social, Mobile, Analytics and Cloud, I-SMAC 2019*, 572–576. 10.1109/I-SMAC47947.2019.9032438

Nekouie, A., & Moattar, M. H. (2018). Missing value imputation for breast cancer diagnosis data using tensor factorization improved by enhanced reduced adaptive particle swarm optimization. *Journal of King Saud University Computer and Information Sciences.*

Nguyen, T., & Shirai, K. (2013). *Text Classification ofTechnical Papers Basedon Text Segmentation.* Natural Language Processing and Information Systems.

Niranjan, M., Madhukar, N., Ashwini, A., Muddsar, J., & Saish, M. (2017). IOT Based Industrial Automation. *IOSR Journal of Computer Engineering (IOSR-JCE),* 36-40.

Nookhao, S., Thananant, V., & Khunkhao, T. (2020). Development of IoT Heartbeat and Body Temperature Monitoring System for Community Health Volunteer. *2020 Joint International Conference on Digital Arts, Media and Technology with ECTI Northern Section Conference on Electrical, Electronics, Computer and Telecommunications Engineering, ECTI DAMT and NCON 2020,* 106–109. 10.1109/ECTIDAMTNCON48261.2020.9090692

Oikonomidi. (2020). *Impact of Big Data Analytics in Industry 4.* Academic Press.

Öztürk, Ş., Ahmad, R., & Akhtar, N. (2020). Variants of Artificial Bee Colony algorithm and its applications in medical image processing. *Applied Soft Computing, 97,* 106799. doi:10.1016/j.asoc.2020.106799

Palanisamy, R., Hiteshkumar, M. K., Sahasrabuddhe, R., Puranik, J. A., & Vaidya, A. (2019). IoT based patient monitoring system. *International Journal of Recent Technology and Engineering, 8*(2), 2559–2564. doi:10.35940/ijrte.B1304.0982S1119

Panja, A. K., Karim, S. F., Neogy, S., & Chowdhury, C. (2022). A novel feature based ensemble learning model for indoor localization of smartphone users. *Engineering Applications of Artificial Intelligence, 107,* 104538. doi:10.1016/j.engappai.2021.104538

Parvathy, V. S., Pothiraj, S., & Sampson, J. (2021). Automated internet of medical things (iomt) based healthcare monitoring system. In *Cognitive Internet of Medical Things for Smart Healthcare* (pp. 117–128). Springer. doi:10.1007/978-3-030-55833-8_7

Patton, M. (2015). *US health care costs rise faster than inflation.* Retrieved from Forbes: https:// scholar. google. com/scholar

Penang Institute. (2020). *Smart City Technologies Take on COVID-19.* https://penanginstitute.org/publications/issues/smart-city-technologies-take-on-covid-19/

Pham, Q. V., Nguyen, D. C., Mirjalili, S., Hoang, D. T., Nguyen, D. N., Pathirana, P. N., & Hwang, W. J. (2021). Swarm intelligence for next-generation networks: Recent advances and applications. *Journal of Network and Computer Applications, 191,* 103141. doi:10.1016/j.jnca.2021.103141

Philip, N. Y., Rodrigues, J. J. P. C., Wang, H., Fong, S. J., & Chen, J. (2021). Internet of Things for In-Home Health Monitoring Systems: Current Advances, Challenges and Future Directions. *IEEE Journal on Selected Areas in Communications, 39*(2), 300–310. doi:10.1109/JSAC.2020.3042421

Phillips, A. (2021). *A History and Timeline of Big Data*. www.techtarget.com/whatis/feature/A-history-and-timeline-of-big-data

Ping, G., Chunbo, X., Yi, C., Jing, L., & Yanqing, L. (2014). Adaptive ant colony optimization algorithm. *2014 International Conference on Mechatronics and Control (ICMC)*, 95-98. 10.1109/ICMC.2014.7231524

Pourpanah, F., Shi, Y., Lim, C. P., Hao, Q., & Tan, C. J. (2019, July). Feature selection based on brain storm optimization for data classification. *Applied Soft Computing*, *80*, 761–775. doi:10.1016/j.asoc.2019.04.037

Pretz, K. (2013). *The Next Evolution of the Internet*. Retrieved 2018/3/11 from http://theinstitute.ieee.org/technology-focus/ technology-topic/the-next-evolution-of-the-internet

Priya, S., Selvakumar, S., & Velusamy, R. L. (2021). Evidential theoretic deep radial and probabilistic neural ensemble approach for detecting phishing attacks. *Journal of Ambient Intelligence and Humanized Computing*, 1–25.

Punitha Ponmalar, P., & Vijayalakshmi, C. R. (2019, December). Aggregation in IoT for Prediction of Diabetics with Machine Learning Techniques. In *International conference on Computer Networks, Big data and IoT* (pp. 789-798). Springer.

Qasem, S. N., & Shamsuddin, S. M. (2011). Radial basis function network based on time variant multi-objective particle swarm optimization for medical diseases diagnosis. *Applied Soft Computing*, *11*(1), 1427–1438. doi:10.1016/j.asoc.2010.04.014

Qi, X., Zhu, S., & Zhang, H. (2017). A hybrid firefly algorithm. *2017 IEEE 2nd Advanced Information Technology, Electronic and Automation Control Conference (IAEAC)*, 287-291. 10.1109/IAEAC.2017.8054023

Quintana, Y., Darren, F. A. H. Y., Crotty, B., Ruchira, J. A. I. N., Kaldany, E., Gorenberg, M., ... Safran, C. (2018). Infosage: Supporting elders and families through online family networks. *AMIA ... Annual Symposium Proceedings - AMIA Symposium. AMIA Symposium*, *2018*, 932. PMID:30815136

Radanliev, P., De Roure, D. C., Nurse, J. R., Montalvo, R. M., & Burnap, P. (2019). *The Industrial Internet of Things in the Industry 4.0 supply chains of small and medium sized enterprises*. University of Oxford.

Rafael, A. (2020, April 6). Health Surveillance during covid-19pandemic. *BMJ (Clinical Research Ed.)*, *369*, m1373. doi:10.1136/bmj.m1373

Raghuvanshi, A., Singh, U. K., & Joshi, C. (2022). A review of various security and privacy innovations for IoT applications in healthcare. *Advanced Healthcare Systems: Empowering Physicians with IoT-Enabled Technologies*, 43–58.

Rahmatizadeh, S., Valizadeh-Haghi, S., & Dabbagh, A. (2020). The role of artificial intelligence in management of critical COVID-19 patients. *J. Cell. Mol. Anes.*, *5*(1), 16–22.

Ramos, G. N., Hatakeyama, Y., Dong, F., & Hirota, K. (2009). Hyperbox clustering with Ant Colony Optimization (HACO) method and its application to medical risk profile recognition. *Applied Soft Computing*, *9*(2), 632–640. doi:10.1016/j.asoc.2008.09.004

Ramzan, M., & Ahmad, M. (2014). Evolution of data mining: An overview. *2014 Conference on IT in Business, Industry and Government (CSIBIG),* 1-4. 10.1109/CSIBIG.2014.7056947

Ranga Suria, Narasimha Murty, & Athithan. (2014). *A ranking-based algorithm for detection of outliers in categorical data.* Academic Press.

Ratta, P., Kaur, A., Sharma, S., Shabaz, M., & Dhiman, G. (2021). Application of blockchain and internet of things in healthcare and medical sector: Applications, challenges, and future perspectives. *Journal of Food Quality*. doi:10.1155/2021/7608296

Raviteja, K., & Supriya, M. (2020). Greenhouse Monitoring System Based on Internet of Things. *Lecture Notes in Electrical Engineering*, *637*, 581–591. doi:10.1007/978-981-15-2612-1_56

Ray & Saeed. (2018). Applications of Educational Data Mining and Learning Analytics Tools in Handling Big Data in Higher Education. *Applications of Big Data Analytics Trends, Issues, and Challenges.*

Reddy, Kumar Reddy, Lakshmanna, Kaluri, Rajput, Srivastava, & Baker. (2020). *Analysis of Dimensionality Reduction Techniques on Big Data.* Academic Press.

Reddy, M. A., Reddy, B. M., Mukund, C. S., Venneti, K., Preethi, D. M. D., & Boopathi, S. (2023). Social Health Protection During the COVID-Pandemic Using IoT. In *The COVID-19 Pandemic and the Digitalization of Diplomacy* (pp. 204–235). IGI Global. doi:10.4018/978-1-7998-8394-4.ch009

Reisman, M. (2017). EHRs: The challenge of making electronic data usable and interoperable. *Pharm Ther*, *42*(9), 572. PMID:28890644

Renuka Devi, K., & Balasamy, K. (2022). Securing Clinical Information Through Multimedia Watermarking Techniques. In D. Samanta & D. Singh (Eds.), *Handbook of Research on Mathematical Modeling for Smart Healthcare Systems* (pp. 86–109). IGI Global. doi:10.4018/978-1-6684-4580-8.ch005

Rezaee, M. J., Eshkevari, M., Saberi, M., & Hussain, O. (2021). GBK-means clustering algorithm: An improvement to the K-means algorithm based on the bargaining game. *Knowledge-Based Systems*, *213*, 106672. doi:10.1016/j.knosys.2020.106672

Rghioui, A., Naja, A., Mauri, J. L., & Oumnad, A. (2021). An IOT based diabetic patient monitoring system using machine learning and node MCU. *Journal of Physics: Conference Series*, *1743*(1), 012035. doi:10.1088/1742-6596/1743/1/012035

Rhmann, W., Pandey, B., & Ansari, G. A. (2022). Software effort estimation using ensemble of hybrid search-based algorithms based on metaheuristic algorithms. *Innovations in Systems and Software Engineering*, *18*(2), 309–319. doi:10.100711334-020-00377-0

Ricci, S. (2018). Lightweight Ring Signatures for Decentralized Privacy-preserving Transactions. *Proceedings of the 15th International Joint Conference on e- Business and Telecommunications*, 526–531.

Rostami, M., Berahmand, K., Nasiri, E., & Forouzandeh, S. (2021). Review of swarm intelligence-based feature selection methods. *Engineering Applications of Artificial Intelligence*, *100*, 104210. doi:10.1016/j.engappai.2021.104210

Ruan, S. (2020). Likelihood of survival of coronavirus disease 2019. *The Lancet. Infectious Diseases*, *20*(6), 630–631. doi:10.1016/S1473-3099(20)30257-7 PMID:32240633

Ru, L., Zhang, B., Duan, J., Ru, G., Sharma, A., Dhiman, G., Gaba, G. S., Jaha, E. S., & Masud, M. (2021). A Detailed Research on Human Health Monitoring System Based on Internet of Things. *Wireless Communications and Mobile Computing*, *2021*, 1–9. doi:10.1155/2021/5592454

Rupert, D. J., Moultrie, R. R., Read, J. G., Amoozegar, J. B., Bornkessel, A. S., Donoghue, A. C., & Sullivan, H. W. (2014). Perceived healthcare provider reactions to patient and caregiver use of online health communities. *Patient Education and Counseling*, *96*(3), 320–326. doi:10.1016/j.pec.2014.05.015 PMID:24923652

S., P. K., Sampath, B., R., S. K., Babu, B. H., & N., A. (2022). Hydroponics, Aeroponics, and Aquaponics Technologies in Modern Agricultural Cultivation. In *Trends, Paradigms, and Advances in Mechatronics Engineering* (pp. 223–241). IGI Global. doi:10.4018/978-1-6684-5887-7.ch012

Sağ, T., & Çunkaş, M. (2015). Color image segmentation based on multiobjective artificial bee colony optimization. *Applied Soft Computing*, *34*, 389–401. doi:10.1016/j.asoc.2015.05.016

Saha, B. C., R, D., A, A., Thrinath, B. V. S., Boopathi, S., J. R., & Sudhakar, M. (2022). *IoT based smart energy meter for smart grid*. Academic Press.

Saha, A., Rajak, S., Saha, J., & Chowdhury, C. (2022). A Survey of Machine Learning and Meta-heuristics Approaches for Sensor-based Human Activity Recognition Systems. *Journal of Ambient Intelligence and Humanized Computing*, 1–28. doi:10.100712652-022-03870-5

Sainadh, A. V. M. S., Mohanty, J. S., Teja, G. V., & Bhogal, R. K. (2021, May). IoT Enabled Real-Time Remote Health Monitoring System. In *2021 5th International Conference on Intelligent Computing and Control Systems (ICICCS)* (pp. 428-433). IEEE. 10.1109/ICICCS51141.2021.9432103

Samikannu, R., Koshariya, A. K., Poornima, E., Ramesh, S., Kumar, A., & Boopathi, S. (2023). Sustainable Development in Modern Aquaponics Cultivation Systems Using IoT Technologies. In *Human Agro-Energy Optimization for Business and Industry* (pp. 105–127). IGI Global. doi:10.4018/978-1-6684-4118-3.ch006

Sampath, B. C. S., & Myilsamy, S. (2022). Application of TOPSIS Optimization Technique in the Micro-Machining Process. In Trends, Paradigms, and Advances in Mechatronics Engineering (pp. 162–187). IGI Global. doi:10.4018/978-1-6684-5887-7.ch009

Santosh, K. C. (2020). AI-driven tools for coronavirus outbreak: Need of active learning and cross-population train/test models on multitudinal/multimodal data. *Journal of Medical Systems*, *44*(5), 1–5. doi:10.100710916-020-01562-1 PMID:32189081

Sanzgiri, A., & Dasgupta, D. (2016). Classification of insider threat detection techniques. *Proceedings of the 11th Annual Cyber and Information Security Research Conference*, 1–4.

Sarangi, S. K., Panda, R., Priyadarshini, S., & Sarangi, A. (2016). A new modified firefly algorithm for function optimization. *2016 International Conference on Electrical, Electronics, and Optimization Techniques (ICEEOT)*, 2944-2949. 10.1109/ICEEOT.2016.7755239

Sasa, M., Dongqing, L., Jia, X., & Xingqiao, F. (2009). Research on Continuous Function Optimization Algorithm Based on Swarm-Intelligence. *2009 Fifth International Conference on Natural Computation*, 61-65. 10.1109/ICNC.2009.9

Schranz, M., Di Caro, G. A., Schmickl, T., Elmenreich, W., Arvin, F., Şekercioğlu, A., & Sende, M. (2021). Swarm intelligence and cyber-physical systems: Concepts, challenges and future trends. *Swarm and Evolutionary Computation*, *60*, 100762. doi:10.1016/j.swevo.2020.100762

Selvakumar, S., Adithe, S., Isaac, J. S., Pradhan, R., Venkatesh, V., & Sampath, B. (2023). A Study of the Printed Circuit Board (PCB) E-Waste Recycling Process. In Sustainable Approaches and Strategies for E-Waste Management and Utilization (pp. 159–184). IGI Global.

Shaik, M. A., & Verma, D. (2022). Prediction of heart disease using swarm intelligence-based machine learning algorithms. *AIP Conference Proceedings*, *2418*(1), 020025. Advance online publication. doi:10.1063/5.0081719

Shen, Y. (2018). Research on Swarm Size of Multi-swarm Particle Swarm Optimization Algorithm. *2018 IEEE 4th International Conference on Computer and Communications (ICCC)*, 2243-2247. 10.1109/CompComm.2018.8781013

Shi, Y. (2011). Brain storm optimization algorithm. In Advances in Swarm Intelligence, Vol. 6728, lecture notes in computer science. Springer. doi:10.1007/978-3-642-21515-5_36

Shunmugapriya, P., & Kanmani, S. (2017). A hybrid algorithm using ant and bee colony optimization for feature selection and classification (AC-ABC Hybrid). *Swarm and Evolutionary Computation*, *36*, 27–36. doi:10.1016/j.swevo.2017.04.002

Sindhu, P. (2015). A Survey of Tools and Applications in Big Data. Academic Press.

Singh, P., Singh, A. P., & Gupta, A. (2021). Design Strategies for Mobile Ad-hoc Network to Prevent from Attack. In *Proceedings of the 3rd International Conference on Advanced Computing and Software Engineering*. SCITEPRESS - Science and Technology Publications. 10.5220/0010566800003161

Singh, I., Kumar, N., Srinivasa, K. G., Maini, S., Ahuja, U., & Jain, S. (2021). A multi-level classification and modified PSO clustering based ensemble approach for credit scoring. *Applied Soft Computing*, *111*, 107687. doi:10.1016/j.asoc.2021.107687

Singh, P., Verma, S., & Kavita. (2019). Analysis on Different Strategies Used in Blockchain Technology. *Journal of Computational and Theoretical Nanoscience*, *16*(10), 4350–4355. doi:10.1166/jctn.2019.8524

Sinha, P., Singh, R., Roy, R., & Singh, P. (2022). Education and Analysis of Autistic Patients Using Machine Learning. *2022 International Conference on Emerging Smart Computing and Informatics (ESCI),* 1-6. 10.1109/ESCI53509.2022.9758322

Slama, D., Puhlmann, F., Morrish, J., & Bhatnagar, R. M. (2015). *Enterprise IoT: Strategies and Best practices for connected products and services*. O'Reilly Media, Inc.

Smailhodzic, E., Hooijsma, W., Boonstra, A., & Langley, D. J. (2016). Social media use in healthcare: A systematic review of effects on patients and on their relationship with healthcare professionals. *BMC Health Services Research*, *16*(1), 442. doi:10.118612913-016-1691-0 PMID:27562728

Soni, J., Ansari, U., Sharma, D., & Soni, S. (2011). Predictive data mining for medical diagnosis: An overview of heart disease prediction. *International Journal of Computer Applications*, *17*(8), 43–48. doi:10.5120/2237-2860

Sriram. (n.d.). *Security challenges of big data computing*. Academic Press.

Stavrotheodoros, S., Kaklanis, N., Votis, K., Tzovaras, D., & Astell, A. (2022). A hybrid matchmaking approach in the ambient assisted living domain. *Universal Access in the Information Society*, *21*(1), 53–70. doi:10.100710209-020-00756-1

Stone, D., Michalkova, L., & Machova, V. (2022). Machine and Deep Learning Techniques, Body Sensor Networks, and Internet of Things-based Smart Healthcare Systems in COVID-19 Remote Patient Monitoring. *American Journal of Medical Research (New York, N.Y.)*, *9*(1), 97. doi:10.22381/ajmr9120227

Subha, S., Inbamalar, T. M., R, K. C., Suresh, L. R., Boopathi, S., & Alaskar, K. (2023, February). A Remote Health Care Monitoring system using internet of medical things ({IoMT}). *IEEE Explore*. doi:10.1109/ICIPTM57143.2023.10118103

Sultana, N., & Tamanna, M. (2021). Exploring the benefits and challenges of Internet of Things (IoT) during Covid-19: A case study of Bangladesh. *Discover Internet of Things*, *1*(1), 20. doi:10.100743926-021-00020-9

Suresh Kumar, Kumar, Gupta, Shrivastava, Kumar, & Jain. (2022). IoT Communication for Grid-Tie Matrix Converter with Power Factor Control Using the Adaptive Fuzzy Sliding (AFS) Method. *Scientific Programming*, 3.

Suresh, R. M., & Padmajavalli, R. (2007). An Overview of Data Preprocessing in Data and Web Usage Mining. *2006 1st International Conference on Digital Information Management*, 193-198. 10.1109/ICDIM.2007.369352

Suryanarayana, G., & Prakash, K. (2022). Novel dynamic k-modes clustering of categorical and non categorical dataset with optimized genetic algorithm based feature selection. *Multimedia Tools and Applications*, *81*(17), 1–20. doi:10.100711042-022-12126-5

Syed, L., Jabeen, S., Manimala, S., & Alsaeedi, A. (2019). Smart healthcare framework for ambient assisted living using IoMT and big data analytics techniques. *Future Generation Computer Systems*, *101*, 136–151. doi:10.1016/j.future.2019.06.004

Szabo, N. (n.d.). Formalizing and Securing Relationships on Public Networks. *First Monday*, *2*(9). https://journals.uic.edu/ojs/index.php/fm/article/view/548 doi:10.5210/fm.v2i9.548

Tabei, F., Gresham, J. M., Askarian, B., Jung, K., & Chong, J. W. (2020). Cuff-less blood pressure monitoring system using smartphones. *IEEE Access : Practical Innovations, Open Solutions*, *8*, 11534–11545. doi:10.1109/ACCESS.2020.2965082

Tang, Liu, & Pan. (n.d.). *A Review on Representative Swarm Intelligence Algorithms for Solving Optimization Problems: Applications and Trends.* Academic Press.

Tang, B., Bragazzi, N. L., Li, Q., Tang, S., Xiao, Y., & Wu, J. (2020). An updated estimation of the risk of transmission of the novel coronavirus (2019-nCov). *Infectious Disease Modelling*, *5*, 248–255. doi:10.1016/j.idm.2020.02.001 PMID:32099934

Tang, C.-P., Huang, T. C.-K., & Wang, S.-T. (2018). The Impact of Internet of Things Implementation on Firm Performance. *Telematics and Informatics*, *35*(7), 2038–2053. doi:10.1016/j.tele.2018.07.007

Thibaud, M., Chi, H., Zhou, W., & Piramuthu, S. (2018). Internet of Things (IoT) in high-risk Environment, Health and Safety (EHS) industries: A comprehensive review. *Decision Support Systems*, *108*, 79–95. doi:10.1016/j.dss.2018.02.005

Thirunavukkarasu & Wadhawa. (n.d.). Analysis and comparison study of data mining algorithms using Rapidminer. *International Journal of Computer Science, Engineering and Applications.*

Thirunavukkarasu, K., Singh, A. S., Irfan, M., & Chowdhury, A. (2018). Prediction of Liver Disease using Classification Algorithms. *2018 4th International Conference on Computing Communication and Automation (ICCCA),* 1-3. 10.1109/CCAA.2018.8777655

Thirunavukkarasu, K., Singh, A. S., Rai, P., & Gupta, S. (2018). Classification of IRIS Dataset using Classification Based KNN Algorithm in Supervised Learning. *2018 4th International Conference on Computing Communication and Automation (ICCCA),* 1-4. 10.1109/CCAA.2018.8777643

Ting, D. S. W., Carin, L., Dzau, V., & Wong, T. Y. (2020, April). Digital Technology and COVID19. *Nature Medicine*, *459–461*(4), 459–461. Advance online publication. doi:10.103841591-020-0824-5 PMID:32284618

Tomar, D., & Agarwal, S. (2013). A survey on Data Mining approaches for Healthcare. *International Journal of Bio-Science and Bio-Technology*, *5*(5), 241–266. doi:10.14257/ijbsbt.2013.5.5.25

Trojovský, P., Dhasarathan, V., & Boopathi, S. (2023). Experimental investigations on cryogenic friction-stir welding of similar ZE42 magnesium alloys. *Alexandria Engineering Journal*, *66*(1), 1–14. doi:10.1016/j.aej.2022.12.007

Tsai, Huang, & Chiang. (2014). *A Novel Spiral Optimization for Clustering*. Academic Press.

van Doremalen, N., Bushmaker, T., Morris, D. H., Holbrook, M. G., Gamble, A., Williamson, B. N., Tamin, A., Harcourt, J. L., Thornburg, N. J., Gerber, S. I., Lloyd-Smith, J. O., de Wit, E., & Munster, V. J. (2020). Aerosol and surface stability of SARS-CoV-2 as compared with SARS-CoV-1. *The New England Journal of Medicine*, *382*(16), 1564–1567. doi:10.1056/NEJMc2004973 PMID:32182409

Vanitha, S. K. R., & Boopathi, S. (2023). Artificial Intelligence Techniques in Water Purification and Utilization. In *Human Agro-Energy Optimization for Business and Industry* (pp. 202–218). IGI Global. doi:10.4018/978-1-6684-4118-3.ch010

Vega-Márquez, B., Nepomuceno-Chamorro, I. A., Rubio-Escudero, C., & Riquelme, J. C. (2021). OCEAn: Ordinal classification with an ensemble approach. *Information Sciences*, *580*, 221–242. doi:10.1016/j.ins.2021.08.081

Vennila, T., Karuna, M. S., Srivastava, B. K., Venugopal, J., Surakasi, R., & B., S. (2023). New Strategies in Treatment and Enzymatic Processes. In *Human Agro-Energy Optimization for Business and Industry* (pp. 219–240). IGI Global. doi:10.4018/978-1-6684-4118-3.ch011

Verity, R., Okell, L. C., Dorigatti, I., Winskill, P., Whittaker, C., Imai, N., Cuomo-Dannenburg, G., Thompson, H., Walker, P. G. T., Fu, H., Dighe, A., Griffin, J. T., Baguelin, M., Bhatia, S., Boonyasiri, A., Cori, A., Cucunubá, Z., FitzJohn, R., Gaythorpe, K., ... Ferguson, N. M. (2020). Estimates of the severity of coronavirus disease 2019: A model-based analysis. *The Lancet. Infectious Diseases*, *20*(6), 669–677. doi:10.1016/S1473-3099(20)30243-7 PMID:32240634

Verma, A., Prakash, S., Srivastava, V., Kumar, A., & Mukhopadhyay, S. C. (2019). Sensing, controlling, and IoT infrastructure in smart building: A review. *IEEE Sensors Journal*, *19*(20), 9036–9046. doi:10.1109/JSEN.2019.2922409

Vijay Kumar, G., Bharadwaja, A., & Nikhil Sai, N. (2018). Temperature and heart beat monitoring system using IOT. *Proceedings - International Conference on Trends in Electronics and Informatics, ICEI 2017*, 692–695. 10.1109/ICOEI.2017.8300791

Walls, A. C., Park, Y. J., Tortorici, M. A., Wall, A., McGuire, A. T., & Veesler, D. (2020). Structure, function and antigenicity of the SARS-CoV-2 spike glycoprotein. *Cell*, *18*(2), 281–292. doi:10.1016/j.cell.2020.02.058 PMID:32155444

Wang, Q., Qiu, Y., Li, J. Y., Zhou, Z. J., Liao, C. H., & Ge, X. Y. (2020). A unique protease cleavage site predicted in the spike protein of the novel pneumonia coronavirus (2019-nCoV) potentially related to viral transmissibility. *Virologica Sinica*, *20*(3), 1–3. doi:10.100712250-020-00212-7 PMID:32198713

Wang, S., Wang, J., Wang, X., Qiu, T., Yuan, Y., Ouyang, L., Guo, Y., & Wang, F.-Y. (2018). Blockchain-powered parallel healthcare systems based on the ACP approach. *IEEE Transactions on Computational Social Systems*, *5*(4), 942–950. doi:10.1109/TCSS.2018.2865526

Wang, Y., Zhang, D., Du, G., Du, R., Zhao, J., Jin, Y., Fu, S., Gao, L., Cheng, Z., Lu, Q., Hu, Y., Luo, G., Wang, K., Lu, Y., Li, H., Wang, S., Ruan, S., Yang, C., Mei, C., ... Wang, C. (2020). Remdesivir in adults with severe COVID-19: A randomised, double-blind, placebo-controlled, multicentre trial. *Lancet*, *395*(10236), 1569–1578. doi:10.1016/S0140-6736(20)31022-9 PMID:32423584

Wei, X., & Feifan, Y. (2009). Swarm Intelligence in Modeling Adaptive Behavior of the Industry Cluster. *2009 WRI Global Congress on Intelligent Systems*, 213-217. 10.1109/GCIS.2009.50

Wen, T., Liu, H., Lin, L., Wang, B., Hou, J., Huang, C., Pan, T., & Du, Y. (2020). Multiswarm Artificial Bee Colony algorithm based on spark cloud computing platform for medical image registration. *Computer Methods and Programs in Biomedicine*, *192*, 105432. doi:10.1016/j.cmpb.2020.105432 PMID:32278250

WHO. (2016). *Technical package for cardiovascular disease management in primary health care.* https://apps.who.int/iris/handle/10665/252661

WHO. (2022). *Integrated chronic disease prevention and control.* https://www.who.int/chp/about/integrated_cd/en/

Williams, J. (2011). A new roadmap for healthcare business success. *J Healthc Financ Manage Assoc.*, *65*(5), 62–69. PMID:21634269

Winter, A. K., & Hegde, S. T. (2020). The important role of serology for COVID-19 control. *The Lancet. Infectious Diseases*, *20*(7), 758–759. doi:10.1016/S1473-3099(20)30322-4 PMID:32330441

Wood, E., Mohamedally, D., Sebire, N. J., & Visram, S. (2020). *44 Internet of healthcare things (IoHT) handheld device for secure patient data retrieval.* Academic Press.

Woolhandler, S., & Himmelstein, D. U. (2020, July). Intersecting U.S. epidemics: COVID-19 and lack of health insurance. *Annals of Internal Medicine*, *63–64*(1), 63–64. Advance online publication. doi:10.7326/M20-1491 PMID:32259195

World Health Organization. (2020). *Coronavirus disease 2019 (COVID-19): Situation report.* www.who.int/docs/default-source/coronaviruse/situation-reports/20200624

World Health Organization. (n.d.). *Draft landscape of COVID-19 candidate vaccines.* www.who.int/publications/m/item/draft-landscape-of-covid-19-candidate

Xie, Y., Zhang, J., Wang, H., Liu, P., Liu, S., Huo, T., Duan, Y.-Y., Dong, Z., Lu, L., & Ye, Z. (2021). Applications of Blockchain in the Medical Field: Narrative Review. *Journal of Medical Internet Research*, *23*(10), e28613. doi:10.2196/28613 PMID:34533470

Xu , L. D., He , W., & Li , S. (2014). Internet of Things in Industries: A Survey. *IEEE Transactions on Industrial Informatics*, *10*(4), 2233–2243. doi:10.1109/TII.2014.2300753

Xu, G. (2020). IoT-Assisted ECG Monitoring Framework with Secure Data Transmission for Health Care Applications. *IEEE Access : Practical Innovations, Open Solutions*, *8*, 74586–74594. doi:10.1109/ACCESS.2020.2988059

Yamin, M., Alsaawy, Y., & Alkhodre, B., A., & Abi Sen, A. A. (. (2019). An innovative method for preserving privacy in Internet of Things. *Sensors (Basel)*, *19*(15), 3355. doi:10.339019153355 PMID:31370150

Yang, J., Qu, L., Shen, Y., Shi, Y., Cheng, S., Zhao, J., & Shen, X. (2020, June 22). Swarm Intelligence in Data Science: Applications, Opportunities and Challenges. *Lecture Notes in Computer Science*, *12145*, 3–14. doi:10.1007/978-3-030-53956-6_1

Yang, Z., Zhou, Q., Lei, L., Zheng, K., & Xiang, W. (2016). An IoT-cloud Based Wearable ECG Monitoring System for Smart Healthcare. *Journal of Medical Systems*, *40*(12), 1–11. doi:10.100710916-016-0644-9 PMID:27796840

Yekkala, S. D., & Jabbar, M. A. (2017). Prediction of heart disease using ensemble learning and Particle Swarm Optimization. *2017 International Conference On Smart Technologies For Smart Nation (SmartTechCon),* 691-698. 10.1109/SmartTechCon.2017.8358460

Yin, Zeng, Chen, & Fan. (2016). The Internet of Things in healthcare: An overview. *Journal of Industrial Information Integration, 1*, 3–13. doi:10.1016/j.jii.2016.03.004

Yitong, L., Mengyin, F., & Hongbin, G. (2007). A Modified Particle Swarm Optimization Algorithm. *2007 Chinese Control Conference*, 479-483. 10.1109/CHICC.2006.4347362

Yom-tov, E. (n.d.). *Ebola data from the Internet: An Opportunity for Syndromic Surveillance or a News Event?* Categories and Subject Descriptors. doi:10.1145/2750511.2750512

Young, S. D., Mercer, N., Weiss, R. E., Torrone, E. A., & Aral, S. O. (2018). Using social media as a tool to predict syphilis Prev. *Preventive Medicine*, *109*, 58–61. doi:10.1016/j.ypmed.2017.12.016 PMID:29278678

Yu, Liu, & Wang. (2013). *An automatic method to determine the number of clusters using decision-theoretic rough set.* Academic Press.

Yu, N., Li, W., Kang, Q., Xiong, Z., Wang, S., Lin, X., Liu, Y., Xiao, J., Liu, H., Deng, D., Chen, S., Zeng, W., Feng, L., & Wu, J. (2020). Clinical features and obstetric and neonatal outcomes of pregnant patients with COVID-19 in Wuhan, China: A retrospective, single-centre, descriptive study. *The Lancet. Infectious Diseases*, *20*(5), 559–564. doi:10.1016/S1473-3099(20)30176-6 PMID:32220284

Yupapin, P., Trabelsi, Y., Nattappan, A., & Boopathi, S. (2023). Performance Improvement of Wire-Cut Electrical Discharge Machining Process Using Cryogenically Treated Super-Conductive State of Monel-K500 Alloy. *Iranian Journal of Science and Technology. Transaction of Mechanical Engineering*, *47*(1), 267–283. doi:10.100740997-022-00513-0

Zhang, G., Mei, Z., Zhang, Y., Ma, X., Lo, B., Chen, D., & Zhang, Y. (2020). A noninvasive blood glucose monitoring system based on smartphone PPG signal processing and machine learning. *IEEE Transactions on Industrial Informatics*, *16*(11), 7209–7218. doi:10.1109/TII.2020.2975222

Zhang, H., Gao, M., & Zhang, X. (2010). Improved hybrid particle swarm optimization algorithm. *2010 Sixth International Conference on Natural Computation*, 2642-2646. 10.1109/ICNC.2010.5583000

Zhang, J., Zhu, X., Wang, W., & Yao, J. (2014). A fast restarting particle swarm optimizer. *2014 IEEE Congress on Evolutionary Computation (CEC),* 1351-1358. 10.1109/CEC.2014.6900427

Zhang, Z. Z., & Lin, X. (2021). An Improved Artificial Bee Colony with Self-Adaptive Strategies and Application. *2021 International Conference on Computer Network, Electronic and Automation (ICCNEA),* 101-104. 10.1109/ICCNEA53019.2021.00032

Zheng, Yang, Zhang, Chatzimisios, Yang, & Xiang. (2016). *Big Data-Driven Optimization for Mobile Networks toward 5G*. Academic Press.

Zhou, X., & Ye, J. (2011). Y. Feng Tuberculosis surveillance by analyzing google trends. *IEEE Transactions on Biomedical Engineering*, *58*(8), 2247–2254. doi:10.1109/TBME.2011.2132132 PMID:21435969

Zhu & Tang. (2010). Overview of swarm intelligence. In *2010 International Conference on Computer Application and System Modeling (ICCASM 2010)* (vol. 9). IEEE.

Zhu, H., Wu, C. K., Koo, C. H., Tsang, Y. T., Liu, Y., Chi, H. R., & Tsang, K. F. (2019). Smart healthcare in the era of internet-of-things. *IEEE Consumer Electronics Magazine*, *8*(5), 26–30. doi:10.1109/MCE.2019.2923929

Zhu, Y., & Tang, X. (2010). Overview of swarm intelligence. *2010 International Conference on Computer Application and System Modeling (ICCASM 2010),* 400-403. 10.1109/ICCASM.2010.5623005

About the Contributors

Arumugam Suresh Kumar graduated in Computer Science and Engineering (B.E) from Periyar University, India in 2003. Master's (M.E) in Computer Science and Engineering from Anna University, India in 2010. He has been awarded Ph.D in Computer Science and Engineering from Anna University, Chennai in 2017. He is having 18+ Teaching and Research experience in various institutions, and presently working as Professor in the department of Computer Science and Engineering at Jain (Deemed to be) University, Bangalore. He has published 20 SCI articles and more than 30 Scopus articles in peer reviewed journals. He has published 7 Indian Patent and received 1 Innovation Grand patent from Germany Patent. He has actively participated as reviewers in some of the international journals and member of IEEE, IAENG and CSI societies. His main research interest is in the area of Wireless Sensor Network, Internet of Things, Artificial Intelligence and Machine Learning.

Utku Kose received the B.S. degree in 2008 from computer education of Gazi University, Turkey as a faculty valedictorian. He received M.S. degree in 2010 from Afyon Kocatepe University, Turkey in the field of computer and D.S. / Ph. D. degree in 2017 from Selcuk University, Turkey in the field of computer engineering. Between 2009 and 2011, he has worked as a Research Assistant in Afyon Kocatepe University. Following, he has also worked as a Lecturer and Vocational School - Vice Director in Afyon Kocatepe University between 2011 and 2012 and as a Lecturer and Research Center Director in Usak University between 2012 and 2017. Currently, he is an Assistant Professor in Suleyman Demirel University, Turkey. His research interest includes artificial intelligence, machine ethics, artificial intelligence safety, optimization, the chaos theory, distance education, e-learning, computer education, and computer science.

Sachin Sharma is currently an Associate Dean, International Affairs and Professor, Department of Computer Science and Engineering at Graphic Era Deemed to be University, Dehradun, UK, India. He is also Co-founder and Chief Technology officer (CTO) of IntelliNexus LLC, Arkansas, USA based company. He also worked as a Senior Systems Engineer at Belkin International, Inc., Irvine, California, USA for two years. He received his Philosophy of Doctorate (Ph.D.) degree in Engineering Science and Systems specialization in Systems Engineering from University of Arkansas at Little Rock, USA with 4.0 out 4.0 GPA and M.S. degree in Systems engineering from University of Arkansas at Little Rock with 4.0 out 4.0 GPA and He received his B.Tech. degree from SRM University, Chennai including two years at University of Arkansas at Little Rock, USA as an International Exchange Student. His research interests include wireless communication networks, IoT, Vehicular ad hoc networking and network security.

S. Jerald Nirmal Kumar is working as an Associate Professor in Sharda University, I have completed my B.E(CSE) at Anna university in 2005 and MTech at Veltech Technical University in 2011 and Doctor of Philosophy in CSE at Anna University in 2021 in the domain of cloud and network security, I have 13 years of experience among 11 years of teaching and 2.2 years in Industry. I have completed my OBE certification in Swayam NPTEL, and Wipro 10 X certification for Teaching Learning Process. I have published 5 SCI and 2 Scopus and 1 Book chapter and 3 patents and edited 2 books and also played role as a session chair for International Conference My area of research is cloud computing security and Network security with Machine Learning. I am a life member in Indian society for technical education and a member of professional bodies like IFERP, IEANG, and IRED.

* * *

C. V. Suresh Babu is a pioneer in Content Development. A true entrepreneur, He floated Anniyappa Publications, a company which is very active in bringing out books related to Computer Science and Management. Dr. C. V. Suresh Babu has also ventured into SB Institute, a centre for knowledge transfer. He holds Ph.D in Engineering Education from National Institute of Technical Teachers Training & Research, Chennai along with seven Master degrees in various disciplines such as Engineering, Computer Applications, Management, Commerce, Economics, Psychology, Law and Education. He also has the UGC-NET/SET qualifications in the disciplines of Computer Science, Management, Commerce and Education to his credit. Currently, Professor, Department of Information Technology, School of Computing Science, Hindustan Institute of Technology and Science, (Hindustan University), Padur, Chennai, Tamil Nadu, India Personal blog: .e2f99afb-1a1c-43c5-978b-f2cacc9d88ea

Sampath Boopathi () completed his undergraduate in Mechanical Engineering and postgraduate in the field of Computer-Aided Design. He completed his Ph.D. from

Anna University and his field of research includes Manufacturing and optimization. He published 60 more research articles in Internationally Peer-reviewed journals, one Patent grant, and three published patents. He has 16 more years of academic and research experiences in the various Engineering Colleges in Tamilnadu, India.

Aarthi Chelladurai obtained her Bachelor's degree in Electronics and Communication Engineering and obtained her Master's degree in VLSI Design from Sona College ofTechnology. She obtained her Ph.D in Information and Communication Engineering from Anna University in 2019. Her specializations include VLSI and Networking.

Aparna Chelladurai obtained her Bachelor's degree in Information Technology from Anna University in 2005.Then she obtained her Master's degree in Computer Science & Engineering from Mahendra Engineering College in 2010. She obtained her Ph.D in Information and Communication Engineering from Anna University in 2020. Her specializations include Data mining, Networking and Networking. Her current research interests are spatial data mining, co located pattern recognition and pattern mining.

N. Yuvaraj, received the B.E. degree in Computer Science Engineering from Coimbatore Institute of Engineering and Technology, Anna University, Tamil Nadu, India, in 2010 and the M.E. degree in Computer Science engineering from Sri Shakthi Institute of Engineering and Technology, Anna University, Tamil Nadu, India, in 2012. I have completed Ph.D. degree in Computer Science engineering at St. Peter's Institute of Higher Education and Research, Chennai, India, in 2020. His research interests include Data Mining, Wireless Sensor Networks, Mobile Computing, Machine and Deep Learning. He filed and published 2 International Patents, 12 Indian Patents, also wrote 2 Text Books and also published 13 Book Chapters in Springer, Academic Press, John Wiley and Sons. Also published 85 research papers in SCI, Scopus, International and National Conferences.

Jeyaprabhavathi Perumal received the B.Sc., degree in Physics from Madurai Kamaraj University, Madurai, Tamil Nadu, India, in 1996 and the M.Sc., degree in Computer Science from Madurai Kamaraj University, Madurai, Tamilnadu, Inida, in 1998. She has 20 plus years of hands-on experience in Teaching & Education Management as a Lecturer and exclusive Seven years as a Faculty Head in the private international university at London and Four years as a Curriculum Manager in FE and currently working as a Senior lecturer and program team leader at Arden University. She is a member of society for education and training. Her research interests include Cloud Computing, Big Data, Blockchain, Data Mining, Artificial

Intelligence, Machine and Deep Learning techniques. She has published several research papers in leading international journals and Book Chapters indexed in SCI/SCI-E, Scopus. She has attended many International and National Conferences.

Srivastava is a student at Graphic Era Deemed to be University pursuing Bachelor's of Technology in Computer Science.

Ananya Srivastava is a student at Graphic Era University pursuing Bachelor's of Technology in Computer Science.

Sakshi Srivastava is a student at Graphic Era Deemed to be University Dehradun, India pursuing Bachelor's of Technology in Computer Science.

Radha Subramani obtained her Bachelor's degree in Computer Science & Engineering from Periyar University in 2004.Then she obtained her Master's degree in Computer Science & Engineering from Mahendra Engineering College in 2010. She obtained her Ph.D in Information and Communication Engineering from Anna University in 2020. Her specializations include Data mining, Networking and Networking. Her current research interests are spatial data mining, co located pattern recognition and pattern mining

Index

A

B

C

D

E

Printed in the United States
by Baker & Taylor Publisher Services